608

Human cells in *in vitro* pharmaco-toxicology

DG XII
Science, Research & Development

Human cells in *in vitro* pharmaco-toxicology

Present status within Europe

Edited by

Vera Rogiers
Walter Sonck
Elizabeth Shephard
Antoine Vercruysse

Dept.
of Toxicology

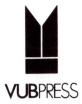

VUBPRESS

Group for
reflection on
the quality of
life and
environment

Book design: Walter Sonck
Cover design: Danny Somers

© Copyright 1993, VUBPRESS - Brussels
ISBN 90 5487 041 9   NUGI 743
D/1993/1885/182

All rights reserved; no part of this publication may be reproduced, stored in any retrieval system, or transmitted in any form or by any means, electronic, mechanical, photocopying, recording, otherwise without prior written permission of the publisher.

The work presented in this book is the result of years of intensive work by many European scientists, from both the academic and industrial spheres, who are active in the field of in vitro research concerned with the testing of drugs and chemicals.

Being a member of the 'Group for the reflection on the quality of life and environment', I would like to express my pride in being able to support this European initiative.

My sincere gratitude goes to the organizers of this European Symposium, in particular to Prof. Vera Rogiers, the European Community, DG XII, for financial support for in vitro research, to the scientists who have contributed to this book and to all those investigators who have dedicated their working lives to the development of systems that will refine, reduce and replace the use of animals in pharmaco-toxicological research.

H.R.H. Prince Laurent of Belgium
Founder of the 'Group for the reflection on the quality of life and environment'*

---

* Secretariate :
   E. Tombeur
   Rue de la Duchesse 34 Bte 4
   B-1200 Brussels

Preface

Scientists working in pharmaco-toxicology are facing a dilemma: on the one hand they are confronted with the growing demand to use less animals in research and testing of drugs but on the other hand they are facing increasing stringent regulatory standards to guarantee product safety for man and the environment. Will *in vitro* pharmaco-toxicology as we know it to-day, based on the 3R's and using cells and tissues of nearly exclusively non-human origin, provide a possible solution to this dilemma or is the more difficult approach of using, whenever possible, human derived materials, necessary to solve the growing conflict? This book does not provide the answer but rather initiates the discussion at the Community level. The text is unique in the sense that it is the first to cover the present status, within Europe, of the use of human derived cells in pharmaco-toxicology. Before a discussion can begin we need an exact knowledge of the progress within this field: e.g. what are the technical possibilities at present, advantages and disadvantages, the regulatory aspects and the laboratories involved.

Authors of the various chapters of this book are scientists involved in the day to day development and use of *in vitro* models for pharmaco-toxicological purposes. They have been requested, on the occasion of a European Symposium*, to write 'a state of the art' article on the cell type they are particulary familiar with and to focus on human-derived cells. They have been asked to present an overview of the existing 'human' literature in order to provide the reader with a picture of the present situation.

Since most of our *in vitro* knowledge and experience is gained through *in vitro* experimentation with cells and tissues isolated from animals, in particular rodents, it is inevitable that most chapters will discuss some of the basic results and background information obtained through the use of non-human derived cells.

The material presented in this book clearly demonstrates that important information can be gained through the use of *in vitro* experiments involving primary cultures of human derived cells. It is the clear wish of scientists from both the academic and industrial worlds to have a more readily available source of human cells and tissues for experimental purposes. It is evident that the EC has to take responsibility for the availibility of human material for pharmaco-toxicological research. Discussions should be begin that will lead to an efficient and ethical legislation on the use of human derived cells and tissues for experimental purposes, other than transplantation.

The editors

---

* A symposium 'Human cells in pharmaco-toxicology' was held in Brussels on September 23-24, 1993. The realisation of this symposium and the proceedings book were possible thanks to the EC pilot project BMH*-CT92-0005-BE

Contents

Foreword ... v

Preface ... vi

1. The significance and applicability of human tissues and cells as *in vitro* models in toxicology ... 1
   B.J. Blaauboer

2. *In vitro* systems to study fibroblast functions ... 11
   B. Eckes and T. Krieg

3. Three-dimensional reconstructed human skin for *in vitro* pharmaco-toxicology ... 27
   B. Coulomb and L. Dubertret

4. Keratinocytes and reconstructed epidermis for *in vitro* pharmacological and toxicological testing ... 45
   H. Merk, F. Jugert and S. Frankenberg

5. Use of human skin models in the study of retinoic acid metabolism and lipid synthesis, effects of liarozole ... 61
   H. Vanden Bossche, G. Willemsens, H. Schreuders, M.-C. Coene, C. Van Hove and W. Cools

6. Cultures of human hepatocytes in *in vitro* pharmaco-toxicology ... 77
   V. Rogiers

7. Potential of freshly isolated and cryopreserved human hepatocytes in drug research and development ... 117
   R. Rahmani, G. de Sousa, F. Marre, F. Nicolas and M. Placidi

8. Human models for the *in vitro* assessment of neuro-toxicity ... 139
   C.K. Atterwill and W.M. Purcell

9. Interference of sesquiterpenoid unsaturated dialdehydes with neuronal transduction studied in human neuroblastoma cells 169
A. Forsby, M.I. Andres and E. Walum

10. Human immune cells and *in vitro* immunotoxicity testing 185
I. Kimber and M. Cumberbatch

11. Human kidney cells in *in vitro* pharmaco-toxicology 197
S. Kastner, M. Soose and H. Stolte

12. Isolated human heart cells 239
M. Borgers and L. Ver Donck

13. Human chondrocyte culture in pharmaco-toxicological research 253
M. Adolphe, B. Benoit, G. Verbruggen and E.M. Veys

14. Use of human pulmonary cells in pharmaco-toxicology 265
B. Nemery and P.H.M. Hoet

15. Research and testing in pharmaco-toxicology with human intestinal cells 283
F. Zucco and A. Stammati

16. Legislation and regulation on the use of cells from human origin in pharmaco-toxicology 305
A. Vercruysse

17. Pharmaceutical research initiatives of the EC 309
G.N. Fracchia

18. Obtaining human tissues for research and testing: practical problems and public attitudes in Britain 315
J. Gurney and M. Balls

1

The significance and applicability of human tissues and cells as *in vitro* models in toxicology

B. J. Blaauboer

Research Institute of Toxicology (RITOX), Utrecht University
P.O. Box 80.176, 3508 TD Utrecht (The Netherlands).

Introduction

Man is exposed to an enormous amount of chemical compounds present in his environment. Foodstuffs that are taken up do not only contain nutrients but also substances that are considered to be non-nutrients. Such xenobiotics can either be of natural origin, e.g. components of plants, or of man-made origin, such as agrochemicals or environmental pollutants. Other natural or synthetic chemicals can be found in the air that we inhale and in goods and products coming into contact with our skin.

Chemicals have always been present in our *milieu exterieur*. However, in our industrialized society the demand for an ever increasing number of chemicals has increased such exposure to a great extent. This calls for a good understanding of the hazards these chemicals might represent. This is especially the case for all those compounds that are produced, handled or applied for defined purposes, e.g. in industry, as agrochemicals, as drugs for the treatment of human and animal diseases, in the production and use of foodstuffs or other consumer products. Hazard evaluation must not be restricted to man-made chemicals, since the toxicological risks represented by natural compounds are not be underestimated [1].

It is the responsibility of toxicologists to provide the knowledge that forms the basis of risk evaluation and to provide society with the information needed to handle chemicals in a safe way. Special attention is needed for the use of compounds as medicines. The purpose of drug application is to achieve a beneficiary effect in a patient. Therefore, it is implicated that medicines have a biological activity at the applied dose levels. A thorough evaluation of beneficiary effects as well as unwanted effects is necessary before a drug can be released on the market.

In both pharmacology and toxicology, two fields of interest can be distinguished. One area is concerned with understanding why and how chemicals can have a certain wanted or unwanted biological activity. The other area concentrates on the determination of the doses or concentrations at which pharmacological or toxicological effects occur. In both areas much of the data has been derived from experiments with laboratory animals. However, an increasing number of model systems at a level of integration lower than the intact organisms have been developed, especially when the mechanisms of action of compounds are studied. Such systems are normally derived from animal tissues. The use of human-derived *in vitro* systems is still limited. Data produced either in experiments performed with intact animals or with animal-derived *in vitro* models will therefore have to be extrapolated to the human situation.

Interspecies extrapolation

The use of animal data to predict the pharmacological or toxicological activities of compounds in man is always prone to some degree of uncertainty. Important sources of uncertainty can be found in qualitative or quantitative differences between physiological processes in animals and man. As an example, differences in body size between rat and man implies a different ratio between body weight and body volume, resulting in different metabolic needs. Extrapolation of dose levels, calculated per kg body weight, can therefore result in erroneous predictions with regard to the distribution and metabolism of the compound under study. Furthermore, other biokinetic parameters, like uptake, distribution, biotransformation and excretion may also differ [2]. These deviations may result in dissimilarities in the concentration at the site of action. Furthermore, there can be wide species differences in the mode of action of compounds. Examples are compounds that are carcinogenic in man but not in rodents [3], or *vice versa* [4], and the skin effects (chloracne) of some dioxins in man that do not occur in rodents [5].

Other difficulties arise from the fact that extrapolations have to be carried out from a rather small, but homogeneous, group of laboratory animals to the very heterogeneous human general population. Therefore, in risk assessment of chemicals one tries to overcome these uncertainties by introducing safety factors. For example, no(toxic) effect levels determined in an animal experiment are divided by a given factor and the result is used in setting safety standards.

Although there is an increasing interest in expanding knowledge with regards to pharmacology and toxicology in species other than man, still the main activity in both scientific areas is directed towards humans. To overcome the difficulties of extrapolating data from one species to another, an obvious choice seems to be to perform studies, if possible, in the 'target species', i.e. the species that will be exposed and in which the risk of such an exposure has to be evaluated. If human pharmacology and toxicology are considered, studies performed in man would give the most appropriate results. However, it is obvious that a compound of which no data exist on its biological activity cannot be tested in man. The risk of encountering unwanted effects would be ethically unacceptable. Therefore, there still is a heavy reliance on experimental models making use of animals. Here too, however, there are ethical considerations: animal use should be well justified and if alternatives are available these should be preferred [6].

The advancement of cell and tissue culture techniques provides an enormous potential for biomedical research as a whole and for pharmacology and toxicology in particular. While such *in vitro* methods are particularly suitable for studying mechanistic aspects of biological activity, their use in risk assessment presents yet another problem of extrapolation from *in vitro* data to the situation in the intact organism.

In vitro - *in vivo* extrapolation

Data obtained in *in vitro* experiments are not directly applicable to the *in vivo* situation. One drawback is the absence of the *in vivo* biokinetics [7,8]. This can lead to a misinterpretation of *in vitro* data. For example, the concentrations employed in such methods may be irrelevant to the *in vivo* situation. One possibility is that cells are exposed to much lower concentrations *in vivo*, because the compound cannot easily reach the cells. An overestimation of the compound's biological activity for the cell type under study will be the result. Otherwise, compounds can accumulate in certain organs, tissues or cell types and then an *in vitro* model system may lead to an underestimation of biological properties of the compound under study [9].

Moreover, *in vitro* systems comprising intact cells can be used to study the biological activity of chemicals in a number of ways. Test parameters may either be related to cellular functioning in a more general way or be more relevant for specific functions of the cell type under study. If, for example, the cytotoxicity of compounds is studied, one can pay attention to effects on functions present in practically all cell types, the so-called housekeeping functions such as the maintenance of cellular integrity or energy supplies. In this case it is relatively unimportant which cell type is used as a model system. In contrast, the biological effects on more specific cellular functions can only be studied if the relevant targets are present [8].

These factors call for an integration of data on the mechanisms of action of compounds and on their biokinetic behaviour in studies of biological activity. It is clearly obvious that a great number of data can be derived from *in vitro* experiments, provided that the results are interpreted in the context of the *in vivo* situation. For instance, knowledge of physico-chemical data, such as volatility, solubility, reactivity etc. can not only be used for an estimation of exposure to a chemical, but can also be incorporated into predictions of the biokinetic behaviour as well. Properties such as lipophilicity, molecular size, ionisation and binding to proteins, are of importance in an estimation of the compound's reactivity and its ability to cross biomembranes. Passive uptake from the *milieu exterieur*, distribution, accumulation and excretion, will for the most part be governed by these properties. These characteristics can all be determined in non-animal systems. To characterize the cellular biokinetic behaviour of compounds, uptake and subcellular distribution can be measured in various cell types. The choice of cells and culture systems to be used in such studies should be based on knowledge of possible uptake mechanisms (e.g. carrier-mediated uptake) and of the physiological role of cells, tissues and organs *in vivo*.

Biotransformation plays a pivotal role in the biological activity of many compounds. This is especially true for compounds of which metabolites have a higher activity than the parent compound. *In vitro* systems, especially those derived from the liver, can be used to elucidate metabolic pathways and to characterize the enzyme systems involved [10]. Studies with subcellular fractions, such as microsomes, can provide important qualitative data. Systems comprising intact cells, such as shaking cultures or primary cultures, permit a detailed study of biotransformation reactions under physiological intracellular conditions, while the extracellular environment can be manipulated easily [11]. Compilation of a data set derived from a battery of different *in vitro* and other non-animal experiments can be the basis for a prediction of the *in vivo* biokinetic behaviour as well as the biological activity of a compound. The use of computerised model systems describing *in vivo* biokinetics can be a very powerful tool in this respect. Such physiologically-based biokinetic model systems are now in development in pharmacology and toxicology [12,13].

Currently, a programme for the application of *in vitro* test systems in chemical hazard assessment, including the above-mentioned factors is in development [14]. In this scheme, set up by the European Research Group for Alternatives in Toxicity Testing (ERGATT) a battery of non-animal tests will be performed within eight areas of research: basal cytotoxicity, irritancy, developmental toxicity, hepatotoxicity, nephrotoxicity, immunotoxicity, neurotoxicity and biokinetics. This scheme will be used to evaluate the toxic hazard of a set of chemicals, chosen as calibration compounds for one of the tests in the battery. Also included are a number of chemicals from the OECD test programme on High Production Volume Chemicals, thus providing the possibility of testing the compounds *in vitro* in parallel with the standard *in vivo* testing performed in the OECD programme.

The use of human cells and tissues

As mentioned above, the most reliable data on a compound's human pharmacology or toxicology would be that derived from experiments with man. Full-scale testing of compounds with unknown biological properties in man is hardly possible, because of ethical considerations. The fast development in cell and tissue culture techniques may provide the possibility of studying compounds in *in vitro* systems derived from man. This conference was organised to compile data on the current possibilities with regards the use of human-derived systems in toxicology. Such data will also be of importance in other areas of the biomedical sciences, e.g. in pharmacology.

A review of the relevant literature shows that many studies were and are being performed with cell lines derived from human tissues. The vast majority of these studies are performed with the aim of a better understanding of physiological processes. There is a trend towards the use of genetically-modified cell lines. However, practically none of these studies was used for toxicological risk evaluation.

For an understanding of a compound's effect in an intact organism, the *in vitro* model system should have as many characteristics of the *in vivo* situation as possible. This would imply that freshly isolated cells or primary cultures will have advantages over cell lines. However, freshly isolated cells have their disadvantages also. Shortly after isolation of, for example, hepatocytes the cells do not exactly have their normal physiological state [15] and need a certain amount of time to recover from the damage caused by the isolation procedure [16]. Another disadvantage of many systems employing freshly isolated cells is the lack of intercellular connections. Furthermore, the cells can only be kept in culture for several hours. Taking these limitations into account, short-term experiments can be performed with suspension cultures, but the study of phenomena taking more than a few hours is not possible.

Cultures of many cell types can be maintained for much longer periods. For example, hepatocytes can be kept in such cultures for up to several weeks. However, during culture a number of functions specific for the cell type under study can be reduced or lost [17,18], changes which can be interpreted as dedifferentiation. Despite these drawbacks, the use of freshly isolated cells or cells in primary cultures seem to have advantages over the use of cell lines. During this conference emphasis will be laid on the application of human-derived cells in primary culture. Employment of *in vitro* systems derived from different animals may greatly increase the possibilities of interspecies extrapolations. It allows a comparison of, for example, mechanisms of action between species. Furthermore, data derived from experiments with animal cells can be compared with *in vivo* animal data. If no *in vivo* data in the other animal species (e.g. man) exists, extrapolation can now follow two routes: 1; from *in vivo* animal data to man and 2; from *in vitro* human data to man [7]. This would then give the extrapolation of data a more scientific basis, since mechanistic data can be incorporated [8].

Availibility, ethical and legal considerations

During the last few decades there has been an enormous increase in the technical possibilities for employing primary cultures of many cell types derived from a wide variety of animal species. These advancements were made possible by increased knowledge in surgical techniques, cell biology and cell culture. For example, cell isolation from laboratory animals can be performed after optimal preparation of the animal and technically there are no limits on the availability of animals.

This is obviously not the case for human tissues or cells. In a number of cases human tissues can be obtained by biopsy [19], but the amount of tissue will be limited. Another source for human tissues is material obtained from patients donating organs for transplantation. In both cases the achievement of optimal conditions for cell isolation and culture is not the highest priority.

Donation of human tissues for transplantation purposes is well organized in Europe. Ethical and legal procedures exist, making it possible to employ a wide array of tissues, e.g. blood, kidney, heart, liver, skin and cornea. In a number of cases those tissues that cannot be used for transplantation for technical or logistic reasons are available for cell isolation and research in other areas. Up to now, no unity exists in ethical and legal procedures with regards to the acquirement and application of human tissues for scientific research. In many western countries the trade in materials of human origin or their use for commercial purposes is explicitly excluded by legislation. In the USA, a number of commercially operating institutions exist that offer human-derived tissue or cell cultures for testing procedures, including toxicological screening of compounds. These institutions are not allowed to pay for the acquirement of human material and only charge customers for the 'value added' by development and processing.

It would be highly desirable to have a more widespread public debate on the feasibility of using human tissues for research, such as toxicity studies, and on the ethical and legal issues connected with this. This debate should result in internationally implemented and uniform legislation. This is of importance since international cooperation in science and trade is increasing. Such trends towards an international agreement on the acceptability of *in vitro* methods in toxicology can also be seen with respect to the validation of these methods [20].

Conclusions

There is an obvious need, scientifically and ethically, to implement human tissues and cells in the study of effects of xenobiotics. The incorporation of such model systems would imply important improvements in toxicological risk evaluations. Technically, for many cell types and tissues this is now possible as a result of the fast developments in cell biology and culture. However, the availability of human tissues for purposes other than transplantation is very limited. The implementation and international acceptance of new legislation for this scientifically very promising area is highly desirable.

References

1. Jelenik C.F., Pohland A.E. and Wood G.E. Review of mycotoxin contamination. Worldwide occurrence of mycotoxins in foods and feeds - an update. Journal of the Association of Official Analytical Chemists 1989;72:223-230.
2. Relius H.W. Extrapolation from animals to man: prediction, pitfalls and perspectives. Xenobiotica 1987;17:255-265.
3. Rao M.S. and Reddy J.K. The relevance of peroxisome proliferation and cell proliferation in peroxisome proliferator-induced hepatocarcinogenesis. Drug Metabolism Reviews 1989;21:102-110.
4. Van Raalte H.G.S. and Grasso P. Hematological, myelotoxic, clastogenic, carcinogenic and leukemogenic effects of benzene. Regulatory Toxicology and Pharmacology 1982;2:153-176.
5. Kimbrough R. Skin lesions in animals and humans: a brief overview. In: Banbury Report 18: Biological mechanisms of dioxin action (Poland A. and Kimbrough R., eds.) Cold Spring Harbor Laboratory, New York, 1984:357-365.
6. Frazier J.M. and Goldberg A.M. Alternatives to and reduction of animal use in biomedical research, education and testing. Alternatives to Laboratory Animals 1990;18:65-74.
7. Blaauboer B.J., Wortelboer H.M. and Mennes W.C. The use of liver cell cultures derived from different mammalian species in *in vitro* toxicological studies: implementation in extrapolation models? Alternatives to Laboratory Animals 1990;18:251-258.
8. Flint O.P. *In vitro* toxicity testing: purpose, validation and strategy. Alternatives to Laboratory Animals 1990;18:11-18.
9. Smith L.L. and Nemery B. Cellular specific toxicity in the lung. In: Selectivity and molecular mechanisms of toxicity (De Matteis F. and Lock E.A., eds.) McMillan, London, 1987:3-26.
10. Chenery R.J. The utility of hepatocytes in drug metabolism studies. Progress in Drug Metabolism 1988;11:217-265.
11. Moldeus P. Comparison of model systems for metabolism. In: Drug Metabolism: From Molecule to Man (Benford D.J., Bridges J.W. and Gibson G.G., eds.) Taylor & Francis, London, 1987:309-316.
12. Zwart A., Arts J.H.E., Kolkman-Houweling J.M. and Schoen E.D. Determination of concentration-time-mortality relationships to replace LC_{50} values. Inhalation Toxicology 1990;2:105-117.

13. Conolly R.B. and Andersen M.E. Biologically based pharmacodynamic models: Tools for toxicological research and risk assessment. Annual Reviews in Pharmacology and Toxicology 1991;31:503-523.
14. Walum E., Balls M., Bianchi V., Blaauboer B., Bolcsfoldi G., Guillouzo A., Moore G.A., Odland L., Reinhardt C. and Spielmann H. ECITTS: an integrated approach to the application of *in vitro* test systems to the hazard assessment of chemicals. Alternatives to Laboratory Animals 1992;20:406-428.
15. Sirica A.E. and Pitot H.C. Drug metabolism and effects of carcinogens in cultured hepatic cells. Pharmacology Reviews 1980;31:205-228.
16. Van de Werve G. Isolation and characteristics of hepatocytes. Toxicology 1980;18:179-185.
17. Paine A.J. The maintenance of cytochrome P-450 in rat hepatocyte culture: some applications of liver cell cultures to the study of drug metabolism, toxicity and the induction of the P-450 system. Chemico-Biological Interactions 1990;74:1-31.
18. Guguen-Guillouzo C., Clement B., Baffet G., Beaumont C., Morel-Chany E., Glaise D. and Guillouzo A. Maintenance and reversibility of active albumin secretion by adult rat hepatocytes co-cultured with another liver epithelial cell type. Experimental Cell Research 1983;143:47-54.
19. Gómez-Lechón M.J., Lopez P., Donato M.T., Montoya A., Laurrauri A., Giminez P., Trullenque R., Fabra R. and Castell J.V. Culture of human hepatocytes from small surgical liver biopsies. Biochemical characterization and comparison with *in vivo*. In Vitro Cellular and Developmental Biology 1990;26:67-74.
20. Balls M., Blaauboer B., Brusick D., Frazier J., Lamb D., Pemberton M., Reinhardt C., Roberfroid M., Rosenkranz H., Schmid B., Spielmann H., Stammati A.-L. and Walum E. Report and recommendations of the CAAT/ERGATT workshop on the validation of toxicity test procedures. Alternatives to Laboratory Animals 1990;18:303-337.

2
In vitro systems to study fibroblast functions

B. Eckes and T. Krieg

Department of Dermatology, University of Cologne,
Joseph-Stelzmann Straße 9, 50931 Köln (Germany).

Introduction

Fibroblasts represent a poorly characterized cell type which is present in most tissues of the organism. Although fibroblasts can be maintained in cell culture for a long time, not much is known about their differentiation state *in vivo*. Some evidence exists that fibroblasts are present in various types, specific for a certain tissue. So, tendon fibroblasts differ from skin fibroblasts, and in skin distinct fibroblasts have been isolated from papillary and reticular dermis. In addition, based on recent publications by Bayreuther [1], it can be concluded that fibroblasts represent a stem cell system and that they undergo a distinct terminal differentiation allowing to characterize several fibroblasts subtypes which have been numbered I through VII. Some of these characteristics can be kept also under *in vitro* conditions for some time. In addition, several attempts have been made to develop *in vitro* systems which resemble some aspects of the *in vivo* situation and which allow to study fibroblast function and their modulation by pharmacologic agents.

Fibroblasts have a variety of different functions which include the migration and recognition of certain chemotactic agents. This enables fibroblasts to follow a concentration gradient and migrate directionally. Fibroblasts can also proliferate according to external signals, e.g. cytokines; they can recognize distinct domains of the extracellular matrix molecules and attach to them. Fibroblasts can construct lattices formed from collagen fibrils, and probably they are responsible for wound contraction *in vivo*. Finally, fibroblasts are mainly responsible for synthesis and degradation of the extracellular matrix and also for the remodeling of the tissue following damage. All these different functions play an important role for many biological and pathological events. They regulate morphogenesis and development, control wound healing, tissue repair and scar formation. There is a strong demand to develop pharmacologic agents which modulate these functions. There is also the need to screen for side effects of drugs which could potentially interfere with wound healing or tissue repair. This requires the establishment and characterization of *in vitro* systems which allow to study the various fibroblast functions, to quantify them, and to investigate the influence of drugs under conditions similar to the *in vivo* situation.

Migration and chemotaxis

Luring fibroblasts from the surrounding tissue into an area of injury is a crucial event during wound healing. *In vitro*, the directional movement of fibroblasts along a concentration gradient can be studied using a Boyden chamber [2-5]. Here the cells migrate through a polycarbonated filter towards a chemoattractant. This system also allows to investigate and quantify random migration, when identical concentrations of chemoattractants are supplied to both chambers.

Numerous substances have already been identified to display strong chemotactic activity for fibroblasts. These include several cytokines such as platelet-derived growth factor (PDGF), epidermal growth factor (EGF), fibroblast growth factor (FGF) and transforming growth factor-β (TGF-β) [6-7]. Additional modulation of fibroblast migration can be achieved by substances which do not possess intrinsic activity, but regulate the cellular response to other chemoattractive substances. Here, interferon-α (IFN-α) and interferon-γ (IFN-γ) have been shown to reduce the responsiveness of fibroblasts toward other chemoattractants [8,9]. Similar effects have been reported to occur after treatment with retinoids and corticosteroids [10].

Besides cytokines, extracellular matrix proteins and even more proteolytic fragments derived from these molecules (e.g. fibronectin, collagens) have been found to exert strong chemotactic activities. The degree of tissue damage resulting in the formation of proteolytic fragments determines therefore the quantity of chemotactic substances and regulates the migration of fibroblasts into the damaged area. A similar regulatory loop has been found to control the activity of some cytokines. Interleukin-1 (IL-1) has a high chemotactic activity in low concentrations, whereas at high concentrations it induces fibroblast proliferation (Fig. 1). By releasing IL-1, fibroblasts are therefore lured from the surrounding tissue following the concentration gradient into the injured area where high concentrations of IL-1 are present. Chemotactic activity is therefore reduced and IL-1 acts mainly as an inducer of fibroblast proliferation, which is required after the cells have invaded the damaged tissue [11].

In many situations fibroblasts have to pass through extracellular matrix, which could act as a barrier. Therefore, the classic Boyden chamber reflects the *in vivo* situation only to a certain extent, and a modified assay has been developed which allows to introduce extracellular matrix components as barriers [12]. The cells are seeded on top of a lattice formed by an interstitial collagen or by basement membrane proteins. Fibroblasts then recognize a chemoattractive substance in the lower chamber and start to migrate through the barrier toward the chemoattractant. Several factors have already been recognized which modulate the interaction of the cells with different barriers. This can result in a markedly increased penetration of the cells although their chemotactic response is not altered.

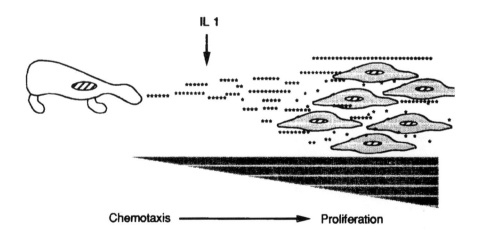

Figure 1:
Biphasic effect of IL-1 on fibroblasts.
A concentration gradient of interleukin-1 (*) elicits fibroblast migration at low, and fibroblast proliferation at high concentrations.

Attachment of fibroblasts to various matrix proteins

A prerequisite for fibroblast-matrix interaction is the recognition of certain biologically active domains in the large multidomain extracellular matrix proteins by cellular receptors. Several of these have been identified, and they were found to be specific for distinct proteins. Fibronectin is probably the best characterized protein which acts as an attachment protein for fibroblasts. However, fibroblasts can also adhere to collagens I, III, IV, to laminin and also glycosaminoglycans [13].

Various factors were found to influence fibroblast attachment; so cytokines are able to up- or downregulate fibroblast receptors. Induction of collagen synthesis in fibroblasts by ascorbic acid has also been shown to increase fibroblast attachment. Several *in vitro* assays are available to monitor and quantify fibroblast attachment to various substances, and to investigate the influence of pharmacologic agents.

Proliferation of fibroblasts

Control of fibroblast proliferation plays an important role during the formation of granulation tissue, the development of hypertrophic scars, of keloids and also in fibrotic reactions. *In vivo*, proliferation of fibroblasts is mainly controlled by cytokines and growth factors, e.g. IL-1, FGF, PDGF, tumor necrosis factor (TNF) and TGF-β [14]. These are released by immune cells, by epithelial cells, or even by fibroblasts. The influence of various cytokines can be investigated in *in vitro* systems. Here, the combination of cell biological procedures and molecular biological techniques will in addition allow to differentiate between a direct effect of these cytokines and an indirect activity by modulating the expression of a cytokine receptor on the cell surface (Fig. 2).

In these systems, specific culture conditions including type and concentration of serum, duration of cultures, number of passages and cell density are critical. In addition, *in vivo* fibroblasts are in close contact with other cells, and much more complex interactions have to be considered. Therefore combined culture systems have been developed, in which 2 or 3 different cell types are kept in close contact, are then exposed to cytokines or pharmacologic agents, and the proliferation of fibroblasts in these systems is followed.

Lattice contraction by fibroblasts

In search of an *in vitro* culture system for fibroblasts that reflects the physiological environment of cells more closely than monolayer cultures, Bell *et al.* [15] established three-dimensional matrices reconstituted mainly of collagen I fibrils. Fibroblasts seeded into such matrices are able to contract the initially loose fibrillar collagen network to a dense, dermis-like structure. This contraction process occurs time-dependently and has a duration of a few hours to 1 day. The rate of lattice contraction is directly proportional to the number of cells which populate the matrix, and varies inversely with the protein concentration in the matrix. The addition of serum is indispensable for contraction to proceed.

Fibroblasts can be maintained in such three-dimensional collagenous environments over long periods of time, e.g. several weeks to a few months, provided replenishment of nutrients and serum occurs [16].

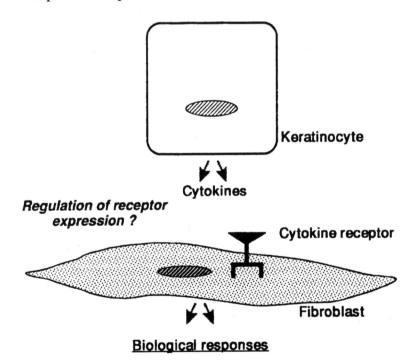

Figure 2:
Cell-cell interaction modulates the biological response of fibroblasts. Cell-cell interactions are frequently mediated by cytokines which can only become active when their corresponding receptor is expressed on the target cell.

Short-term culture, however, has provided more evidence elucidating the mechanism of contraction. Inhibition experiments showed that an intact cytoskeleton as well as ongoing protein synthesis are mandatory [15,17]. It has been suggested that contraction results from migration of fibroblasts through the lattice, attachment to collagen fibrils via integrin receptors, and subsequent organization of collagen fibres into bundles. This physical rearrangement of the matrix involves tractional forces which can be measured in appropriate experimental set-ups, and which provide a suitable parameter for quantitative studies [18]. In addition, quantification is easily achieved by plotting the gel diameter against the time of lattice culture.

Numerous substances have been included in this system and shown to modulate the contraction process. These include physiologically active agents like TGF-β and PDGF which could both be shown to stimulate contraction [19,20], and pharmacologic agents like glucocorticoids which inhibit lattice contraction in a linear, dose-dependent fashion [21].

In summary, three-dimensional collagen lattices populated by fibroblasts are regarded as a suitable *in vitro* system to study the mechanisms operating in the process of wound contraction (Fig. 3). Unlike other culture systems, it allows the quantification of contractile forces exerted by fibroblasts as well as the investigation and measurement of drug action pertinent to the pathogenesis or treatment of fibrosis and diseases involving dysregulated wound healing.

Matrix production

Fibroblasts are the main resident cells in skin responsible *in vivo* for the tightly controlled processes of matrix deposition on one hand, and on the other of matrix degradation during tissue remodeling.

In vitro, the accumulation of newly synthesized matrix molecules has been studied in detail using fibroblast monolayer cultures derived from tissue explants [22-24]. These represent a well-characterized system that allows monitoring of a number of cellular functions simultaneously. In specific, the biosynthesis of matrix molecules and its modulation by biologically active substances can be studied applying a wide range of technical approaches which give insight not only into the nature and quality of products synthesized, but - in part - also allow quantitative assessment of biosynthetic capacities (Figs. 4 and 5). These studies include the application of protein chemistry using e.g. metabolic protein labelling, immunochemistry trying to detect specific antigens by radio-immunoassays, as well as molecular biology relating to measurement of cell proliferation and transcriptional activity.

Monolayers do not allow, however, to study the interaction of fibroblasts with a surrounding extracellular matrix which *in vivo* constitutes the physiological three-dimensional environment, communicating with the cells via specific receptors, eliciting cascades of signalling pathways, thereby modulating numerous cellular functions including the synthesis of matrix macromolecules. Table I summarizes the most abundant constituents of extracellular matrix which interact with cells in skin.

Studies based on the collagen lattice as a model to investigate cell-extracellular matrix interaction clearly demonstrated differential

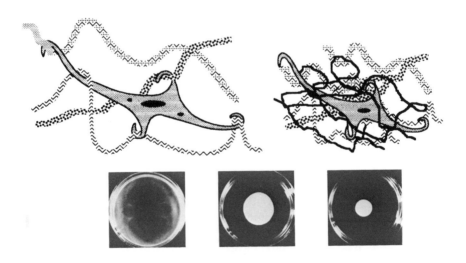

Figure 3 :
Collagen lattice as a model for wound contraction. Collagen lattices are prepared by seeding fibroblasts into a suspension of collagen fibers (lower left). During a few hours, the cells organize and contract the matrix to a dense, tissue-like structure (lower middle and right). The upper scheme depicts this process, showing a fibroblast attaching to various matrix molecules.

REGULATION OF COLLAGEN SYNTHESIS BY TGF-ß

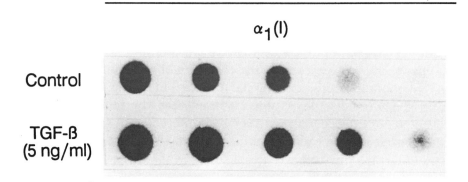

Figure 4:
Induction of collagen synthesis by TGF-β. RNA was isolated from fibroblast monolayers which were treated with 5 ng/ml TGF-β (lower) and from untreated controls (upper), and applied in decreasing amounts to a filter. This dot blot was hybridized to a probe specific for the alpha-1 chain of collagen I. TGF-β clearly leads to increased steady-state levels of collagen I mRNA.

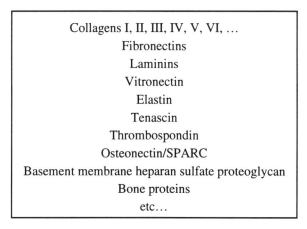

Table I:
Components of the extracellular matrix interacting with cells. List of the most frequently occurring extracellular matrix (ECM) macromolecules which surround and interact with all types of cells via specific cell surface receptors, thereby modulating cellular response.

regulation of matrix components. As shown in Table II, the cell-matrix interaction leads to specific downregulation of collagens I and III, whereas others are simultaneously upregulated. Collagen VI provides an excellent example for differential subunit regulation within one final multimeric protein. These studies also demonstrate that cytoskeletal components such as actin, but also others not listed here which relate to matrix contraction are clearly regulated [25-28].

Three-dimensional fibroblast culture models like the floating collagen

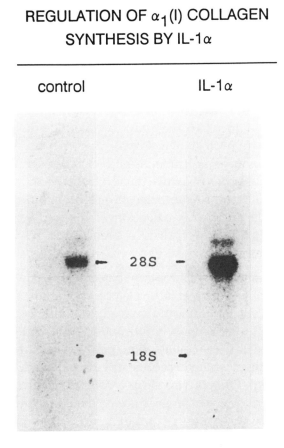

Figure 5 :
Induction of collagen synthesis by IL-1 alpha. RNA was isolated from fibroblast monolayer which were treated with IL-1 (right) and from untreated controls (left). Northern blots were hybridized to a collagen alpha-1 (I)-specific cDNA. IL-1 alpha increases the level of both alpha-1 transcripts.

lattice described above, have yielded insight into the regulation of collagen production by fibroblasts, in specific of collagen I. On the protein level, as well as on the transcriptional level, collagen I is reduced to less than 10% compared to monolayer cultures. Downregulation of collagen I has been shown to be regulated on a pretranslational level, involving both transcriptional and posttranscriptional control mechanisms [29]. Owing to the fact that collagen production in this system is reduced to very low basal levels, this model is well-suited to study the mode of action of fibrogenic agents like TGF-β, known to enhance collagen production, and associated *in vivo* with the induction of fibrosis in various tissues [30-32].

As also shown in Table II, the interaction of fibroblasts with a three-dimensional collagen matrix induces the synthesis of high levels of collagenase. Applying molecular biological techniques, the mechanism of induction was elucidated. The collagenase gene contains an upstream regulatory element which interacts with the nuclear protein complex AP-1 and thereby leads to increased transcription of the gene [33]. Analysis of the culture supernatant revealed a much more efficient conversion of latent to active enzyme, as well as secretion, when compared to monolayer cultures. As with collagen synthesis induction, this system represents a sensitive tool to study the action of substances which reduce collagenase synthesis or activation, and might therefore be of importance in the investigation of the pathogenesis of tumor formation and metastasis, and in tissue remodeling during development and wound repair.

An *in vitro* system which reflects even better the physiology of skin than the above described collagen lattice is one combining several cell types in co-culture, therefore allowing to study not only cell-matrix, but in addition cell-cell interactions [34]. Fibroblasts and endothelial cells are seeded together into a collagenous matrix, constituting a dermal equivalent, on top of which keratinocytes are cultured, constituting the epidermal moiety of this *in vitro* skin equivalent. It had been known that co-culture of keratinocytes on postmitotic mouse or human fibroblastic cells is required to support human keratinocyte growth at clonal densities in serum containing medium. Exposing the 'epidermis' of this organotypic co-culture system to air has been suggested to result in a more physiologic flow of nutrients, which leads to an improvement of tissue architecture and induction of terminal differentiation. This complex model system has been designed to study the specific interaction between epidermal and mesenchymal compartments.

Each of the individual cells in this system is subject to complex regulatory circuits elicited by the intercellular communication. Obviously the pattern of biologically active substances released from each individual cell type may be different from the pattern of the identical cell type cultured in another system, due to the pattern of synergizing or inhibitory substances released by neighbouring cell types.

Studying this net effect is of special importance in the testing of pharmacologic agents which in less complex systems yield differential

	monolayer	collagen lattice
α1(I)	100	5
α2(I)	100	5
α1(III)	100	6
α1(VI)	100	290
α2(VI)	100	250
α3(VI)	100	100
Fibronectin	100	100
β-Tubulin	100	100
β-Actin	100	8
Collagenase	100	2300
Il-6	100	1300
Decorin	100	300

Table II :

Differential regulation of matrix components in fibroblast monolayers and collagen lattices. Embedding fibroblasts into a three-dimensional collagenous matrix results in up- and downregulation of a number of matrix constituents, including collagens, cytokines, enzymes, proteoglycans, and cytoskeletal scaffold proteins. The values shown here are based on Northern and dot blot analyses, representing pretranslational controls. Values for monolayers are set at 100%. Most interesting is coordinated downregulation of collagens I and III, with simultaneous strong induction of interstitial collagenase, and subunit regulation (collagen VI).

responses by the individual cell types, e.g. proliferation in the epidermal, but growth arrest in the dermal compartment.

An example which illustrates nicely the importance of feedback control arising from cells interacting with each other and the matrix is the application of retinoic acid to the skin equivalent (Fig. 6). Here, the substance induces synthesis of TGF-β in keratinocytes, inducing proliferation and collagen synthesis in fibroblasts [35].

Fig. 7 describes the different monolayer and combined culture systems that can be established from skin biopsies, and which are used to

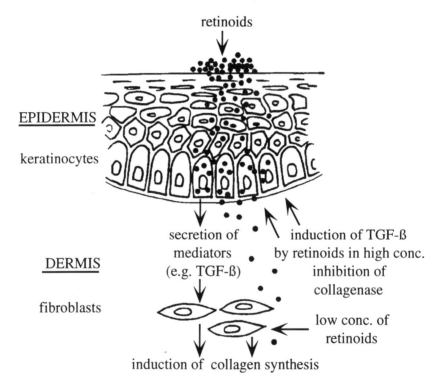

Figure 6 :
Differential effect of retinoids in skin. Application of retinoids to the skin surface leads to a concentration gradient of the substance in skin. At high concentrations in the basal cell layer of the epidermis, it induces secretion of mediators like TGF-β in keratinocytes. In addition, high retinoid concentrations in the epidermis and in the upper dermis lead to inhibition of collagenase. As the concentration is decreased in lower layers of the dermis, synthesis of collagen in fibroblasts is induced by low retinoid concentrations and also by TGF-β secreted by the epidermal cells.

investigate the action of pharmacologic agents in skin. Thus skin biopsies can be taken into short-term organ culture or processed directly, as for in situ hybridization and immunohistochemistry. Alternatively, the dermis can be separated from the epidermis, and fibroblasts and keratinocytes are studied individually in monolayers or combined in co-culture which takes into account cell-cell interactions. Matrix proteins, e.g. laminin, fibronectin, and collagen can be extracted and purified from the dermis and combined with fibroblasts in a dermal equivalent (collagen lattice) which allows to study cell-extracellular matrix interactions. Finally, combination of several cell types and matrix leads to an *in vitro* reconstituted skin model which is a fairly close

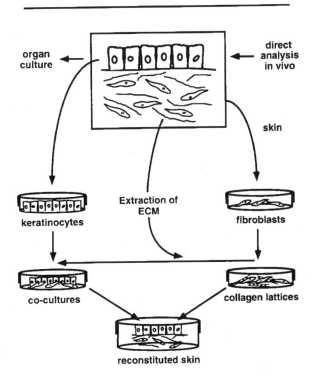

Figure 7 :
In vitro cell culture models derived from skin. Skin biopsies (in box) can be used to establish monolayer cultures of epidermal and dermal cell types, as well as combined cultures to study cell-cell and cell-matrix interactions. For details, see text.

approximation to the organ 'skin'.

In summary, it appears reasonable to use simple systems containing few variables to assess major effects of substances under investigation, and to dissect the molecular mechanism of action, before proceeding to more and more complex systems like organotypic co-culture of several cell types in different matrix environments which are better suited to study net effects.

References

1. Bayreuther K., Rodemann H.P., Hommel R., Dittmann K., Albiez M. and Francz P.I. Human skin fibroblasts differentiate along a terminal cell lineage. Proceedings of the National Academy of Sciences of the USA 1988;85:5112-5116.
2. Boyden S. The chemotactic effect of mixtures of antibody and antigen on polymorphonuclear lymphocytes. Journal of Experimental Medicine 1962;115:453-462.
3. Postlethwaite A.E., Snyderman R. and Kang A.H. The chemotactic attraction of fibroblasts to a lymphocyte-derived factor. Journal of Experimental Medicine 1976;144:1188-1203.
4. Lauffenberger P.A. and Zigmon S.H. Chemotactic factor concentration gradients in chemotaxis assay systems. Journal of Immunological Methods 1981;49:45-60.
5. Mensing H., Pontz B.F., Müller P.K. *et al.* A study on fibroblast chemotaxis using fibronectin and conditioned medium as chemoattractants. European Journal of Cell Biology 1983;29:268-273.
6. Seppä H., Grotendorst G., Seppä S., Schiffman E. and Martin G.R. Platelet-derived growth factor is chemotactic for fibroblasts. Journal of Cell Biology 1982;92:584-588.
7. Chen T.L., Bates R.L., Xu Y., Ammann A.J. and Beck L.S. Human recombinant transforming growth factor-$\beta 1$ modulation of biochemical and cellular events in healing of ulcer wounds. Journal of Investigative Dermatology 1992;98:428-435.
8. Adelmann-Grill B.C., Hein R., Wach F. and Krieg T. Inhibition of fibroblast chemotaxis by recombinant human interferon-gamma and interferon-alpha. Journal of Cellular Physiology 1987;130:270-275.
9. Hein R., Mensing H., Müller P.K., Braun-Falco O. and Krieg T. Effect of vitamin A and its derivatives on collagen production and chemotactic response of fibroblasts. British Journal of Dermatology 1984;111:37-44.
10. Hein R., Mauch C., Hatamochi A. and Krieg T. Influence of corticosteroids on chemotactic response and collagen metabolism of human skin fibroblasts. Biochemical Pharmacology 1988;37:2723-2729.

11. Heckmann M., Adelmann-Grill B.C., Hein R. and Krieg T. Biphasic effect of IL-1-alpha on dermal fibroblasts: enhancement of chemotactic responsiveness at low concentrations and of mRNA expression for collagenase at high concentration. Journal of Investigative Dermatology 1993;100:780-784.
12. Albini I., Iwamoto Y., Kleinmann H.K. et al. Invasive activity and chemotactic response to growth factors by Kaposi's sarcoma cells. Cancer Research 1987;47:3239-3245.
13. Ruoslahti E. and Pierschbacher M. Arg-Gly-Asp: A versatile cell recognition signal. Cell 1986;44:517-518.
14. Kang A.H. Fibroblast activation. Laboratory and Clinical Medicine 1978;92:1-4.
15. Bell E., Ivarsson B. and Merrill C. Production of a tissue-like structure by contraction of collagen lattices by human fibroblasts of different proliferative potential in vitro. Proceedings of the National Academy of Sciences of the USA 1979; 76:1274-1278.
16. Nakagawa S., Pawelek P. and Grinnell F. Long-term culture of fibroblasts in contracted collagen gels: effects on cell growth and biosynthetic activity. Journal of Investigative Dermatology 1989;93:792-798.
17. Guidry C. and Grinnell F. Studies on the mechanism of hydrated collagen gel reorganization by human skin fibroblasts. Journal of Cell Science 1985;79:67-81.
18. Delvoye P., Wiliquet P., Leveque J.L., Nusgens B.V. and Lapière C.M. Measurement of mechanical forces generated by skin fibroblasts in a three-dimensional collagen gel. Journal of Investigative Dermatology 1991;97:898-902.
19. Montesano R. and Orci L. Transforming growth factor β stimulates collagen-matrix contraction by fibroblasts: implications for wound healing. Proceedings of the National Academy of Sciences of the USA 1988; 85:4894-4897.
20. Gullberg D., Tingström A., Thuresson A.C., Olsson L., Terracio L., Borg T.K. and Rubin K. $\beta 1$ integrin-mediated collagen gel contraction is stimulated by PDGF. Experimental Cell Research 1990;186:264-272.
21. Coulomb B., Dubertret L., Bell E. and Touraine R. The contractility of fibroblasts in a collagen lattice is reduced by corticosteroids. Journal of Investigative Dermatology 1984;82:341-344.
22. Goldring M.B. and Krane S.M. Modulation by recombinant IL-1 of synthesis of types I and III collagens and associated procollagen levels in cultured human cells. Journal of Biological Chemistry 1987;262:16724-16729.
23. Hämäläinen L., Oikarinen J. and Kivirikko K.I. Synthesis and degradation of type I procollagen mRNAs in cultured human fibroblasts and the effect of cortisol. Journal of Biological Chemistry 1985;260:720-725.
24. Ignotz R.A. and Massague J. TGF-β stimulates the expression of fibronectin and collagen and their incorporation into the extracellular matrix. Journal of Biological Chemistry 1986;261:4337-4342.
25. Mauch C., Hatamochi A., Scharffetter K. and Krieg T. Regulation of collagen synthesis within a three-dimensional collagen gel. Experimental Cell Research 1988;178:493-503.

26. Mauch C., Adelmann-Grill B., Hatamochi A. and Krieg T. Collagenase gene expression in fibroblasts is regulated by a three-dimensional contact with collagen. FEBS Letters 1989;250:301-305.
27. Heckmann M., Aumailley M., Hatamochi A., Chu M.L., Timpl R. and Krieg T. Down-regulation of alpha-3 (VI) chain expression by gamma-interferon decreases synthesis and deposition of collagen type VI. European Journal of Biochemistry 1989;182:719-726.
28. Eckes B., Hunzelmann N., Ziegler-Heitbrock H.W.L., Urbanski A., Luger T., Krieg T. and Mauch C. Interleukin-6 expression by fibroblasts grown in three-dimensional gel cultures. FEBS Letters 1992;298:229-232.
29. Eckes B., Mauch C., Hüppe G. and Krieg T. Downregulation of collagen synthesis in fibroblasts within three-dimensional collagen lattices involves transcriptional and posttranscriptional mechanisms. FEBS Letters 1993; 318:129-133.
30. Roberts A.B., Sporn M.B., Assoian R.K., Smith J.M., Roche N.S., Wakefield L.M., Heine U.I., Liotta L.A., Falanga V., Kehrl J.H. and Fauci S. Transforming growth factor type beta: rapid induction of fibrosis and angiogenesis *in vivo* and stimulation of collagen formation *in vitro*. Proceedings of the National Academy of Sciences of the USA 1986;83:4167-4171.
31. Border W.A. and Ruoslahti E. Transforming growth factor β1 induces extracellular matrix formation in glomerulonephritis. Cell Differentiation 1990;32:425-432.
32. Kulozik M., Hogg A., Lankat-Buttgereit B. and Krieg T. Co-localization of transforming growth factor β2 with alpha-1 (I) procollagen mRNA in tissue sections of patients with systemic scleroderma. Journal of Clinical Investigation 1990;186:917-922.
33. Angel P., Imagawa M., Chiu R., Stein B., Imbra R.J., Rahmsdorf H.J., Jonat C., Herrlich P. and Karin M. Phorbol ester-inducible genes contain a common cis element recognized by a TPA-modulated trans-acting factor. Cell 1987;49:729-739.
34. Asselineau B., Bernard B.A., Bailly C. and Darmon Y.M. Epidermal morphogenesis and induction of the 67 kD keratin polypeptide by culture of human keratinocytes at the liquid-air-interface. Experimental Cell Research 1985;159:536-539.
35. Stumpenhausen G., Kulozik M., Hein R., Oono T., McLane J., Bryce G.F., Mauch C. and Krieg T. The influence of retinoids on chemotaxis and connective tissue synthesis of fibroblasts. In: Cell and tissue culture models in dermatological research. (Bernd A., Bereiter-Hahn J., Hevert F. and Holzmann H., eds.) Springer-Verlag, Berlin, Heidelberg, 1993:241-248.

3

Three-dimensional reconstructed human skin for *in vitro* pharmaco-toxicology

B. Coulomb* and L. Dubertret**

INSERM 312, Laboratoire de Pharmacologie Cutanée
* Hôpital Henri Mondor, 94010 Créteil (France)
** Hôpital St Louis, 75010 Paris (France)

Introduction

The skin is a barrier organ that serves many essential functions, including limiting water loss and protecting against physical, chemical and microbiological agents. Pharmaco-toxicological studies on skin are thus of prime importance to prevent any diminution of these functions, or to restore them. In addition, alterations expressed at the level of the skin can disclose a more general disease.

The skin is formed by an association of two tissues: the epidermis, which is mainly composed of keratinocytes and appendices (hairs and glands), and the dermis.

The epidermis provides the first line of protection through the presence of its three cell types, keratinocytes, melanocytes and Langerhans cells (Fig. 1).

The keratinocytes form 95% of the epidermal cell population. The structure and vital properties of the epidermis depend on keratinocyte differentiation. From a germinative layer, keratinocytes differentiate, migrate to the skin surface and finally form a waterproof horny layer directly in contact with air. The germinative layer of keratinocytes is separated from the dermis by an acellular structure, the basement membrane.

Melanocytes are responsible for skin pigmentation and so play an essential role in photoprotection.

The Langerhans cells play a major role in the recognition of substances that have been able to pass through the horny layer. They are responsible for antigen presentation to keratinocytes and blood cells, and make the skin an important element of the immune system.

Under the epidermis is the dermis, a connective tissue made up of an extracellular matrix interspersed mainly with fibroblasts (Fig. 1).

The dermis has long been considered a supply and support tissue for the epidermis. Nerves and vessels end in the dermis and the surrounding fibroblasts secrete macromolecules (collagen, elastin and proteoglycans) on which the mechanical quality of the skin depends. However, it is now also known that the dermis controls the development of the epidermis during embryogenesis [1] and its growth and differentiation during adulthood [2,3,4].

From this description, it is clear that both the barrier functions of the skin and normal cell differentiation depend on multiple interactions between various cells types, and also between these cells and the extracellular matrix.

Pharmacological research has thus been undertaken with the purpose of finding ways of maintaining or restoring the quality and differentiation of the skin and, more specifically, the epidermis. However, the scope of any *in vivo* study of the human skin is limited for obvious ethical reasons and animal models are sometimes poorly predictive.

It is clear, therefore, that dermatological research needs to develop and

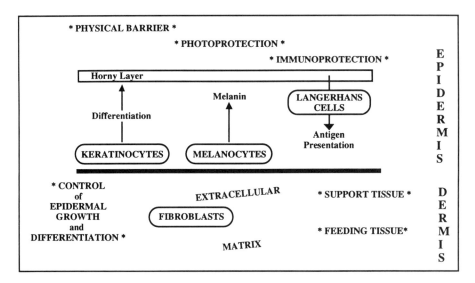

Figure 1 :
Schematic representation of the anatomy and physiology of the skin.

improve *in vitro* models. The advantages of these models include a reduction in the number of living animals used and the possibility of using human cells. Nevertheless, before such models are used extensively in the field of normative toxicological and pharmacological testing, they need to be correlated to the *in vivo* state, firstly to mimic the animal model that has been replaced, and secondly (and most critically) to be predictive for humans.

Two complementary lines of research into the *in vitro* pharmaco-toxicology of the skin are being undertaken: one aims to define *in vitro* models in relation to existing animal models, the other aims to reconstruct skin *in vitro* (with more or less complexity and with normal or pathological cells), in order to identify what are the cell-cell or cell-matrix interactions that are of major importance for cell behaviour and cell response to drugs.

Several skin cell culture models have progressively been developed. The first models used skin samples, either simply to keep them alive, or to enable study of cell behaviour in an organized tissue (organotypic culture), or to use them as a source of skin cells [5,6,7,8]. In the case of the latter, epidermal cells, dermal cells or both could be observed whilst they migrate out of the skin explant and progressively cover the culture substrate.

However, as was discussed previously, the skin is a complex organ and the aim soon became to separate the various cell types from one another, thereby eliminating the multiple interactions existing in the tissue *in vivo* or in the skin explants *in vitro*.

The next development, which is where we are now, is to recreate in controlled conditions *in vitro*, the cell-cell and cell-matrix interactions that exist *in vivo* and that are lost in classical culture systems. This concept of organogenesis *in vitro* (Fig. 2) consists of the recovery of *in vivo* cell behaviour, due to the re-establishment of a physiological environment. A simplified human skin was the first organ to be reconstructed *in vitro* [9] and was composed, as *in vivo*, of a dermis and an epidermis from the recombination of the three basic skin components, fibroblasts, collagen and keratinocytes. Our laboratory has been developing this model for a number of years with a view to both grafting in humans and evaluating the physiology, pathophysiology and pharmacology of the human skin. Whatever the *in vitro* skin model, the reconstruction usually needs two steps. The first one is the reconstruction of a dermal substrate (dermal equivalent), and the second is the covering of this substrate by keratinocytes that will form an epidermis (skin equivalent).

Dermal equivalent

The first model used to study the dermis was simple fibroblast monolayers. Later, the development of three-dimensional cultures within collagen matrices [10] reproduced *in vivo* cell/matrix interactions and, consequently, *in vivo*-like fibroblast differentiation. In addition, fibroblast contractility could be studied.

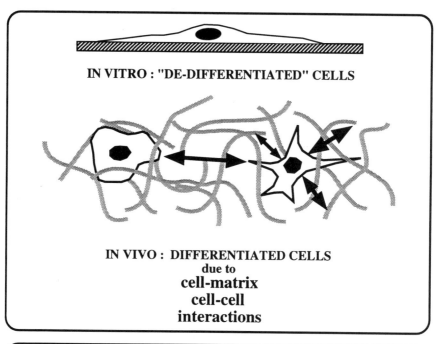

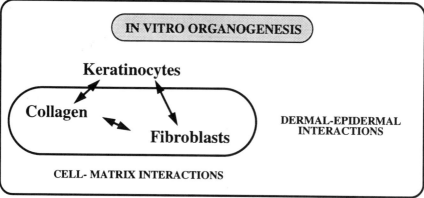

Figure 2 :
In vitro organogenesis

Regulation of fibroblast division in the dermal equivalent.

Whereas fibroblasts cultivated in monolayers divide until they reach confluency, in dermal equivalents they remain well-separated and are also growth-regulated [11].
Changes in fibroblast numbers in the dermal equivalent thus depend on their interactions with the collagen matrix. Fibroblast growth kinetics depend on the density of the cells seeded: from 4×10^4 to 10^5 cells/ml, proliferation is inversely proportional to the number of cells seeded, and cell density reaches a similar point after a few weeks, whatever the density at the time of seeding.
This suggests that the dermal equivalent is an experimental model for studying the cell-cell and cell-matrix interactions responsible for the control of cell growth homeostasis and its modifications by pharmacological agents at a tissue level [12].

Fibroblast morphogenesis.

The dermal equivalent system makes it possible to study the different steps of fibroblast morphogenesis from the spherical shape observed when forming the gel to the bipolar shape similar to that observed *in vivo*. The speed of this morphogenesis increases with fibroblast density, showing that it is dependent on cell to cell interactions. However, a slow but complete morphogenesis can be achieved by a single fibroblast alone in a collagen gel [13].

Fibroblast contraction.

The dermal equivalent model can be used for quantitative studies of collagen fibril condensation by fibroblasts, an important function expressed during wound healing. The rate and extent of contraction is measured by monitoring the decrease in the diameter of the dermal equivalent. Contraction has been shown to be proportional to the initial fibroblast concentration and inversely proportional to the collagen concentration [10].
Contraction is also sensitive to pharmacological treatment. When dexamethasone or hydrocortisone (2.5×10^{-4} M to 1.5×10^{-5} M) are added to the culture medium, in the presence of an inhibitor of cell division that does not affect the cytoskeleton (e.g. 1µg/ml of cytosine arabinoside), the ability of fibroblasts to contract the collagen matrix is inhibited in a

linear, dose-dependent fashion [14]. However, the effect of hydrocortisone is completely reversible, while that of dexamethasone is not. Even if the inhibition of collagen matrix contraction by fibroblasts and its reversibility is related to the therapeutic efficiency of these steroids, their mechanism of action cannot be explained in terms of contraction alone.

Contraction of the dermal equivalent results from several phenomena that can occur simultaneously or independently. It depends not only on the way they spread within and attach to the matrix [15], but also on the fibroblasts themselves, i.e. their state of division and differentiation and, of course, contractility potential. By way of an example, when fibroblast divisions are strongly stimulated by acidic fibroblast growth factor (aFGF), the speed of collagen contraction is strongly reduced, despite the increased number of fibroblasts. In fact, mitotic fibroblasts contract collagen fibers less efficiently [16]. Consequently, the speed of collagen contraction is not a function of the number of fibroblasts, but of the number of fibroblasts able to interact with the collagen matrix. This result suggests that aFGF might be of therapeutic value in reducing the excessive contraction which can occur during wound healing.

Forces developed by fibroblasts in the collagen matrix can be measured [17], together with their variations in response to disease or pharmacological treatment [18]. In addition, when the contraction of collagen gels is mechanically restrained, the fibroblasts under tension are more active in terms of biosynthetic activity, supporting the hypothesis that mechanical information transmitted from the matrix to the cell modulates cell behaviour [19].

According to whether it contracts in restrained conditions or not, the dermal equivalent can thus be considered as a pharmacological model for either a resting tissue or one that is reorganizing, as occurs, for example, during wound healing.

Fibroblast differentiation in the dermal equivalent.

As we have seen, with regard to morphology and proliferation, fibroblasts in the dermal equivalent behave as *in vivo*. This is also true for other differentiation criteria that can also be important for assessing reactions to pharmacological treatment.

In the human skin, the fibroblast cell membrane is permeable to diaminobenzidine (DAB), making it possible to visualize the activity of a key enzyme for arachidonic acid metabolism, prostaglandin H synthetase. This enzymatic activity is clearly expressed in the perinuclear envelope and in the endoplasmatic reticulum. Conversely, human skin fibroblasts cultivated in monolayer became impermeable to DAB and do not express prostaglandin H synthetase activity. In the dermal equivalent, the same fibroblasts, previously cultivated in monolayer, recover an *in vivo*-like cell membrane permeability to DAB, and 80% of these cells express a strong prostaglandin H synthetase activity.

Thus, two important cell functions, cell membrane permeability and prostaglandin H synthetase activity, expressed *in vivo*, disappear in monolayer and reappear in the dermal equivalent [20].

We have previously seen that when 1ng/ml aFGF was added to the culture medium in the presence of heparin (a factor that stabilizes aFGF), even though the number of fibroblasts in the dermal equivalents increased clearly after 1 and 3 weeks of culture relative to controls, the contraction of the collagen matrix was inhibited [16]. This phenomenon could be explained by the unavailability of dividing fibroblasts for matrix contraction. In addition, these experiments also throw light on the phenomenon of fibroblast maturation, since, when dermal equivalents were treated with aFGF at various times, the enhancement of fibroblast numbers peaked at around the third week and then fell progressively to control values by the fifth week [16]. This indicates that the differentiation and/or maturation of fibroblasts can modify the response to pharmacological agents, and the dermal equivalent provides a way to assess these phenomenons.

The importance of fibroblast origin and culture conditions are illustrated in the following example. The activity of 5α-reductase, an enzyme involved in the metabolism of testosterone, is 5- to 6-fold higher in skin biopsies taken in the pubis than in the arm. Initially present in monolayers, it disappears completely after several passages. Interestingly, fibroblasts from the pubis recover 5α-reductase activity when they are incorporated into the dermal equivalent, whereas fibroblasts from the arm do not [21]. This shows that fibroblasts are able to 'remember' their original localization, but that the expression of this memory depends on the culture conditions. The dermal equivalent thus offers a potential tool for the study of skin endocrinology.

Conclusion.

The dermal equivalent is a three-dimensional culture model that takes into account cell/matrix interactions and fibroblast contractility, parameters which cannot be evaluated in monolayers and are difficult to assay *in vivo*. In addition, fibroblasts recover differentiation characteristics similar to those *in vivo*, for example membrane permeability and enzyme expression, but also matrix component synthesis [22,23,24].

Another model consists in cultivating fibroblasts in a nylon mesh. Fibroblasts synthesize their own matrix leading to a three-dimensional tissular stucture [25]. The absence of exogenous extracellular matrix makes this culture model an important tool for fibrilogenesis studies and its pharmaco-toxicological modulations.

The dermal equivalents are thus important pharmacological models, but just as importantly, they are effective living substrates for epidermal cells.

Epidermis

In addition to allowing the recovery of dissociated cells [8,26,27], the use of a feeder layer of 3T3 fibroblasts permitted the maintenance and subcultivation of keratinocytes (seeded at low densities), which was a major breakthrough [28]. This was followed by the development of a defined culture medium [29].

Two strategies were used in parallel, the first aimed at optimizing keratinocyte proliferation [28,29], and the second one at promoting epidermal differentiation [30,31,32]. Fibroblasts and collagen were both found to be involved in promoting the growth and differentiation of keratinocytes. Indeed, a lethally irradiated feeder layer of either fibroblasts [28] or dermis [33] supports the subcultivation of keratinocytes and increases their life span. Collagen improves cell attachment and plating efficiency [34], and appears to be essential for basal lamina formation [35,36]. In addition, a vital dermis, as well as diffusible dermal products, have been shown to be necessary for normal epidermal growth and differentiation [4].

Dermal equivalents and their associated differentiated fibroblasts and collagen thus form a practical living substrate for keratinocytes.

Keratinocyte differentiation.

The reconstruction of simplified human skin *in vitro* involves, as *in vivo*, the association of a dermis and an epidermis. Initially, the epidermis was made from dissociated keratinocytes [37,38] which were seeded onto the dermal equivalent once fibroblast-mediated contraction had stabilized. In this way, a stratified epidermis formed at the surface of the dermal equivalent. Differentiation was improved when keratinocytes were cultured at the air-liquid interface [31]. The disadvantage of this seeding method is that epidermal growth is difficult to quantify.

We have thus developed another method of epidermalization which permits the quantification of epidermal growth and provides the large numbers of samples necessary for pharmacological experiments [39]. The keratinocyte source consists of small biopsies of either superficial skin or epidermis placed on the surface of the dermal equivalent. Keratinocytes grow out from both types of biopsies and divide: an epidermis thus spreads gradually over the surface of the dermal equivalent, a situation very similar to that which occurs during wound healing, except that the cells grow outwards from the biopsy, rather than inwards from the edges of the wound.

This new epidermis can differentiate as *in vivo*, with the formation of cuboid basal cells, keratohyalin granules, membrane-coating granules and the expression of high-molecular-weight keratins characteristic of terminal differentiation [39].

In vitro *model of epidermal aging.*

Like human diploid fibroblasts [40], human diploid keratinocytes have a finite life span and their growth potential falls with donor age [28], confirming that aging leads to at least a loss of proliferative capacity. In addition, in the Rheinwald and Green model, keratinocytes from sun-exposed skin have a shorter life span, and their plating efficiency is reduced [41]. This supports the view that accumulated damage due to UV irradiation *in vivo* increases cell senescence.

We have used epidermalized dermal equivalents made with biopsies from both pre-auricular (sun-exposed) and post-auricular (unexposed) skin from 40- to 65-year-old women undergoing face-lifts [42] and found that sun exposure *in vivo* strongly reduced epidermal growth *in vitro*, not only in terms of a decrease in the proliferation potential of the keratinocytes, but also in their migration.

Two parameters which are known to diminish with age (responsiveness to growth factors *in vitro* [41] and the rate of wound healing [43]) are taken into account in this model, along with the presence of epidermal growth factor (EGF) in the culture medium and the outgrowth of keratinocytes from the biopsy.

Having shown that sun-exposed and unexposed keratinocytes behave differently in the skin equivalent, the next step was to obtain differential responses to pharmacological agents according to cellular aging. We chose to study retinoic acid, which attenuates the *in vivo* changes induced by sunlight [44,45] and found that it reduced the proliferation of keratinocytes with normal growth potential in our model but not that of keratinocytes with a lower growth potential due to *in vivo* sun exposure. The main action of retinoic acid was to inhibit migration. These observations have important implications for the long-term use of retinoids in the treatment of aging skin (although the inflammatory phenomenon observed *in vivo* is clearly absent *in vitro*).

In conclusion, living human skin equivalents permit the effects of epidermal aging and pharmacological agents to be evaluated in terms of keratinocyte proliferation and migration.

In vitro *model of pigmentation.*

We found that not only keratinocytes but also melanocytes grew out from foreskin punch biopsies, even in the absence of agents such as 12-O-tetradecanoyl-phorbol-13-acetate (TPA) and specific growth factors such as basic fibroblast growth factor (bFGF) which are usually required for the culture of human skin melanocytes [46]. Although numerous around the biopsy, their number progressively decreased towards the edges of the newly formed epidermis.

In addition, melanocyte migration is enhanced by irradiation with UVB or treatment with 8-methoxypsoralen (8-MOP) plus UVA, suggesting that growth factors secreted by fibroblasts and keratinocytes (perhaps stimulated by UV irradiation) are important for melanocyte growth [46].

Dermal-epidermal interactions.

The importance of cell-to-cell communication is being increasingly stressed in physiology and pathophysiology. Indeed, organogenesis during embryonic life and the maintenance of tissue organisation in adulthood depend on such exchanges.

Skin equivalent models, consisting of fibroblasts (mesenchymal origin) and keratinocytes (ectodermal origin), provide a way of studying dermal-epidermal interactions *in vitro*. Both elements of the reconstructed skin can be modulated and analysed separately, permitting their reciprocal influence to be investigated (Fig. 3).

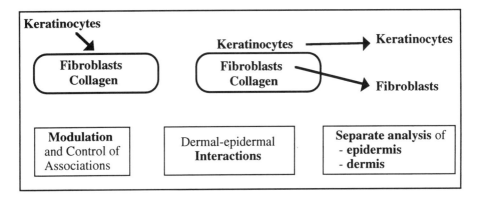

Figure 3 :
Dermal-epidermal interactions.

Influence of normal fibroblasts on the epidermis.

To investigate the influence of normal fibroblasts on keratinocytes, we modulated the dermal-epidermal composition of the skin-equivalents. Epidermal outgrowth from biopsies taken from a single donor was compared on four substrates, these being collagen gel, collagen gel containing fibroblasts lysed by osmotic shock, week-old dermal equivalents in which fibroblasts were lysed after having contracted the collagen matrix and, finally, dermal equivalents containing viable fibroblasts. No epidermal growth occurred on the cell-free collagen gel. In the presence of lysed fibroblasts, growth was significantly stronger on the contracted collagen matrix than on the collagen gels, clearly showing the importance of the degree of substrate organization. Growth was further enhanced when the reorganized matrix contained viable fibroblasts (i.e. the dermal equivalent). A similar enhancement was obtained in the presence of fibroblast-conditioned medium, showing that fibroblasts regulate epidermal growth not only by organizing the extracellular matrix, but also by secreting diffusible growth-promoting factors [2].

We have found that fibroblasts grown in the dermal equivalent secrete immunoreactive molecules with the same physicochemical characteristics as 'mature' insulin-like growth factor 1 (IGF1) and that this secretion is stimulated by the addition of human growth hormone (hGH), EGF or FGF. The influence of the extracellular matrix is further underlined by the fact that fibroblasts cultivated in monolayers only appear to synthesize an IGF1 precursor [47]. Given the presence of a specific IGF1 receptor at the surface of keratinocytes and the fact that keratinocyte division and differentiation are induced when this receptor is activated, the skin equivalent model can be used to study the involvement of IGF1 in dermal-epidermal interactions.

Influence of psoriatic fibroblasts on the epidermis.

Psoriasis is a human skin disease characterized by an inflammatory process in the dermis, keratinocyte hyperproliferation and incomplete keratinization. Interestingly, the maintenance of psoriatic lesions after grafting on nude mice is dependent on the presence of the psoriatic dermis [48]. We used the skin equivalent model to study various combinations of psoriatic and normal fibroblasts and keratinocytes grown in the presence of human AB serum. The most striking result was that psoriatic fibroblasts, even those from non-involved regions, were able to stimulate the proliferation of normal keratinocytes [49]. Psoriasis can thus be considered as a disease of dermal-epidermal interactions. This *in vitro* psoriasis model thus provides a way of determining whether or not a given pharmacological treatment acts via its effect on the disturbed dermal-epidermal interactions. In addition, the importance of systemic factors can be evaluated by using serum from normal and psoriatic donors.

Dermal-epidermal interactions and pharmacology

The role of fibroblasts in the effect of a given pharmacological treatment can be determined by comparing the responses of keratinocytes grown on dermal equivalents in which the fibroblasts are viable or have been lysed by osmotic shock.

Fibroblasts modulate the effect of retinoids on the epidermis.

In another study, skin equivalents containing viable or lysed fibroblasts were treated with the following three retinoids at 10^{-6}M and 10^{-7}M: retinoic acid as a reference molecule; isotretinoin (13-*cis* retinoic acid), a drug used for the treatment of severe acne, and acitretin, a drug which improves psoriasis by reducing epidermal proliferation in affected skin. In the absence of viable fibroblasts, retinoic acid and isotretinoin stimulated epidermal growth. Conversely, acitretin inhibited epidermal growth. The opposing effects between the two isomers (retinoic acid and isotretinoin) on the one hand, and the aromatic compound (acitretin) on the other hand, are in keeping with their different therapeutic effects. When similar experiments were performed with skin equivalents containing viable fibroblasts, the same opposition between the retinoids was observed, confirming the apparent structure-effect relationship. However, a curious phenomenon occurred: the effects of retinoic acid and isotretinoin on epidermal growth were reversed and the inhibitory action of acitretin disappeared. This demonstrated very clearly that the effects of retinoids on epidermal growth are modulated by dermal fibroblasts [50] (Fig. 4).

Interestingly, despite its effective inhibition of epidermal proliferation in affected psoriatic skin *in vivo*, acitretin had no effect on the growth of normal keratinocytes in the presence of normal viable fibroblasts in the skin equivalent.

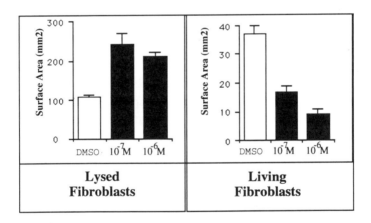

Figure 4:
Influence of fibroblasts on the effects of retinoic acid on epidermal growth

In vivo predictiveness for human pharmacology

There are several possible explanations for the discrepancies between the *in vivo* effects of acitretin on psoriatic lesions and those observed in the skin equivalent model. Firstly, the inhibitory effect of acitretin *in vivo* is observed in psoriatic lesions but not in unaffected skin [51] and, in the previous study, both the fibroblasts and the keratinocytes were normal. Secondly, fetal calf serum was used in these cultures and, as we know from our studies on psoriasis, the nature of the serum is crucial in determining the cellular response.

To investigate the influence of retinoids on the abnormal dermal-epidermal interactions in psoriasis, we performed experiments with acitretin, psoriatic fibroblasts and pooled AB serum from healthy donors. Again, epidermal growth was stimulated in the presence of psoratic fibroblasts, but acitretin no longer had an inhibitory effect. These results show that even if the effects of acitretin on epidermal growth are modulated by fibroblasts, its therapeutic action on the psoriatic epidermis is not [52].

Other experiments were performed with normal fibroblasts and serum from psoriatic patients before and after etretinate therapy (acitretin is the main metabolite of etretinate). Acitretin concentrations were measured in the serum of treated patients and the same concentrations were added to aliquots of serum obtained before treatment. The remaining pretreatment serum served as a control. The serum of retinoid-treated patients and acitretin-supplemented serum taken before treatment inhibited epidermal growth to a similar extent. Furthermore, the individual *in vitro* results paralled the observed *in vivo* efficacy [52].

In the presence of psoriatic serum, the inhibition observed with acitretin was similar with psoriatic and normal fibroblasts, whereas no effect occurred in the presence of human AB serum or fetal calf serum.

In conclusion, the predictiveness of the response in this model depended on psoriatic serum factors, suggesting that the antipsoriatic effect of acitretin *in vivo* occurs mainly via modifications of these factors. The living skin equivalent can thus be considered suitable for screening retinoids for antipsoriatic efficacy in the conditions described above.

Conclusion

As we have seen, these three-dimensional reconstructed human skin models can be used to study not only the dermis and epidermis simultaneously or separately, but also various cell associations (normal/pathological cells, for instance) and dermal-epidermal interactions. It is clear that skin equivalents are suitable for testing the effects of certain chemicals and pharmaceuticals *in vitro*.

However, it must be borne in mind that the results obtained with *in vitro* reconstructed organs vary enormously according to the culture conditions and that their extrapolation to the *in vivo* situation should be made with the utmost care.

With the ability to reproduce *in vivo*-like fibroblast and keratinocyte differentiation, the addition of other cellular and extracellular components to the skin equivalent (for example, immunocompetent cells, endothelial cells and elastin) will enable the study of a wider range of pathological states and the production of models more predictive of drug efficacy and toxicity in humans.

A major aim is to identify, among the multiple interactions, those interactions that are of major pharmacological or toxicological significance and to derive relatively simple, but highly predictive, models for use in the screening of diverse products for pharmacological, toxicological and cosmetic properties.

References

1. Sengel P. Epidermal-dermal interactions during formation of skin and cutaneous appendages. In: Biochemistry and physiology of the skin (L. Goldsmith, ed.) Oxford University Press, NY/Oxford, 1983:102-131.
2. Coulomb B., Lebreton C. and Dubertret L. Influence of human dermal fibroblasts on epidermalization. Journal of Investigative Dermatology 1989;92:22-125.
3. Karasek M. Growth and differentiation of transplanted epithelial cells. Journal of Investigative Dermatology 1968;51:247-252.
4. Mackenzie I.C. and Fusenig N.E. Regeneration of organized epithelial structure. Journal of Investigative Dermatology 1983;81:189s-194s.
5. Flaxman B.A. and Harper R.A. Primary cell culture for biochemical studies of human keratinocytes. British Journal of Dermatology 1975;92:305-309.
6. Halprin K.M., Lueder M. and Fusenig N.E. Growth and differentiation of postembryonic mouse epidermal cells in explants cultures. Journal of Investigative Dermatology 1979;72:88-98.
7. Karasek M. *In vitro* cultures of human skin epithelial cells. Journal of Investigative Dermatology 1966;47:533-540.
8. Prunieras M., Delecluse C. and Regnier M. The culture of skin. A review of theories and experimental methods. Journal of Investigative Dermatology 1976;67:58-65.
9. Bell E., Sher S., Hull B., Merrill C., Rosen S., Chamson A., Asselineau D., Dubertret L., Coulomb B., Lapière C., Nusgens B. and Neveux Y. The reconstitution of a living skin. Journal of Investigative Dermatology 1983;81:2s-10s.
10. Bell E., Ivarsson B. and Merrill C. Production of a tissue-like structure by contraction of collagen lattices by human fibroblasts of different proliferative potential *in vitro*. Proceedings of the National Academy of Sciences of the USA 1979;76:1274-1278.

11. Sarber R., Hull B., Merrill C., Soranno T. and Bell E. Regulation of proliferation of fibroblasts of low and high population doubling levels grown in collagen lattices. Mechanisms of Ageing and Development 1981;17:107-117.
12. Coulomb B., Lebreton C. and Dubertret L. Regulation of fibroblasts divisions in a human dermal equivalent culture model. Journal of Investigative Dermatology 1986;87:34.
13. Ochonisky S. Morphogénèse des fibroblastes en matrice tridimensionnelle de collagène: Rôle du sérum et des Fibroblast Growth Factors. Effet d'un peptide de synthèse contenant la séquence R-G-D. Mémoire de DEA 1990. Université Pierre et Marie Curie, Paris.
14. Coulomb B., Dubertret L., Bell E. and Touraine R. The contractility of fibroblasts in a collagen lattice is reduced by corticosteroids. Journal of Investigative Dermatology 1984;82:341-344.
15. Gillery Ph., Maquart F.X. and Borel J.P. Fibronectin dependence of the contraction of collagen lattices by human skin fibroblasts. Experimental Cell Research 1986;167:29-37.
16. Dubertret L., Brunner-Ferber F., Misiti J., Thomas K.A. and Dubertret M.L. Activities of human acidic fibroblast growth factor in an *in vitro* dermal equivalent. Journal of Investigative Dermatology 1991;97:793-798.
17. Delvoye P., Lévêque J.L. and Lapière Ch. Mechanical forces are developed by fibroblasts in a three-dimensional collagen lattice. Journal of Investigative Dermatology 1986;87:135.
18. Delvoye P., Colige A. and Lapière Ch. Isometric traction developed by fibroblasts in a collagen gel: a model for pharmacological studies. Journal of Investigative Dermatology 1988;91:393.
19. Lambert Ch., Mauch C., Nusgens B., Krieg Th. and Lapière Ch. Regulation of collagen and collagenase genes expression in cultured fibroblasts by their interaction with the surrounding connective tissue. Journal of Investigative Dermatology 1990;95:477.
20. Coulomb B., Dubertret L., Bell E., Merrill C., Fosse M., Breton-Gorius J., Prost C. and Touraine R. Endogenous peroxidases in normal human dermis: a marker of fibroblast differentiation. Journal of Investigative Dermatology 1983;81:75-78.
21. Boudou Ph. Mise au point du dosage radio-enzymatique de la testosterone 5a reductase au niveau de la peau. Application à l'expression de cette activité par des fibroblastes 'in vivo' et 'in vitro'. Mémoire de DEA 1986. Université René Descartes, Paris.
22. Mauch C., Hatamochi A., Scharffetter K. and Krieg Th. Regulation of collagen synthesis in fibroblasts within a three-dimensional collagen gel. Experimental Cell Research 1988;178:493-503.
23. Mauch C., Adelmann-Grill B., Hatamochi A. and Krieg Th. Collagenase gene expression in fibroblasts is regulated by a three-dimensional contact with collagen. FEBS Letters 1989;250:301-305.
24. Nusgens B., Merrill C., Lapiere C. and Bell E. Collagen biosynthesis by cells in a tissue equivalent matrix *in vitro*. Collagene Related Research 1984;4:351-364.

25. Fleishmajer R., Contard P., Schwartz E., MacDonald D., Jacobs L. and Sakai L. Elastin-associated microfibrils in a three-dimensional fibroblasts culture. Journal of Investigative Dermatology 1991;97: 638-643.
26. Cruickshank C.N.D., Cooper J.R. and Hooper C. The cultivation of cells from adult epidermis. Journal of Investigative Dermatology 1960;34:339-342.
27. Regnier M., Delecluse C. and Prunieras M. Studies on guinea pig skin cell culture. I. Separate cultures of keratinocytes and dermal fibroblasts. Acta Dermato-Venereologica 1973;53:241-247.
28. Rheinwald J.G. and Green H. Serial cultivation of strains of human epidermal keratinocytes: the formation of keratinizing colonies from single cells. Cell 1975;6:331-344.
29. Boyce S.T. and Ham R.G. Calcium regulated differentiation of normal human epidermal keratinocytes in chemically defined clonal culture and serum-free serial culture. Journal of Investigative Dermatology 1983;81:33s-40s.
30. Prunieras M., Regnier M. and Woodley D. Methods for cultivation of keratinocytes with an air-liquid interface. Journal of Investigative Dermatology 1983;81:38s-33s.
31. Asselineau D., Bernard B., Bailly C. and Darmon M. Epidermal morphogenesis and induction of the 67kD keratin polypeptide by culture of human keratinocytes at the liquide-air interface. Experimental Cell Research 1985;159:536-539.
32. Basset-Seguin N., Culard J.F., Kerai C., Bernard F., Watrin A., Demaille J. and Guilhou J.J. Reconstituted skin culture: a simple method with optimal differentiation. Differentiation 1990;44:232-238.
33. Woodley D., Didierjean L., Regnier M., Saurat J. and Prunieras M. Bullous pemphigoid antigen synthesized *in vitro* by human epidermal cells. Journal of Investigative Dermatology 1980;75:148-151.
34. Holbrook K.A. and Hennings H. Phenotypic expression of epidermal cells *in vitro*: A review. Journal of Investigative Dermatology 1983;81:11s-24s.
35. Hirone T. and Taniguchi S. Basal Lamina formation by epidermal cells in cell culture. Biochemistry of normal and abnormal epidermal differentiation. Current problems in Dermatology (Vol. ed. I.A. Bernstein and M. Seiji, Series ed. J.N.H. Mali), 1979;10:159-169.
36. Lillie J.H., MacCallum D.K. and Jepsen A. Fine structure of subcultivated stratified squamous epithelium grown on collagen rafts. Experimental Cell Research 1980;125:153-165.
37. Bell E., Ehrlich H.P., Sher S., Merrill C., Sarber R., Hull B., Nakatsuji T., Church D. and Buttle D. Development and use of a living skin equivalent. Journal of Plastic and Reconstructive Surgery 1981;67:386-392.
38. Bell E., Erlich H.P., Buttle D. and Nakatsuji T. Living tissue formed *in vitro* and accepted as a skin-equivalent tissue of full thickness. Science 1981;211:1052-1054.
39. Coulomb B., Saiag Ph., Bell E., Breitburd F., Lebreton C., Heslan M. and Dubertret L. A new method for studying epidermalization *in vitro*. British Journal of Dermatology 1986;114:91-101.
40. Hayflick L. The limited *in vitro* lifetime of human diploid cell strains. Experimental Cell Research 1965;37:614-636.

41. Gilchrest B.A. *In vitro* assessment of keratinocyte aging. Journal of Investigative Dermatology 1983;81:184s-189s.
42. Coulomb B., Lebreton C. and Dubertret L. Quantitative *in vitro* evaluation of keratinocytes growth after *in vivo* light induced aging. Journal of Investigative Dermatology 1989;92:415.
43. Grove G.L. Age-related differences in healing of superficial skin wounds in humans. Archives of Dermatological Research 1982;272:381-385.
44. Kligman A.M., Grove G.L., Hirose R. and Leyden J.J. Topical tretinoin for photoaged skin. Journal of the American Academy of Dermatology 1986;15:836-859.
45. Weiss J.S., Ellis C.N., Headington J.T., Tincoff T., Hamilton T.A. and Voorhees J.J. Topical tretinoin improves photoaged skin. A double-blind vehicle-controlled study. JAMA 1988;259:527-532.
46. Bertaux B., Morlière P., Moreno G., Courtalon A., Massé J.M. and Dubertret L. Growth of melanocytes in a skin equivalent model *in vitro*. British Journal of Dermatology 1988;119:503-512.
47. Aractingi S., Coulomb B., Lebreton C., Corvol M.T. and Dubertret L. Production of insulin like growth factor (IGF1) by dermal fibroblast culture. Journal of Investigative Dermatology 1989;92:396.
48. Fraki J.E., Brigagaman R.A. and Lazarus G.S. Transplantation of psoriatic skin onto nude mice. Journal of Investigative Dermatology 1983;80:31s-35s.
49. Saiag Ph., Coulomb B., Lebreton C., Bell E. and Dubertret L. Psoriatic fibroblasts induce hyperproliferation of normal keratinocytes in a skin equivalent model *in vitro*. Science 1985;230:669-672.
50. Sanquer S., Coulomb B., Lebreton C. and Dubertret L. Human dermal fibroblasts modulate the effects of retinoids on epidermal growth. Journal of Investigative Dermatology 1990;95:700-704.
51. Lassus A. Systemic treatment of psoriasis with an oral retinoic acid derivative (RO 10-9359). British Journal of Dermatology 1980;102:195-202.
52. Sanquer S., Coulomb B., Lebreton C. and Dubertret L. Influence of psoriatic fibroblasts and serum on the response of normal keratinocytes to acitretin. Dermatologica 1990;181:353.

4
Keratinocytes and reconstructed epidermis for *in vitro* pharmacological and toxicological testing

H. Merk, F. Jugert and S. Frankenberg

University of Cologne, Department of Dermatology,
Joseph-Stelzmann-Straße 9, 50931 Köln (Germany).

Introduction

Increasing awareness of the toxic effects of environmental agents on the human population has focused attention on those structures, such as the skin, that function as interfaces between the body and its environment. The human skin is both a physical and biochemical barrier to the absorption and penetration of potentially damaging compounds within the environment. It consists of two main tissues: the epidermis and the dermis.

The dermis is mainly responsible for the remarkably resistant, tough, yet pliable and membranous character of the skin, making it well suited for a passive role in protection. Additionally, it has become known that the cells of the connective tissue play an important role in the three dimensional assembly, migration and support of cells, as well as in the synthesis of the extracellular matrix and wound healing. The role of this tissue and the use of cell culture systems in the study of skin pharmacology and toxicology is summarized by Eckes and Krieg in this issue.

The epidermis consists of a basal layer of germinating keratinocytes (which make up 90% of all cells in this tissue) in direct and tight apposition to the underlying dermis and a variable number of differentiating squamous cells which are in a continuous movement outwards towards the skin surface [1]. Here, the stratum corneum is formed, which is the critical structure for epidermal barrier function. The keratinocytes have turned out to be a very metabolically active cell type with the capability to metabolize xenobiotics [2].

Since keratinocytes can be isolated from human skin and grown in tissue culture conditions they are an excellent system to perform studies related to skin pharmacology and toxicology. In vitro models have important advantages: reproducibility, control over assay conditions, moderate costs, ability to construct dose-response curves, and the possibility of testing highly toxic compounds, including carcinogens for which there is an obvious limitation with regard to in vivo testing. Conversely, animal experiments tend to be more expensive and time consuming and the extrapolation of data to man is limited due to various species differences with regard to, for example, drug metabolizing enzymes [2,3].

In vitro system	Endpoint	References
Human fibroblasts and keratinocytes	Neutral red incorporation Cellular protein	29,32 37-39
Human keratinocytes	[^{3}H]Uridine incorporation Cellular protein	40-44
Skin organ culture (human, guinea pig, rabbit)	[^{14}C]Leucine incorporation Cellular vacuole formation	45,46
Cell-free macromolecular mixture (SKINTEX)	Cellular vacuole formation Physical/chemical reaction	51,52
Human keratinocytes	Cell growth inhibition and enzyme and ion leakage	47,48
3T3 fibroblasts XB-2 keratinocytes	Neutral red uptake MTT cleavage Hexosamidase leakage Colony area, cell number Keratin staining	49
Keratome skin in diffusion chamber Fibroblast culture with keratin/agar overlay	Amino acid uptake Enzyme release Histochemistry [^{3}H]Thymidine uptake Chromium release	50

Table I :
In vitro systems for assays of cutaneous irritancy (according to ref. 6)

The historical development of the use of keratinocytes in skin toxicology and skin pharmacology was reviewed by Prunieras and Delescluse [4]. The role of xenobiotic-metabolizing enzymes in keratinocytes and their relationship to the different effects of xenobiotica was examined mainly in studies concerning chemocarcinogenesis [5]. Another field of interest was cutaneous irritancy testing, which was recently reviewed by De Leo [6] and Ponec [7]. Table I summarizes most important *in vitro* systems for assaying cutaneous irritancy under *in vitro* conditions. New developments include the measurement of released cytokines by keratinocytes after incubation with toxic compounds [7]. Also, many different culture systems were developed such as monolayer cultures, as well as skin equivalents consisting of a dermal equivalent made of fibroblasts embedded in collagen and a reconstructed epidermis from keratinocytes [8,9].

For skin pharmacology and toxicology studies such cell systems are especially important and are easily obtainable in a convenient manner. Therefore, we will focus primarily on keratinocytes which are raised from hair follicles [10]. This technique makes it possible to obtain cultures without the necessity of taking biopsies in order to get human keratinocytes. Since these cells express all major cutaneous xenobiotic-metabolizing enzymes in a similar manner (as has been shown from *in vivo* studies) these systems are very promising, especially with regard to studies in skin pharmacology and skin toxicology [11].

Some aspects of xenobiotic-metabolizing enzymes in the skin and in particular in keratinocytes will be summarized before we describe recent progress in the application of keratinocytes in skin toxicology and pharmacology studies, including the possibility of raising keratinocyte cultures, including skin equivalents, from hair follicles.

Skin / keratinocytes as a xenobiotic-metabolizing tissue

Our understanding of the functions of the skin has changed fundamentally in recent years. The skin is not just an inert sheath covering the body but performs a wide range of active metabolic functions. One example is xenobiotic metabolism involving enzymes specific to the skin. The xenobiotic metabolism of the skin differs not only quantitatively but also qualitatively from that of the liver, which is the central organ of xenobiotic metabolism [12].

Xenobiotic metabolism is divided up into several phases. Characteristic enzymes operate in each of these phases which are summarized in Fig. 1.

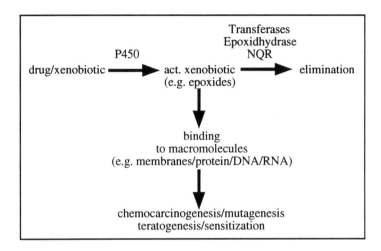

Figure 1 :
Foreign substances such as drugs are mostly metabolised in the first phase by cytochrome P450-dependent enzyme activities to chemically highly reactive metabolites (eg. epoxides). The broad range of possible reactions displayed by P450 in comparison to other enzymes is based on the relatively low substrate specificity and abundance of isoenzymes in this system. The highly reactive intermediates are transformed in the second phase by enzymes such as epoxidhydrases, various transferases and NAD(P)H-quinone reductase (NQR) mostly to organic acids. These are then eliminated through the renal or bilious systems. When a disparity arises between the activating P450 enzymes and the phase 2 enzymes, the highly reactive intermediate may bind to cell macromolecules such as proteins or react with RNA or DNA which can lead to toxic reactions, carcinogenesis or sensitization of the skin.

Cytochrome P450

Many xenobiotics are initially metabolised by the cytochrome P450 mediated mono-oxygenase system. The cytochromes P450 comprise a very large gene superfamily as of December 1992 DNA sequences encoding 221 cytochrome P450 isoenzymes had been cloned. In mammals 10 cytochrome P450 families have been identified on the basis of amino acid sequence [13]. Members of 4 of these families, P450 1, 2, 3 and 4 play a central role in xenobiotic metabolism. P4501A1 is predominant in the skin after pretreatment with polyaromatic hydrocarbons which are present, for example, in coal tar preparations [14]. It has recently been shown that the induction of P4501A1 in human keratinocytes by 2,3,7,8-tetrachlordibenzofuran occurred only after the cells had undergone differentiation following incubation in media containing serum or a high calcium concentration. These results suggest that the expression of P4501A1 in the epidermis changes during epidermal differentiation [15]. It has also been shown that P4502A and P4502B are present in keratinocytes [3,16]. It is thought that, in keratinocytes, P4501A1 is the only cytochrome P450 involved in the metabolism of benzo(a)pyrene and hence in the production of carcinogenic metabolites from this compound [5]. In contrast, in the liver benzo(a)pyrene is also metabolized by other P450 isoenzymes although these cytochromes P450 do not metabolize this chemical to carcinogenic products.

Besides the cytochrome P450-dependent monooxygenases, mentioned above, other enzymes may be of importance such as epoxygenases [17,18,19], playing a role in arachidonic acid metabolism, and transferases [12,20], e.g. UDP-glucuronyltransferases. Both have been identified in keratinocytes.

NAD(P)H-quinone reductase

Another enzyme that has recently attracted much interest is NAD(P)H-dependent quinone reductase (NQR, also called DT-diaphorase, EC 1.6.99.2). While the above-mentioned drug metabolizing enzymes display skin/liver activity ratios of about 1-10%, this reductase has equally high activities in the skin and liver [21]. In inhibition studies, several known inhibitors of dihydrodiol dehydrogenase, aldo-keto and carbonyl reductase activities were used and a similar pattern of inhibition of the basal and induced activity was found in all tissues investigated suggesting a similarity between the NQR in liver and skin, as well as in murine and human keratinocytes (Fig. 2) [27]. Quinones are involved in many toxic reactions of fundamental relevance to dermatology. For example, there are many contact allergens that possess a quinone-type structure or are metabolised into quinones within the skin [22]. Quinones can be transformed to semiquinones, extremely unstable substances that tend to spontaneously oxidize back into quinones, thus releasing oxygen free radicals [23]. This sequence of reactions is called the quinone-redox-cycle and is responsible for the toxicity of quinones (Fig. 3). Quinone reductase reduces quinones to hydroquinones that are relatively stable in comparison to semiquinones. This enzyme system thereby provides a protective mechanism by bypassing the quinone-redox-cycle [24,25]. In consequence, this enzyme not only contributes to xenobiotic metabolism but also protects the cell from oxidative stress [23].

NQR belongs to the aromatic hydrocarbon-responsive [Ah] gene battery. In mice this gene battery includes the genes encoding P4501A1, P4501A2 and NAD(P)H-quinone reductase [26]. There is also a coinduction of these enzymes in human keratinocytes by polyaromatic hydrocarbons, such as benz(a)anthracene (Table II). The NQR activity is dependent on the cell cycle, as a threefold difference in NQR activity was observed

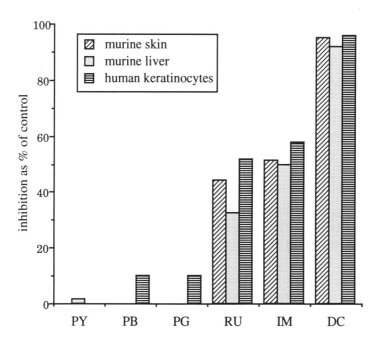

Figure 2 :
Inhibition studies on NQR: there was no inhibition of NQR in murine skin and liver, or in human keratinocytes, by pyrazol (PY), phenobarbital (PB), or hydroxyprogesterone acetate (PG). However, in all tissues the NQR activity was inhibited by rutin (RU), indomethacine (IM), and dicoumarol (DC). This inhibition was dose dependent in a range from 1µM to 100µM (data not shown). The values for inhibition as % of control are presented for 100µM concentrations.

between keratinocytes in proliferating and differentiating phase (Fig. 4) [27]. Several studies revealed that NQR activity is induced by different mechanisms. One mechanism involves Ah-receptor binding leading to the induction of P4501A1, P4501A2 and NAD(P)H quinone reductase gene expression [20]. Petersen and colleagues suggested that a gene located on chromosome 7 encodes a trans-acting regulatory factor that might be a negative effector of the NAD(P)H quinone reductase gene, which is located on murine chromosome 8 [28]. Induction studies with the NAD(P)H quinone reductase promoter, chloramphenicol acetyltransferase fusion genes, have suggested that, in the case of rats, there is a *cis*-acting regulatory element which regulates inducible expression [29]. Our findings of very high NQR activity in human skin and especially human keratinocytes demonstrates the opportunity for further studies relating

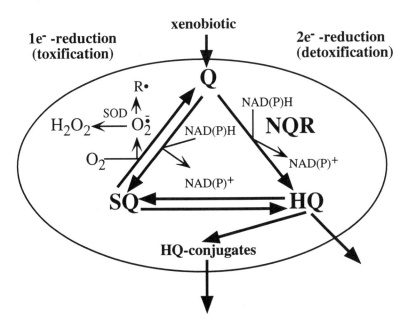

Figure 3 :
The Quinone-Redox Cycle: Most reductases transform quinones (Q) with one electron into semiquinones (SQ). Semiquinones are, however, unstable and tend to spontaneously oxidize back into quinones, which leads to the release of highly reactive (and cell-damaging) oxygen radicals or H_2O_2. The NAD(P)H-quinone reductase (NQR), on the other hand, promotes 2-electron reductions of quinones, thereby forming hydroquinones (HQ) which are more stable and can usually be eliminated. SOD; superoxide dismutase.

to this complex induction mechanism.

Further studies have shown that the widely used antipsoriatic agent dithranol (via its metabolite danthron), as well as coal tar preparations used in dermatology as antiinflammatory agents, are able to induce NQR activity [27]. The semiquinone anthralin is metabolised in the skin to danthron and studies by Giovanni and Yuspa have produced evidence that one of the enzymes involved in this transformation is NAD(P)H-quinone reductase [12]. We have therefore investigated whether any reaction between anthralin and this enzyme occurs and whether anthralin itself induces the NAD(P)H-dependent quinone reductase. In addition, we applied anthralin topically to mice and found that under *in vivo* conditions NAD(P)H-quinone reductase was indeed induced in a dose-dependent manner by anthralin [23]. In further experiments, we addressed the question as to whether the reductase activity is influenced by anthralin itself or by the quinone metabolite, danthron. For this purpose we used human keratinocytes and a photometrical assay for NAD(P)H quinone reductase that produces coloured images of the enzyme activity within the keratinocyte culture [27]. These *in vitro* studies on cell cultures showed that the inducer of NAD(P)H-quinone reductase was not anthralin but danthron [27]. Anthralin must therefore be oxidised to danthron for induction of this enzyme.

	Cyp1a1 activity		Nmo-1 activity
Treatment	7-EROD	AHH	NQR
control	2.14 ± 0.4	7.6 ± 1.8	777.2 ± 38.0
BA	24.8 ± 4.8	36.1 ± 4.3	1319.5 ± 147.8

Table II :
Induction of microsomal Cyp1a1 activities (measured as 7-ethoxyresorufin-O-deethylase (7-EROD) and aryl hydrocarbon hydroxylase (AHH) and cytosolic Nmo-1-activity (measured as NQR), respectively, in human keratinocytes by benzanthracene (BA). Benzanthracene (2mM) was added to the cultures 2 days before harvesting of the cells in a final concentration of 0.1% DMSO during subconfluency. Controls were treated only with 0.1% DMSO. 7-EROD and AHH activity are given as pmol product/min.mg prot. and NQR as nmol product/min.mg prot.

Keratinocytes derived from hair follicles

Recently keratinocyte cultures including models of reconstructed epidermis were raised from a single hair follicle [10]. Randomly plucked anagen hair follicles were washed in Eagle's minimum essential medium (MEM) supplemented with 10% fetal calf serum (FCS), 100 IU/ml penicillin, 100 µg/ml streptomycin and 2.5 µg/ml amphotericin B. After the removal of the bulb the follicles were implanted vertically into the fresh cast dermal equivalent, which consists of normal human epidermal fibroblasts embedded in collagen. It was prepared according to a method originally described by Bell *et al.* [8] and Lenoir *et al.* [10]. After contraction of the gel by the fibroblasts, the culture medium was replaced by a serum-free keratinocyte growth medium to allow the outgrowing

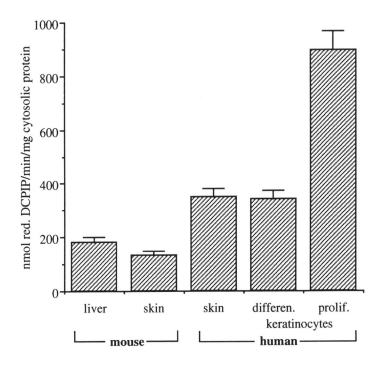

Figure 4:
Comparison of the NQR activity in murine liver and skin and in human skin and keratinocytes. The columns represent the mean value of at least 6 experiments with a variation of less than 10%. Differentiating and proliferating keratinocytes were used. (DCPIP = dichlorophenolindophenol).

keratinocytes to form a monolayer. To induce a multilayered and differentiated epidermis the dermal equivalent was raised to the air-liquid interface on stainless steel grids. The culture medium used after immersion was Eagle's MEM supplemented with 10% FCS, 100 IU/ml penicillin, 100 µg/ml streptomycin, 2.5 µg/ml amphotericin B, 1 mM sodium pyruvate, 1% non-essential amino acids, 2 mM L-glutamine, 0.4 µg/ml hydrocortisone, 5 µg/ml insulin, 10^{-10} M choleratoxin, 10 ng/ml epidermal growth factor, 0.8 mM adenine and 2×10^{-9} M triiodothyronine. The medium was changed twice a week. This technique enabled the establishment of a multilayered reconstituted epidermis with a *stratum corneum* derived from hair follicles. The different levels of differentiation can be recognized by the polygonal shape with loss of polarity in the basal layers and by the cells in the upper layers becoming flattened to the surface, with their long axis arranged parallel to the skin surface. Keratohyalin granule-like structures were absent. Subsequently, the differentiation state of these cells, was monitored by the presence of the differentiation markers filaggrin and cytokeratin 1 (67Kd). It has also been shown that this epidermis possesses drug-metabolizing enzymes such as the cytochrome P450 dependent O-deethylation of 7-ethoxy-resorufin, 7-pentoxyresorufin, and 7-benzoxyresorufin and the reductase activities for NADPH cytochrome c (P450), testosterone 5 alpha, the transferase activities for UDP-glucuronyl and glutathione, the sulfatase activities for steroids and epoxide hydrolase activities. These cells have also been used for skin absorption studies [31]. For the application of this system in dermatopharmacology it is important that xenobiotic metabolizing enzymes such as P4501A1 be present. As is the situation *in vivo*, the cells express only very small amounts of members of the P4501A subfamilly. We have investigated the localization of P4501A1 and shown by immunohistochemical techniques and by catalytic activity measurements (Fig. 5) that this protein is induced in keratinocytes by benz(a)anthracene. Further studies have shown that other cytochrome P450 isoenzymes are also inducible in these cells [11]. The ability to induce cytochromes P450 makes this cell system useful for research in skin pharmacology and toxicology.

We have also demonstrated the dependency of cytochrome P4501A expression on the level of differentiation of keratinocytes *in vitro* [33]. An immunohistochemical examination of normal human skin after topical treatment with the coal tar containing *liquor carbonis detergens in vivo* demonstrated, that P4501A was found only in the basal keratinocytes [16]. The relationship between cell differentiation and P4501A expression

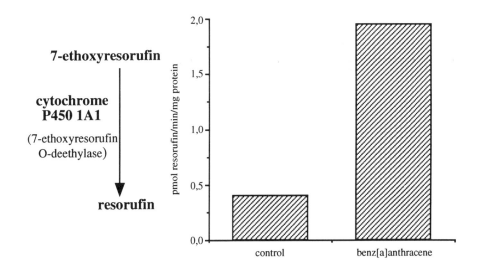

Figure 5 :
7-ethoxyresorufin-deethylase activity is mainly mediated by cytochrome P450 1A1. This enzyme activity is induced in hair follicle derived keratinocytes after the incubation with benzanthracene.

correlates with the finding that cytochrome P450 dependent enzyme activity in isolated skin cells is primarily present in heavier basal cells [34]. This is also in accordance with the finding of Reiners et al. that the constitutive expression of cytochrome P450 in murine keratinocytes can be modulated by the extracellular Ca^{2+} concentration under in vitro conditions and by differentiation under in vivo conditions [35]. It is known that Ca^{2+} concentration plays a crucial role in the differentiation of keratinocytes. It is interesting to speculate about the relationship of cytochrome P450 expression and differentiation processes of the skin, because small molecular substances such as retinoic acid or vitamin D_3, which influence the Ca^{2+} concentration, are synthetized and metabolized by reactions known to be dependent of cytochrome P450 activities [13]. Recently, it has been proposed that drug-metabolizing enzymes, especially cytochromes P450, play a role in the control of steady state levels of small organic oxygenated molecules, such as steroids or retinoids, which act as signals for growth, and differentiation [36]. The linkage between the multiple differentiation levels of keratinocytes, the possibility of characterizing these cells by studying their morphology and the expression of different proteins, as well as their ability to express and support the induction of cytochrome P450 enzymes, suggests that this culture system may be useful for studying not only the problems of skin pharmacology and toxicology but also the relationship between xenobiotic-metabolizing enzymes and cell differentiation processes.

References

1. Eckart R.L. The structure and function of the skin. In: Pharmacology of the skin (Mukhtar H., ed.) CRC Press, Boca Raton, 1992:3-12.
2. Bickers D.R., Kappas A. The skin as a site of chemical metabolism. In: Extrahepatic metabolism of drugs and other compounds (Gram T.E., ed.) MTP Press Limited, Lancaster, 1980:295-318.
3. Mukhtar H., Khan I.U., Haqqi T.M. and Bickers D.R. Polymerase chain reaction based detection of messenger RNA for three gene families of cytochrome P-450 in mammalian epidermis. Journal of Investigative Dermatology 1991;96:581.
4. Prunieras M and Delescluse C. Epidermal cell culture systems in skin pharmacology. British Journal of Dermatology 1984;111:43-57.
5. Bickers D.R., Das M. and Mukhtar H. Pharmacological modification of epidermal detoxification systems. British Journal of Dermatology 1986;115:9-16.
6. De Leo V.A. Cutaneous Irritancy. In: In Vitro Toxicity Testing (Frazier J.M., ed.) Marcel Dekker, New York, 1993:191-203.
7. Ponec M. *In vitro* cultured human skin cells as alternatives to animals for skin irritancy screening. International Journal of Cosmetic Science 1992;14:245-264.
8. Bell E., Ivarsson B. and Merrill C. Production of a tissue-like structure by contraction of collagen lattices by human fibroblasts of different proliferative potential *in vitro*. Proceedings of the National Academy of Sciences of the USA 1979;76:1274-1278.
9. Coulomb B. and Dubertret L. Interactions dermo-epidermiques et pharmacologie cutanée. Pathologique Biologique 1992;40:139-146.
10. Lenoir M.C., Bernard B.A., Pautrat G., Darmon M. and Shroot B. Outer root sheath cells of human hair follicle are able to regenerate a fully differentiated epidermis *in vitro*. Developmental Biology 1988;130:610-620.
11. Frankenberg S., Jugert F.K. and Merk H.F. Multiple cytochrome P450 isozymes present in human hair follicle derived keratinocytes Journal of Investigative Dermatology 1993;100:518.
12. Merk H.F. and Jugert F.K. Metabolic activation and detoxification of drugs and xenobiotica by the skin. In: Dermal and Transdermal Drug Delivery (Gurny R. and Teubner A., eds.) Wissenschaftliche Verlagsgesellschaft, Stuttgart, 1993:91-100.

13. Nelson D.R., Kamataki T., Waxman D.J., Guengerich F.P., Estabrook R.W., Feyereisen R., Gonzalez F.J., Coon M.J., Gunsalus I.C. Gotoh O. et al. The P450 superfamily: Update on new sequences, gene mapping, accession Numbers, early trivial names of enzymes and nomenclature. DNA and Cell Biology 1993;12:1-51.
14. Merk H., Mukhtar H., Kaufmann I., Das M. and Bickers D.R. Human hair follicle benzo(a)pyrene and benzo(a)pyrene 7,8-diol metabolism: Effect of exposure to a coal tar-containing shampoo. Journal of Investigative Dermatology 1987;88:71-76.
15. Berghard A., Gradin K. and Toftgard R. Serum and extracellular calcium modulate induction of cytochrome P-4501A1 in human keratinocytes. Journal of Biological Chemistry 1990;265:21086-21090.
16. Jugert F.K., Frankenberg S., Junginger H. and Merk H.F. Multiple cytochrome P450 isozymes are present in human keratinocytes. 13th European Drug Metabolism Workshop 1992 Bergamo.
17. Fitzpatrick F.A. and Murphy R.C. Cytochrome P-450 metabolism of arachidonic acid: formation and biological actions of 'epoxygenase'-derived eicosanoids. Pharmacological Reviews 1989;40:229-241.
18. Holtzman M.J., Turk J., Pentland A. A regiospecific monooxygenase with novel stereopreference is the major pathway for arachidonic acid oxygenation in isolated epidermal cells. Journal of Clinical Investigation 1989;84:1446-1453.
19. Mukhtar H., Bik D.P., Ruzicka T., Merk H. and Bickers D.R. Cytochrome P-450-dependent omega-oxidation of leukotriene B_4 in rodent and human epidermis. Journal of Investigative Dermatology 1989;93:231-235.
20. Lilienblum W., Irmscher G., Fusenig N.E. and Bock K.W. Induction of UDP-glucuronyltransferase and arylhydrocarbon hydroxylase activity in mouse skin and in normal and transformed skin cells in culture. Biochemical Pharmacology 1986;35:1517.
21. Khan W.A., Das M., Stick S., Javed S., Bickers D.R. and Mukhtar H. Induction of epidermal NAD(P)H: quinone reductase by chemical carcinogens: a possible mechanism for the detoxification. Biochemistry and Biophysical Research Communications 1987;146:126.
22. Benezra C., Sigman C.C., Bagheri D., Fraginals R. and Maibach H.I. Molecular aspects of allergic contact dermatitis. In: Contact Dermatitis (Rycroft R.J.G., Menne T., Frosch P.J. and Benezra C., eds.) Springer, Heidelberg 1992:103-119.
23. Wefers H., Komai T., Talalay P. and Sies H. Protection against reactive oxygen species by NAD(P)H:quinone reductase induced by the dietary antioxidant butylated hydroxyanisole (BHA). FEBS Letters 1984;169:63-66.
24. Prochaska H.J., De Long M.J. and Talalay P. On the mechanisms of induction of cancer-protective enzymes: A unifying proposal. Proceedings of the National Academy of Sciences of the USA 1985;82:8232-8236.
25. Smith M. Quinones as mutagens, carcinogens and anticancer agents: Introduction and overview. Journal of Toxicology and Environmental Health 1985;16:665-672.
26. Robertson J.A., Chen H.-C. and Nebert D.W. NAD(P)H:menadioneoxidoreductase. Journal of Biological Chemistry 1987;201:15794-15799.

27. Merk H.F., Jugert F.K., Bonnekoh B. and Mahrle G. Induction and Inhibition of NAD(P)H:quinone reductase in murine and human skin. Skin Pharmacology 1991;4:183-190.
28. Petersen D.D., Gonzales F.J. and Rapic V. Marked increase in hepatic NAD(P)H:oxidoreductase gene transcription and mRNA levels correlated with a mouse chromosome 7 deletion. Proceedings of the National Academy of Sciences of the USA 1989;86:6699-6703.
29. Borenfreund E. and Puerner J.A. A simple quantitative procedure using monolayer cultures for cytotoxicity assays (HTD/NR-90). Journal of Tissue Culture Methods 1984;9:7-9.
30. Pham M.A., Magdalou J., Siest G., Lenoir M.C., Bernard B.A., Jamoulle J.C. and Shroot B. Reconstituted epidermis: A novel model for the study of drug metabolism in human epidermis. Journal of Investigative Dermatology 1990;94:749-752.
31. Regnier M., Caron D., Reichert U. and Schaefer H. Reconstructed epidermis: A model to study *in vitro* the barrier function of the skin. Skin Pharmacology 1992;5:49-56.
32. Borenfreund E. and Puerner J.A. Toxicity determined *in vitro* by morphological alterations and neutral red absorption. Toxicology Letters 1985;24:119-124.
33. Thiele B., Merk H., Bonnekoh B., Mahrle G. and Steigleder G.K. Epidermal cell growth-dependent arylhydrocarbon-hydroxylase (AHH) activity *in vitro*. Archives for Dermatological Research 1987;279:521-523.
34. Coomes M.W., Norling A.H., Pohl R.J., Muller D. and Fouts J.R. Foreign compound metabolism by isolated skin cells from hairless mouse. Journal of Pharmacology and Experimental Therapeutics 1983;225:770-778.
35. Reiners J.J., Amador R.C. and Pavone A. Modulation of constitutive cytochrome P450 expression *in vivo* and *in vitro* in murine keratinocytes as a function of differentiation and extracellular Ca^{2+} concentration. Proceedings of the National Academy of Sciences of the USA 1990;87:1825-1829.
36. Nebert DW. Growth signal pathways. Nature 1990;47:709-710.
37. Borenfreund E. and Puerner J.A. Cytotoxicity of metals, metal-metal and metal-chelator combinations assayed *in vitro*. Toxicology 1986;39:121-134.
38. Borenfreund E. and Puerner J.A. Short-term quantitative *in vitro* cytotoxicity assay involving an a-9 activating system. Cancer Letters 1987;34:243-248.
39. Babich H., Martin-Alguacil N. and Borenfreund E. Comparisons of the cytotoxicities of dermatotoxicants to human keratinocytes and fibroblasts *in vitro*. In: Progress in Toxicology (Goldberg A.M., ed.) Mary Ann Liebert, New York 1989:Vol.7:153-167.
40. Shopis C.S. Inhibition of uridine uptake by cultured cells: A rapid, sublethal cytotoxicity test. Journal of Tissue Culture Methods 1984;9:19-22.
41. Shopis C.S. and Sathe S. Uridine uptake as a cytotoxicity test: correlations with the Draize test. Toxicology 1984;29:195-206.
42. Shopis C.S., Borenfreund E., Walberg J. and Stark D.M. A battery of potential alternatives to the Draize test: Uridine uptake inhibition, morphological cytotoxicity, macrophage chemotaxis and exfoliative cytology. Food and Chemical Toxicology 1985;23:259-266.

43. Shopis C.S. and Eng B. Rapid cytotoxicity testing using a semi-automated protein determination on cultured cells. Toxicology Letters 1985;26:1-8.
44. Shopis C.S. and Eng B. *In vitro* occular irritancy prediction: assays in seven free media correlate better with *in vivo* data. In: Progress in In Vitro Toxicology (Goldberg A.M., ed.) Mary Ann Liebert, New York, 1988:Vol.6:253-263.
45. Dannenberg A.M., Moore K.G., Schofield B.H., Higuchi K., Kajiki A., Au K.-W., Pula P.J. and Bassett D.P. Two new *in vitro* methods for evaluating toxicity to the skin (employing short-term organ culture): I. Paranuclear vacuolization, seen in glycol methacrylate tissue sections; II. Inhibition of ^{14}C-leucine incorporation. Alternative Methods in Toxicology 1987;5:115-127.
46. Moore K.G., Schofield B.H., Higuchi K., Kajiki A., Au K.-W., Pula P.J., Bassett D.P. and Dannenberg A.M. Two sensitive *in vitro* monitors of chemical toxicity to human and animal skin (in short-term organ culture): I. Paranuclear vacuolization, in glycol methacrylate tissue sections; II. Interference with ^{14}C-leucine incorporation. Journal of Toxicology: Cutaneous and Ocular Toxicology 1986;5:285-302.
47. Von Genderman J., Mol M.A.E. and Wolthus O.L. On the development of skin models for toxicity testing. Fundamental and Applied Toxicology 1985;5:98-111.
48. Mol M.A.E., Von Genderman J. and Wolthus O.L. Cultured human epidermal cells as tool in skin toxicology. Food and Chemical Toxicology 1986;24:519-520.
49. Duffy P.A., Flint O.P., Onton T.C. and Fursey M.J. Initial validation of an *in vitro* test for predicting skin irritancy. Food and Chemical Toxicology 1986;24:517-518.
50. Parish W.E. Relevance of *in vitro* tests to *in vivo* acute skin inflammation: potential *in vitro* applications of skin keratome slices, neutrophils, fibroblasts, mast cells and macrophages. Food and Chemical Toxicology 1985;23:275-285.
51. Gordon V.C., Kelly C.P. and Bergman H.C. SKINTEX® an *in vitro* method for determining dermal irritation. Oral Communication, Congress of Toxicology, Brighton 1989.
52. Goldberg A.M. (ed.) A critical evaluation of alternatives to acute occular irritation testing. Alternative Methods in Toxicology 1987;4:109-110.

5

Use of human skin models in the study of retinoic acid metabolism and lipid synthesis, effects of liarozole

H. Vanden Bossche, G. Willemsens, H. Schreuders, M-C. Coene, C. Van Hove and W. Cools

Division of Medicinal Chemistry and Pharmacology,
Janssen Research Foundation, Turnhoutseweg 30, 2340 Beerse (Belgium).

Introduction

Vitamin A (retinol) is an essential nutrient known to be involved in, e.g., the regulation of cell proliferation and differentiation. Retinol is converted into all-*trans*-retinoic acid (RA; tretinoin) which in, for example, F9 murine embryonal carcinoma cells is 175-times more potent than retinol in inducing differentiation [1]. RA is now generally assumed to mediate retinoid effects in most tissues [2]. However, RA's potency is attenuated by its rapid metabolism [2] into 4-hydroxyretinoic acid, 4-oxoretinoic acid and more polar metabolites [3]. The 4-hydroxylation of RA is mediated by a cytochrome P450-dependent monooxygenase system. Indeed, rat liver P450s 2B1 and 2C7 [4], human liver P4502C8 [5] and rabbit liver P450s 1A2 and 2B4 [6] have been found to metabolize RA and retinol to more polar products, including the 4-hydroxymetabolite. We described that skin epidermal microsomes, prepared from neonatal rats also 4-hydroxylated RA by a P450-dependent pathway [7-8]. After pretreatment with RA or 3-methylcholanthrene (3-MC) the rate of 4-hydroxylation increased about 3- and 4-times, respectively [8]. Other conditions that may induce P450s, such as phenobarbital, pregnenolone 16α-carbonitrile or triacetyloleandomycin pretreatment, enhanced RA metabolism to a much lesser degree [8]. These results suggest that the

P450 form involved in rat epidermal RA metabolism is related to a family of 3-MC inducible P450s, including P4501A2, and differs from that catalyzing RA metabolism in rat liver.

The metabolism of RA in different tissues may be affected not only by exposure of the animal to P450 inducers but also to various P450 inhibitors. For example, ketoconazole and liarozole (Fig. 1) inhibited at micromolar concentrations RA metabolism in rat epidermal [7-8] and liver [9] microsomes. *In vivo*, both imidazole derivatives increased the plasma half-life of exogenously administered RA and enhanced the endogenous plasma levels of the retinoid [10-12].

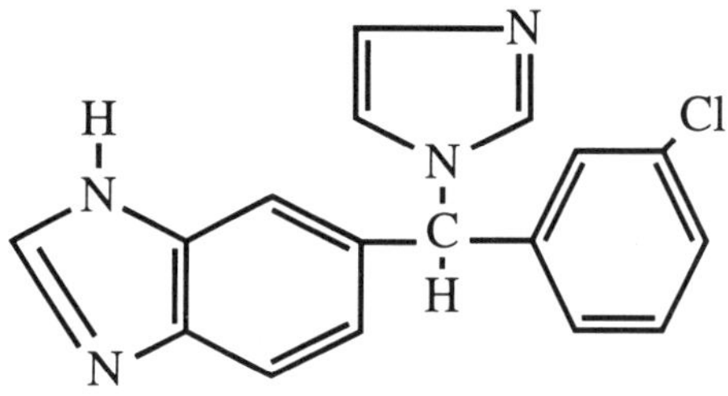

Figure 1 :
Chemical structure of liarozole

Topical all-*trans*-RA (tretinoin) is effective in the treatment of acne vulgaris [2]. Retinoids, particularly the aromatic retinoid, etretinate, are available for the treatment of psoriasis [13]. By inhibiting RA metabolism, treatment with P450 inhibitors, such as liarozole, will result in higher and more sustained tissue levels of RA. Therefore, these P450 inhibitors may exert retinoid-mimetic effects [12] and be of use in the treatment of, among others, psoriasis [14].

Although, RA metabolism in rat epidermal microsomes was sensitive to both ketoconazole and liarozole, the fact that the P450s involved in RA metabolism are species and even tissue specific made it necessary to develop human skin models to evaluate the potency of potential RA metabolism inhibitors. In this paper two such models have been evaluated.

The epidermis is not only a site for RA metabolism it is the major skin site for drug and endogenous substrate metabolism (for a review see Ref. 15). A major function of the epidermis is to form a protective layer, the stratum corneum [16]. Although lipids account for a small percentage of the total stratum corneum weight, they are crucial for the permeability barrier function [17-18]. The sterol synthetic capacity of the skin rivals that of the liver and gastrointestinal tract [17]. Of the sterol synthetic capacity in rodent skin about 75% occurs in the dermis, while the remaining 25% occurs in the viable epidermis [19]. Since the viable epidermis layer comprises only a small fraction of the skin, on a weight basis this fraction can be considered among the most active sites of sterol synthesis in the body [19]. Evidence for a role of cholesterol in the barrier function of the skin has been collected by, e.g., measuring the effects of the 3-hydroxy-3-methylglutaryl coenzyme A (HMG-CoA) reductase inhibitor, lovastatin, on barrier function and repair [16-17,20]. Lovastatin delays barrier recovery after topical aceton treatment of hairless male mice [16] and when applied to intact skin it produces a defect in barrier functions [16-17,20]. Co-application of cholesterol with lovastatin normalizes the rate of barrier repair and blocks the lovastatin-induced barrier disruption and epidermal hyperplasia, demonstrating the importance of cholesterol for skin functions [20]. It should be noted that although cholesterol synthesis initially was reduced in lovastatin-treated epidermis, a compensatory increase in HMG-CoA reductase activity leads to a normalization of epidermal sterol synthesis and content [19]. Rather than reduced cholesterol content, the lovastatin-induced barrier abnormality is associated with a disproportionate increase in fatty acid synthesis leading to altered sterol:fatty acid ratio [19]. Thus, compounds, such as liarozole, with potential use in skin diseases should be evaluated for their effects on sterol and fatty acid synthesis. These effects can be tested on epidermis prepared from neonatal rats and mice. However, the lipid composition of rodent skin differs from that of human skin. In human epidermal lipids sterol esters are present as minor components [21]. In rat skin, however, nearly half of the sterols present are esterified to fatty acids. In contrast to human skin, rat skin is able to cyclise oxidosqualene to $\Delta^{7,24}$ lanostadienol in addition to lanosterol and it also contains an extremely active enzyme which esterifies Δ^7 sterols. Once esterified the methylated Δ^7 sterols are rendered inert for the demethylation enzyme systems [19]. These differences led us to search for *in vitro* skin models.

Material and Methods

Preparation of human skin organ-cultures.

Human skin, taken from patients undergoing plastic surgery, was obtained from local hospitals and transported immediately to the laboratory in sterile 'Transport Medium' (T-medium) containing phosphate buffered saline supplemented with $CaCl_2.2H_2O$ and $MgCl_2.6H_2O$ (PBS, Gibco). T-medium also contained 10 µg gentamycin/ml PBS.

Upon arrival, the skin was washed 3 times with T-medium and, if necessary the adipose tissue was scraped off. Punches of 0.8 cm diameter were obtained with a Keyes' skinpuncher and collected in cold Normal Human Keratinocyte-medium (NHK-medium). NHK-medium contained 3 parts of Dulbecco's Minimum Essential Medium (Gibco) and 1 part Ham's- F12 medium (Flow), 10% fetal calf serum, 2mM L-glutamine, 5 µg gentamycin/ml, 0.4 µg hydrocortisone/ml, 5 µg insuline/ml, 5 µg transferrin/ml, 2.10^{-9} M triiodothyronine (T3), 10^{-10} M cholera toxin, 1.8×10^{-4} M adenine and 10 ng epidermal growth factor/ml.

Skin punches were placed on a Nunc Tissue Culture-insert (diam. 2.5 cm) and cultivated at the air-liquid interface in 6-well plates containing 2 ml NHK-medium/well. After an overnight incubation period at 37°C in a 5% CO_2-humidified atmosphere, the medium was replaced by fresh medium and the experiments were started.

Isolation of human skin epidermis.

About 50 skin-punches were incubated overnight at 4°C in 15 ml PBS without calcium and magnesium, containing 2 ml Dispase II (Boehringer; 24 U/ml). After incubation the epidermis was separated from the dermis using sterile forceps and placed, dermal side down on 2 ml NHK-medium in 6-well plates.

Human Skin equivalents.

The human skin equivalent model ZK1300 (Advanced Tissue Sciences, ATS, La Jolla, USA) was used and processed as described by ATS. In summary: immediately upon receipt, the lid of the 24-well foil-sealed tray containing skin equivalents, was removed. One ml prewarmed (37°C) maintenance medium (kit component) was dispensed under the tissue culture insert, making sure that no air bubbles were trapped underneath the insert. Using sterile forceps, the tissue-equivalents were transferred with the dermis-side down, onto the surface of the tissue culture insert. Prior to the start of the experiments, human skin equivalent cultures were incubated overnight in 1 ml maintenance-medium at 37°C in a 5% CO_2-humidified atmosphere, after which the medium was replaced by 1 ml of fresh medium.

[^{14}C]Acetate incorporation into lipids.

Incubations. The effects of liarozole, dissolved in dimethylsulfoxide (DMSO), on [^{14}C]-acetate incorporation into lipids by human skin organ-cultures, human skin epidermis or human skin equivalent cultures were determined after 2 (epidermis and human skin equivalent cultures) or 3 days (intact skin) of contact with the drug and/or solvent. For these experiments, 5 µCi [2-^{14}C]acetate (S.A. 52 mCi/mmol) together with drug and/or solvent, were added to the medium immediately before insertion of the skin samples. During these incubation periods, the culture medium was not replaced.

Extraction and separation of skin lipids. After incubation, the samples were extracted with 20 ml chloroform/ methanol (2/1, v/v) in a rotatory extractor for 30 minutes. After separation and evaporation of the chloroform layer, 1/8 of the total lipid extract was separated by a TLC-system as described by Vanden Bossche et al. [22] Lipid fractions were localized by autoradiography and the radioactivity determined as described previously [23].

Retinoic acid metabolism in human skin epidermis or human skin equivalents.

Two epidermides (Ø 8 mm) were placed on 2 ml NHK-medium containing 2 µl drug and/or solvent and 1 µCi [11,12-^{3}H(N)]retinoic acid (20 pmol; S.A.: 50.7 Ci/mmol) and incubated for 24 h at 37°C in a 5% CO_2 humidified atmosphere. Blanc values were obtained by incubating boiled skin or medium for 24 h with radiolabelled substrate. The retinoic acid metabolism by human skin equivalents was studied using one human skin equivalent culture incubated in 1 ml maintenance medium containing drug and or solvent, and 1 µCi ^{3}H-RA. After 24 h of incubation, the medium was extracted for 30 min with 5 ml ethylacetate containing 0.005% (w/v) butylated hydroxytoluene (BHT). After evaporation of the organic solvent the samples were analysed by HPLC as described by Van Wauwe et al. [10]. All operations were carried out in a darkened room illuminated with yellow light.

Determination of the epidermal protein content.

The epidermis was washed with bidistilled water, transferred into 1ml of a 1 M sodiumhydroxide solution and sonicated for 15 min in a Branson 3200® sonifier. After homogenization with a Pasteur pipet, 1 ml lysis-buffer [containing 150 mM NaCl, 5 mM EDTA, 50 mM Tris, 62.5 mM sucrose, 0.5% (w/v) Triton-X-100 and 0.5% (w/v) sodium-deoxycholate, pH 7.4] was added and the homogenate sonicated for another 30 min. The homogenate was kept overnight at 4°C. The protein content of the supernatant, obtained after centrifugation at 550 g (10 min), was determined by the Lowry method using bovine serum albumine as standard.

Results and Discussion

Metabolism of retinoic acid by human skin epidermis and skin equivalents

The epidermal fraction prepared from two human skin punches (Ø 8 mm) was incubated for 24 h at 37 °C with [11,12-^{3}H]RA (20 pmol; 1 µCi). After incubation the radioactive products present in the medium and epidermides were analyzed by reverse-phase HPLC. The radioactivity in the remaining substrate and incorporated into the metabolites in the epidermis was below the detection level. Fig. 2 shows a typical HPLC profile of the polar metabolites produced from RA by human epidermis and extracted from the medium. The retention times of the polar products formed after 24 h of incubation corresponded to those of the metabolites formed from RA by hamster liver microsomes [12]. However, it should be noted that we were able to detect trace amounts only of a compound with the same retention time as 4-hydroxyretinoic acid and 4-oxoretinoic acid was not detected. Other experimental conditions are under evaluation to figure out whether the polar metabolites are formed from 4-hydroxyretinoic acid.

Under the present experimental conditions, the amount of product formation from RA was between 8 and 40 h proportional to the time of

incubation (Fig. 3A) and to the number of epidermides used (Fig. 3B). The epidermal fraction prepared from 1 skin punch (Ø 8 mm) contained 0.7 ± 0.1 mg protein (mean ± S.D. of 8 determinations). After 24 h of incubation of 2 epidermal punches 39.8 ± 13.9% of the 20 pmol RA added was metabolized (Fig. 3B). Thus, under the experimental conditions used, the epidermis was capable to metabolize RA at a rate of 5.4 ± 12.9 pmol/24 h/mg protein or about 2 pmol/24 h/cm^2 epidermis.
Advanced Tissue Sciences (La Jolla, California) developed a three-

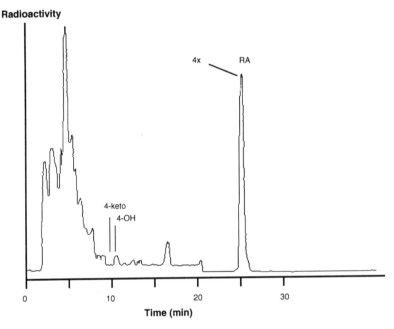

Figure 2 :
Reverse-phase HPLC analysis of RA and radiolabeled metabolites formed by incubation of 2 human epidermides for 24 h with [11,12-^{3}H]RA. The retention times of 4-hydroxyretinoic acid and 4-oxoretinoic acid are marked.

dimensional skin model (skin equivalents) consisting of keratinocytes and fibroblasts derived from human neonatal foreskins [24]. This multi-layered differentiated tissue contains a dermis, epidermis and stratum corneum. Preliminary results indicate that the human skin equivalents metabolize RA at a similar rate as the epidermides. Indeed, after 48 h of incubation 72.8 ± 6.7% (mean ± S.D. of 9 experiments) of the RA added was converted into polar metabolites.

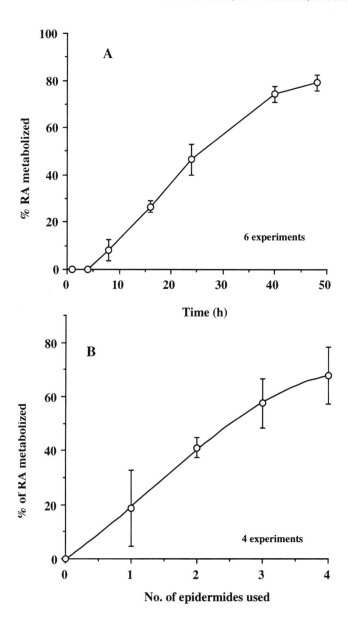

Figure 3 :
A. RA metabolism by 2 human epidermides as a function of time. Results are presented as % of RA metabolized. Number of epidermides : 2.
B. RA metabolism as a function of number of epidermides. Incubation time : 24 h.

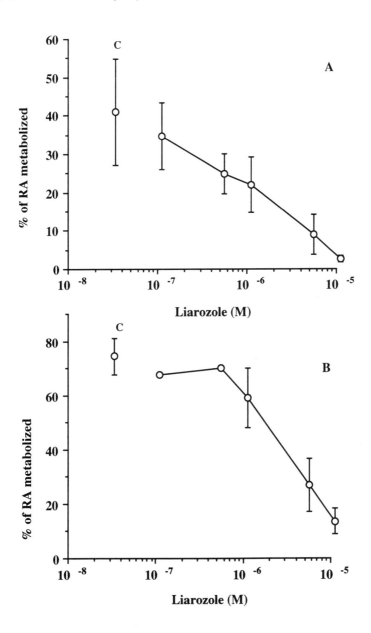

Figure 4 :
Effects of liarozole on RA metabolism by human epidermis (A) and human skin equivalents (B). The results presented in A and B are the mean of 5 and at least 3 experiments, respectively.
A : incubation time : 24 h; number of epidermides : 2
B : incubation time : 48 h.

Effects of liarozole on RA metabolism

Liarozole inhibits the metabolism of retinoic acid in neonatal rat skin epidermal microsomes [7-8], rat [9] and hamster [12] liver microsomes. Incubation of human skin epidermides (Fig. 4A) and human skin equivalents (Fig. 4B) for 24 h or 48 h with liarozole also resulted in a concentration-dependent suppression of RA metabolism. IC_{50}-values calculated from the data presented in Fig. 4A and 4B were 0.8 ± 0.6 µM (5 experiments) and 2.8 ± 1.2 µM (4 experiments), respectively. The somewhat higher IC_{50}-value obtained with the human skin equivalents may be due to the fact that, to reach the epidermis, liarozole had to be transported from the medium through the dermal layer, whereas the epidermides were in direct contact with the liarozole containing medium. As mentioned above RA metabolism is P450-dependent. The fact that liarozole, an inhibitor of some P450-dependent reactions [9], e.g. the 4-hydroxylation of RA, inhibits RA metabolism in human skin models, suggests that human skin RA metabolism may also be P450-dependent. This will be further evaluated by studying the effects of other P450 inhibitors, and by incubating human skin punches under conditions that may induce P450s. The nature of the P450(s) involved will also be determined.

Lipid synthesis

Studies of Slivka [24] indicated that the skin equivalents can be used in the study of testosterone metabolism to dihydrotestosterone (catalyzed by the 5α-reductase) and to more polar metabolites (catalyzed by cytochromes P450). In the present study we evaluated the capability of this skin model to synthesize lipids from [^{14}C]acetate and compared the lipids formed with those synthesized by human skin samples and epidermides prepared from these samples.

Incubations of human skin equivalents for 48 h in the presence of 5 µCi [^{14}C]acetate revealed that about 40% of the total radioactivity present in the lipid extract was incorporated into phospholipids (Table I, Fig. 5). Phosphatidylcholines (PC; ± 27%) and phosphatidylethanolamines (PE; ± 12.5%) accounted for most of the phospholipids synthesized (Table II). The PC:PE ratio of 2.2 resembles the ratio (2.5) found by Tsambaos and Mahtle (cited in Ref. 20) in uninvolved psoriatic epidermis. Most of the radioactivity incorporated into PC was recovered in a fraction with the same Rf-value as dilauroylphosphatidylcholine (DLPC). Similar results were obtained by incubating human skin punches (Tables I-II, Fig. 5). The distribution of radioactivity over the triglycerides- lanosterol-, free fatty acids- and sterol fractions and a fraction with the same Rf-value as ceramides was also similar in both systems (Table I). However, the percentage of radioactivity incorporated into the cholesterol fraction of the lipid extract of the skin equivalents was in some preparations higher than that in extracts from human skin punches, but similar to the % of radioactivity incorporated into cholesterol by the epidermis (Table I, Fig. 5). In the liquid extracts of the latter a much higher percentage of the radioactivity was incorporated in a variety of sofar unidentified

Lipid Fractions*	Radioactivity incorporated as % of total found in the lipid extracts**		
	Human skin 3 days (19)	Human skin epidermis 2 days (6)	Human skin equivalents 2 days (7)
Phospholipids	34.5 ± 6.0	20.7 ± 2.6	42.4 ± 14.4
'Ceramides'	7.2 ± 2.1	12.6 ± 1.1	4.4 ± 1.1
Cholesterol	12.9 ± 2.6	21.5 ± 2.9	23.5 ± 9.4
Lanosterol	1.3 ± 1.1	2.1 ± 0.7	1.5 ± 0.6
Fatty acids (free)	1.7 ± 0.6	3.1 ± 0.7	1.0 ± 0.4
Triglycerides	24.2 ± 6.1	5.8 ± 0.8	18.4 ± 3.5
Sterol esters	2.1 ± 2.2	1.5 ± 0.2	1.1 ± 0.5
Others	15.9 ± 5.6	32.7 ± 3.0	7.7 ± 2.6

Table I :
Lipid synthesis from [^{14}C]acetate.
Tentative identification based on Rf-values of standards. Standards used: Phospholipids: dipalmitoylphosphatidylcholine, dilauroylphosphatidylcholine, dipalmitoylphosphatidyl-N,N-dimethylethanolamine, dipalmitoyl-phosphatidyl-N-methylethanolamine & phosphatidylethanolamine; Ceramides: ceramide III & IV; Fatty acid: oleic acid; Triglyceride: triolein; Sterol ester: cholesterol stearate. Others are unidentified compounds.
** Results are mean values ± S.D. of (n) experiments.

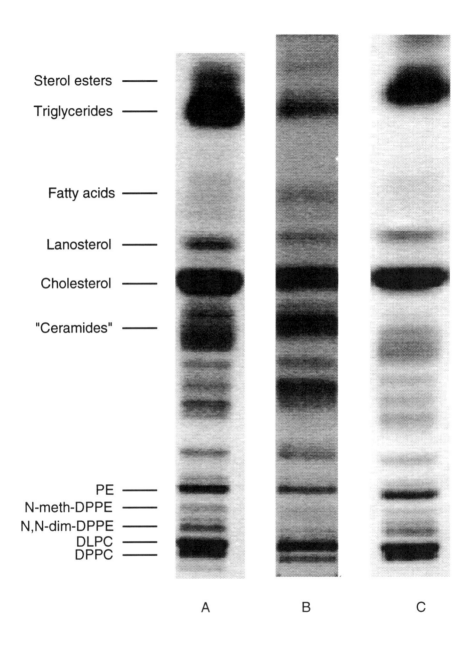

Figure 5 :
TLC of lipid extracts from human skin punches (A), epidermis (B) and skin equivalents (C). Human skin equivalents and human epidermis were incubated for 48 h in the presence of [^{14}C]-acetate; human skin punches were incubated for 3 days.

components. One of these components contained 8.2 ± 1.7% of the radioactivity. In the extracts from skin punches and skin equivalents the fraction with the same Rf-value contained 2.3 ± 1.2% and 1.2 ± 0.3% only. Studies to identify this component(s) are ongoing.

Although there are quantitative differences, the results obtained so far indicate that all three models can be used to evaluate lipid synthesis in skin.

Effects of liarozole on lipid synthesis

Liarozole inhibits in human skin epidermis and skin equivalents the metabolism of retinoic acid. To evaluate possible interactions with lipid synthesis and, thus, with the barrier function of the skin (see introduction) the three skin models were incubated in the presence of increasing concentrations of this imidazole derivative (Table III summarizes the

Lipid Fractions*	Radioactivity incorporated as % of total found in the lipid extracts		
	Human skin 3 days (19)	Human skin epidermis 2 days (6)	Human skin equivalents 2 days (7)
DPPC	6.2 ± 1.2	3.1 ± 0.6	6.5 ± 2.9
DLPC	14.3 ± 4.8	9.0 ± 0.9	21.1 ± 8.1
N,N-dim-DPPE	2.8 ± 1.1	2.0 ± 0.6	2.8 ± 0.7
N-meth-DPPE	0.9 ± 0.3	0.7 ± 0.2	1.1 ± 0.4
PE	7.3 ± 1.2	3.7 ± 0.5	8.6 ± 3.6

Table II :
[14C]Acetate incorporation into different phospholipids.
*Tentative identification based on Rf-values of standards. DPPC: dipalmitoylphosphatidylcholine; DLPC: dilauroylphosphatidylcholine; N,N-dim-DPPE: dipalmitoylphosphatidyl-N,N-dimethylethanolamine; N-meth-DPPE: dipalmitoylphosphatidyl-N-methylethanolamine: PE: phosphatidylethanolamine (nature of the acyl moieties unknown).
** Results are mean values ± S.D. of (n) experiments.

Liarozole	Radioactivity incorporated as % of total found in the lipid extracts*						
(μM)	PL	'Cer.'	Chol.	Lano.	FA	TG	SE
Human skin (4)							
0	27.8	9.1	13.2	1.1	2.0	21.6	4.7
10	27.0	9.2	9.6	1.2	2.4	21.8	5.5
Human epidermis (3)							
0	21.7	11.8	21.4	2.0	3.2	5.3	1.5
10	21.0	14.6	20.2	2.2	3.2	8.2	1.5
Human skin equivalents							
0	51.7	3.3	14.6	1.4	1.4	16.0	1.0
10**	40.5	4.5	12.5	2.1	1.3	24.1	1.3

Table III :
Effects of liarozole on the incorporation of [14C]acetate into lipids.
* Results are mean values of (n) experiments. Only the tentatively identified lipids are listed. PL: phospholipids; 'Cer.': 'ceramides'; Chol.: cholesterol; Lano.: lanosterol; FA: fatty acids; TG: triglycerides; SE: Sterol esters.
** Results are mean values of 2 experiments and are compared with control values obtained with skin equivalent cultures from the same batch.

results obtained in the presence of DMSO and 10 μM liarozole only). Previous studies showed that liarozole is a poor inhibitor of cholesterol synthesis in subcellular fractions of rat liver cells, human liver and hepatoma cells [9]. The results presented here (Table III) indicate that it barely affects cholesterol synthesis in human skin. As shown in Table III, liarozole was up to 10 μM also devoid of effects on phospholipid, triglyceride, 'ceramide', fatty acid, and sterol ester synthesis. Since lipids are crucial for the permeability barrier function of the skin (see introduction), the results obtained at least suggest that oral or topical treatment with liarozole will not affect directly the lipid-dependent properties of the skin.

Conclusions

1. The human skin models presented, especially the epidermal model, can be used to study effects of compounds on the metabolism of retinoic acid. These models may also be used to predict possible side-effects on lipid synthesis. Experiments are ongoing to evaluate their use in the study of the P450-dependent metabolism of other endogenous compounds and of xenobiotics. If skin from cosmetic surgery is locally not available the three-dimensional skin model may be an alternative to the less expensive human skin or epidermal model.
2. Liarozole is a potent inhibitor of retinoic acid metabolism in human skin without interfering with the synthesis of lipids such as cholesterol, which is crucial for the permeability barrier function of the skin.

References

1. Williams J.B. and Napoli J.L. Metabolism of retinoic acid and retinol during differentiation of F9 embryonal carcinoma cells. Proceedings of the National Academy of Sciences of the USA 1985;82:4658-4662.
2. Gilchrest B.A. Retinoid pharmacology and skin. In: Pharmacology of the skin (Mukhtar H., ed.) CRC Press, Boca Raton, 1992:29-38.
3. Roberts A.B. Microsomal oxidation of retinoic acid in hamster liver, intestine, and testis. Annals of the New York Academy of Sciences 1981;359:45-53.
4. Leo M.A. and Lieber C.S. New pathways for retinol and metabolism in liver microsomes. The Journal of Biological Chemistry 1985;260:5228-5231.
5. Leo M.A., Lesker J.M., Raucy J.L., Kim C.-I., Black M. and Lieber C.S. Metabolism of retinol and retinoic acid by human liver cytochrome P450IIC8. Archives of Biochemistry and Biophysics 1989;269:305-312.
6. Roberts E.S., Vaz A.D.N. and Coon M.J. Role of isozymes of rabbit microsomal cytochrome P450 in the metabolism of retinoic acid, retinol and retinal. Molecular Pharmacology 1992;41:427-423.
7. Vanden Bossche H., Willemsens G. and Janssen P.A.J. Cytochrome P450-dependent metabolism of retinoic acid in rat skin microsomes: inhibition by ketoconazole. Skin Pharmacology 1988;1:176-185.
8. Vanden Bossche H. and Willemsens G. Retinoic acid and cytochrome P450. In: Retinoids 10 years on (Saurat J.H., ed.) Karger, Basel, 1991:79-88.
9. Vanden Bossche H. Inhibitors of P450-dependent steroid biosynthesis: from research to medical treatment. The Journal of Steroid Biochemistry and Molecular Biology 1992;43:1003-1021.
10. Van Wauwe J.P., Coene M.-C., Goossens J., Van Nyen G., Cools W. and Janssen P.A.J. Ketoconazole inhibits the *in vitro* and *in vivo* metabolism of all-*trans*-retinoic acid. The Journal of Pharmacology and Experimental Therapeutics 1988;245:718-722.

11. Van Wauwe J.P., Coene M.-C., Goossens J., Cools W. and Monbaliu J. Effects of cytochrome P450 inhibitors on the *in vivo* metabolism of all-*trans*-retinoic acid in rats. The Journal of Pharmacology and Experimental Therapeutics 1990;252:365-369.
12. Van Wauwe J.P., Van Nyen G., Coene M.-C., Stoppie P., Cools W., Goossens J., Borghgraef P. and Janssens P.A.J. Liarozole, an inhibitor of retinoic acid metabolism, exerts retinoic-mimetic effects *in vivo*. The Journal of Pharmacology and Experimental Therapeutics 1992;261:773-779.
13. Goldfarb M.T., Ellis C.N. and Voorhees J.J. Retinoids in dermatology. Mayo Clinics Proceedings 1987;62:1161-1164.
14. Dockx P., Lambert J., De Doncker P., Cauwenbergh G., Janssen P.A.J. Treatment of severe plaque-type psoriasis with oral liarozole (R 75251): an inhibitor of retinoic acid metabolism. Poster presented at the 18th World Congress of Dermatology, June 12-18, 1992, New York, U.S.A.
15. Mukhtar H., Agarwal R. and Bickers D.R. Cutaneous metabolism of xenobiotics and steroid hormones. In: Pharmacology of the skin (Mukhtar H., ed.) CRC Press, Boca Raton, 1992:89-109.
16. Feingold K.R., Mao-Qiang M., Menon G.K., Cho S.S., Brown B.E. and Elias P.M. Cholesterol synthesis is required for cutaneous barrier function in mice. The Journal of Clinical Investigations 1990;86:1738-1745.
17. Elias P.M. and Feingold K.R. Lipid-related barriers and gradients in the epidermis. Annals of the New York Academy of Sciences 1988;548:4-13.
18. Elias P.M. Role of lipids in barrier function of the skin. In: Pharmacology of the skin (Mukhtar H., ed.) CRC Press, Boca Raton, 1992:29-38.
19. Feingold K.R., Brown B.E., Lear S.R., Moser A.H. and Elias P.M. Effect of essential fatty acid deficiency on cutaneous sterol synthesis. Journal of Investigative Dermatology 1986;87:588-591.
20. Feingold K.R., Mao-Qiang M., Proksch E., Menon G.K., Brown B.E. and Elias P.M. The lovastatin-treated rodent: a new model of barrier disruption and epidermal hyperplasia. Journal of Investigative Dermatology 1991;96:201-209.
21. Yardley H.J. and Summerly R. Lipid composition and metabolism in normal and diseased epidermis. Pharmacology and Therapeutics 1981;13:357-383.
22. Vanden Bossche H., Marichal P., Gorrens J., Bellens D., Verhoeven H., Coene M.-C., Lauwers W. and Janssen P.A.J. Interactions of azole derivatives with cytochrome P-450 isozymes in yeast, fungi, plants and mammalian cells. Pesticide Sciences 1987;21:289-306.
23. Vanden Bossche H., Willemsens G., Cools W., Lauwers W. and Le Jeune L. Biochemical effects of miconazole on fungi. II: Inhibition of ergosterol biosynthesis in *Candida albicans*. Chemical-Biological Interactions 1978;21:59-78.
24. Slivka S.R. Testosterone metabolism in an *in vitro* skin model. Cell Biology and Toxicology 1992;8:267-276.

6
Cultures of human hepatocytes in *in vitro* pharmaco-toxicology

V. Rogiers

Vrije Universiteit Brussel, Department of Toxicology, Laarbeeklaan 103, 1090 Brussels (Belgium).

Introduction

The liver is the major site for the uptake of drugs and chemicals, converting them to pharmacologically inactive, active or even toxic metabolites. Biotransformation of xenobiotics and specific liver functions, mostly performed by hepatocytes (parenchymal liver cells) which represent about 65% of the total liver cell population, are difficult to study in the whole organism because other organs and tissues and exogenous and endogenous factors may exert important influences. Consequently, *in vitro* liver systems could represent a valuable tool in pharmaco-toxicology. Several investigators have experimented with isolated perfused livers, liver tissue slices, microsomes, whole homogenates and finally with freshly isolated liver cells and their cultures. Usually cells have been derived from rodents. Since the main objective of human pharmaco-toxicology is not concerned with the knowledge of the mechanism of action and eventual toxicity of drugs and xenobiotics in rodents, but in humans, greater attention should be focused on the isolation, culture and experimental use of human hepatocytes.

Indeed, both qualitative and quantitative interspecies differences exist in drug biotransformation [31,105,106,109,201] making extrapolation of animal data to humans problematic [164]. Furthermore hepatocyte growth factors, controlling liver growth in man and in non-human species, are highly species dependent [91], further highlighting the limitations of extrapolating results obtained with rodents and other species to humans.

Moreover, from agents which are not therapeutically administered to man and from potentially toxic compounds, information on human metabolism or mechanisms of action and toxicity will always remain fragmentary because of obvious ethical considerations. In vitro experimentation, specifically with human cells, could provide suitable data.

The issue of *in vivo/in vitro* extrapolation, however, is not solved and is subject to debate but in the case of drug biotransformation activity, a rather good qualitative *in vivo/in vitro* correlation is found when human freshly isolated or cultured hepatocytes are used as an *in vitro* model [31,60,72,79,101,201].

Other drawbacks such as the lack of reproducibility between different batches of cells and difficulties in standardisation have also not yet been solved [94]. Heterogeneity and genetic polymorphism in the human population also increase the variability.

A positive aspect, however, could be that this variability is an essential component of the risk assessment process. When results are extrapolated from animals to man safety factors for the variability in the human population are used but these are not based on scientific evidence. The use of human cells, however, takes into account this variability on a more realistic basis [94]. Although a lot of progress has been made, the use of human hepatocytes still remains difficult and sometimes unfeasable in several laboratories because of ethical, safety, technical and logistical reasons.

This review summarizes the current knowledge on the isolation of human hepatocytes, their culture and their application in pharmaco-toxicological studies and discusses some perspectives and developments.

Isolation of human hepatocytes

Adult hepatocytes

Cultures of adult human liver cells were first obtained in explant cultures in which peripheral outgrowth of cells was observed around small liver fragments [44,104,107,110,182,187]. These non-perfusion techniques yielded only small amounts of liver cells and a heterogenous cell population, composed mainly of primitive cells, appearing as fibroblasts and undifferentiated epithelial cells, was obtained [76]. Later on, enzymatic methods were used to dissociate biopsy tissue of human liver [13]. In particular collagenase and dispase were utilized as dissociating enzymes [115,132].

The wide application of these methods, however, was restricted by the low yield of hepatocytes obtained. A major progress in primary culture of human hepatocytes was the adaptation of the classic in situ two-step collagenase perfusion technique, initially developed for the isolation of rat hepatocytes, by Berry and Friend [16], into a procedure applicable to human liver.

Pioneering work was carried out by Bojar et al. [25], Reese and Byard [170], Guguen-Guillouzo et al. [74], Strom et al. [199], Ballet et al. [6] and Clément et al. [36]. The availability of human hepatocytes was greatly enhanced with these methods. Recently Ryan et al. [180] have optimized the entire isolation procedure on specimens of surgical hepatic resection resulting in improved yields of hepatocytes.

Most human liver cells obtained by enzymatic perfusion and used for *in vitro* research and testing come either from liver pieces taken from surgical hepatic resections [6,68,90,123,142,161,162,170,199,201], or from hepatic resections during kidney donor operations [90,161,211] or from cadavers [140]. The other most common source is via in situ perfusion of the whole liver of kidney donors [12,25,51,145].

Hepatocytes isolated from surgical biopsies perfused immediately after resection have been compared with cells obtained from donor liver stored in a modified University of Wisconsin (UW) solution for 7± 2 hrs. It seems that the former cells maintained liver specific and non-specific functions better than the latter ones [214].

Human hepatocytes are usually isolated according to the two-step perfusion method mentioned above devised by Berry and Friend [16] and Seglen [188]. Liver species are first perfused with a Ca^{2+}- and Mg^{2+}-free buffer to remove blood and destabilize intercellular contacts followed by perfusion with a Ca^{2+}- and collagenase-containing buffer to degrade the connective tissue of the liver.

Some hepatocytes have been isolated from a whole lobe [84,199] but usually biopsy samples are taken so that the Glisson's capsule is present on all sides except for one cut surface [6,67,77]. Only in isolated cases are several cut surfaces present [180]. The pieces of liver are immediately placed in ice-cold buffer and used within a relatively short time after resection (45 mins reported by Guguen-Guillouzo et al. [73]; 60-120 mins by Gomez-Lechon et al. [67]).

Viable cells could also be obtained 10-20 hrs after organ preservation in

UW solution, containing raffinose and lactobionate [81]. 12 to 24 hrs storage periods at 4°C have also been reported by Ismail et al. [91] by using either UW solution or Euro-Collins according to common procedures in organ transplantation [14,52].

One [51,73,84,170] or more [67,180,199] catheters are introduced into the main portal vein(s). The results are not as good when hepatic veins are used for perfusion [6,73]. The preperfusion buffer is usually a Ca^{2+}-/Mg^{2+}-free Krebs-Ringer buffer, Hank's balanced salt solution or a similar salt solution kept at 37°C.

It is often buffered with 4-(2-hydroxyethyl)-1-piperazineethane sulfonic acid (Hepes), kept at pH 7.4-7.6 and supplemented with EGTA [6,67,170], or EDTA [84,180] and glucose [51,67]. The flow rate, which is related to the weight of the liver pieces, seems to play an important role and readings between 8 to 75 ml/min/catheter have been reported. Recently, a pressure controlled perfusion study has been carried out by Ryan et al. [180], and a variety of flow rates between 2 and 60 ml/min/cannula within the same piece of liver has been reported depending on the geometry of the pieces and the vessel cannulated. Usually, preperfusion continues for 15 to 20 mins without recirculation.

The second perfusion step is carried out with a Hepes buffered solution without a chelating agent but containing 0.05% collagenase (type I) and 5 mM $CaCl_2$, at a flow rate of 40 to 50 ml/min for 15 to 30 mins usually with recirculation [6,67,84,170]. Sometimes all solutions are pregassed in order to obtain saturation with oxygen [90].

At the end of the perfusion, cells are dispersed by various means such as gentle shaking, mincing with scissors or with a metal comb. Cell aggregates can be further dispersed by incubation and gentle shaking in Hepes buffered collagenase solution at 37°C. Often no additional disruption of the tissue is necessary. The cell suspension is then filtered on sterile gauze layers, allowed to sediment and is washed at least twice with culture medium (L15 Leibovitz medium, DMEM, Williams' E,.....) supplemented with albumin 0.2% [6,67,73]. Cells are pelleted by gentle centrifugation at 50-100 g for 1-4 mins. Viability is measured by trypan blue exclusion and is reported to be between 70-90% [67,73].

Under control conditions cell viability rates may strongly depend on various factors related to the premedication and the nutritional status of the donor, the clinical condition of the human liver, (e.g. low-levels of serum bilirubin), the conditions of resection and preservation of the samples before dissociation, efficient oxygenation and glucose supplementation of the perfusion buffers in order to avoid anoxia during isolation and the quality of the collagenase used. The latter factor has been studied by Gomez-Lechon et al. [68] and it appears that high specific activity collagenase should be used in order to reduce perfusion time and concommitant cell destruction. Collagenase with a specific activity of 0.35 U/mg was found to give the best results [68]. In certain techniques mixtures of enzymes are used as dissociating agents such as collagenase, dispase, hyaluronidase and deoxyribonuclease [90].

Fetal hepatocytes

Since the liver of the developing human fetus contains primarily hematopoietic cells with parenchymal cells being present only in small amounts, whole liver is an inappropriate tissue to study the biochemical functions of fetal liver. Between 16-20 weeks of gestation liver tissue contains 45% hematopoietic cells, consisting almost entirely of erythroblasts [202]. It is therefore not easy to isolate viable pure hepatocytes without contamination of other cell types. Studies have been performed on explant cultures of human fetal livers, but the cell population was too heterogeneous, although a good yield of hepatocytes was obtained [153]. More recently enzymatic digestion of human fetal liver has been used with some success.

Livers from human fetuses are obtained at legal abortions between 14-25 weeks of gestation and are used within 2-10 hrs after isolation [147]. The tissue is minced into small fragments [147,160] or sliced [74,218]. After several washes with buffer, enzymatic digestion takes place at 37°C. Nakagami and Ishida [147] describe a two-step digestion with dispase and collagenase (0.1%), whereas Guguen-Guillouzo et al. [74] and Bauer et al. [9] use only collagenase, the former in the presence of 5 mM $CaCl_2$ and in a final concentration of 0.025%; the latter without Ca^{2+} addition but with 0.05% collagenase. 0.1% hyaluronidase and 0.05% collagenase in the presence of 5 mM $CaCl_2$ were tested out with success by Wiebkin et al. [218]. Other reports deal with the use of trypsin (0.1%) [160] or dispase (0.01%) [151]. A more sophisticated technique was proposed by Nagao et al. [146] whereby a 0.05% collagenase solution was injected subcapsularly into the rinsed liver tissue. After enzymatic digestion, cell suspensions are filtered through sterile gauze or nylon screen, centrifuged at a low speed (50 g, 1 min), and washed. The viable hepatocytes are usually resuspended in culture medium supplemented with 10% fetal calf serum (FCS), corticosteroids and insulin [9,74,146].

Culture of functional hepatocytes

Studies on the specific conditions needed for the culture of human hepatocytes are still limited. Most developments and improvements to culture conditions have been obtained using rodent, especially rat hepatocytes, and some of these conditions have been applied to human cells.

An excellent overview of this large field has been given by the Guillouzo's team [75,81] discussing in detail recent advances made in long-term hepatocyte cultures of different species. Four groups of factors seem of utmost importance namely exogenous soluble factors, extracellular matrix components, cell-cell interactions and factors affecting replication of hepatocytes *in vitro*. Although it is beyond the scope of this review to describe all developments made in the culture of non-human hepatocytes, the key developments and their relevance for human hepatocyte culture will be discussed.

Factors of importance in long-term hepatocyte cultures

Exogenous soluble factors. For many years, hepatocytes were cultured on plastic dishes treated for tissue culture or on collagen I coated dishes. The media nearly always contained serum with some other additives. The cells lost their gap junctions in about 12 to 24 hrs and flattened. Dedifferentiation occurred rapidly observed by declining mRNA and protein levels and decreasing liver-specific functions [34,171]. In particular, cytochrome P450-dependent functions were rapidly lost [176]. Attempts to maintain these proteins through modifications of the culture medium by the addition of hormones [46,57], growth factors [82], trace elements [59], special nutrients [71,204], enzyme inducers [8,133,185,205], nicotinamide [158], dimethylsulphoxide [177] and various other substances [157] have met with mixed success. It became clear that maintenance of some specific functions in rat hepatocyte cultures could only be achieved by using serum-free, hormonally defined media as shown by Enat *et al.* [58]. However, the increase in cytochromes P450 was due in part to mRNA stabilization and not to a maintenance of transcription [93].

Very few specific studies on exogenous soluble factors, of particular importance in human hepatocyte cultures, have been carried out. The findings for rat hepatocyte cultures have for the most part simply been extended to human cell cultures.

For human hepatocytes, culture media are either supplemented with fetal calf serum [5,23,70,78,90,211] or do not contain it in order to obtain a better hormonally defined medium [49,118,141,161,162]. Usually, the media also contain insulin and corticosteroids (hydrocortisone or dexamethasone) [5,23,49,70,78,90,118,141]. Other additives may be present such as albumin [49,142,168,210], glucagon, [5,33] δ–aminolaevulinic acid [70], epidermal growth factor [5], pyruvate, aspartate and serine [117], ascorbic acid, glutamine and tryptose phosphate broth [90]. The presence of the amino acid L-ornithine seems to be of importance too since it stimulates, at the pretranslational level, the secretion of transferrin by human hepatocytes in culture [111]. dimethylsulphoxide (DMSO) has also been added to cultures and, although survival of the hepatocytes was improved [210], better enzymatic activity was not observed.

Extracellular matrix. Another factor of importance was found in the extracellular matrix. Although early experiments with rat hepatocyte cultures, extensively reviewed by Guillouzo et al. [81], were disappointing, recent work is more promising.

Matrigel. Matrigel is a laminin- and type IV collagen-rich gel, extracted from the Englebreth-Holm-Swarm mouse sarcoma. Hepatocytes cultured on it remain rounded and grow as single cells or clusters, form irregular cords and remain firmly attached for weeks [20,184]. Matrigel supports long-term transcription of liver specific genes in rat hepatocyte cultures and preserves several of the cytochrome P450 isoenzymes [15,20,30,55,82,184], although not all [82,87]. The maintenance of liver-specific functions is thus not only due to mRNA stabilisation but also to restoration of transcription [192].

It seems to be important that the hepatocytes retain their spherical shape which has been suggested to represent a key element in the preservation of specific hepatocellular functions. The composition and concentration of the extracellular matrix also seems important. It was shown that addition of proteoglycans and glucosaminoglycans to rat hepatocyte cultures on plastic was able to restore transcriptional signals for certain liver specific mRNA's and to induce gap junction formation [62,171]. Addition of diluted laminin to cultures of rat hepatocytes on collagen I was as effective as cultures on diluted matrigel in inducing transcriptional albumin activity [30,220].

Also, a diluted matrigel overlay on cultured adult rat hepatocytes in Williams' E medium was able to preserve phenobarbital-induced responsiveness closely resembling that observed *in vivo* [192], an effect difficult to prove with hepatocytes maintained on matrigel substratum due to the inhibitory effect of the gel on transient gene transfection [159]. Very recently, further evidence for the importance of the chemical composition of the extracellular matrix became available [186]. Indeed, it was shown that laminin and type IV collagen could individually influence the hepatocellular expression of certain genes e.g. Pgp, a plasma membrane protein playing a major role in cellular detoxification by actively pumping xenobiotics out of cells [144]. Furthermore, the biophysical properties (rigid versus soluble) of the extracellular matrix molecules seems also of importance [186].

Data concerning the culture of human cells on matrigel or the use of matrigel overlays and the effects of extracellular matrix composition and medium are not yet available.

Vitrogen. When vitrogen (hydrated collagen) was used at low densities, hepatocyte cultures resembled those using dry collagen in that the cells exhibit a flat extended morphology.

At high densities of vitrogen, however, compact aggregates were formed, maintaining a gene expression pattern ressembling that of rat hepatocytes on Englebreth-Holm-Swarm matrigel [15,217].

Medium composition, as already mentioned before, is of importance since Williams' E [193] and Chee's essential medium [92,217] sustained long-term maintenance of the differentiated state with respect to the response to phenobarbital treatment, which was not the case for modified Weymouth medium [217].

Collagen gel sandwich configuration. When rat hepatocytes are sandwiched between 2 layers of hydrated rat tail tendon collagen, they maintain long-term differentiation with respect to the secretion of albumin [55,108], transferrin, fibrogen, bile salts and urea. Physiological levels are observed for at least 6 weeks [54].

Levels of albumin mRNA, similar to those found in the normal liver were obtained, whereas in a single gel system albumin mRNA levels declined rapidly [53]. The transcription activity is also maintained significantly higher compared to that observed in cells kept in a single gel system. In addition the ultimate rate of albumin production is found to be dependent on the rate of translation, being independent of the type of gel system used [53]. It has been suggested that this stable culture is due to the reinstatement of the cellular polarity of the hepatocytes as a function of the extracellular matrix [55,108].

Indeed, hepatocytes are epithelial cells with distinct apical (bile canalicular) and basal (sinusoidal) surfaces which serve different functions and these cells make contact with the extracellular matrix with both basolateral surfaces.

Human hepatocytes have already been cultured between double layers of collagen [5,180]. The cells demonstrated typical polygonal liver cell morphology and higher albumin secretion for up to 65 days. When exposed to the principal hepatic acute phase response mediators, interleukin-6 and interleukin-1β, an impressive increase in serum amyloid A (positive acute phase proteins) secretion was observed together with a decrease in albumin (negative acute phase protein) secretion, mimicking the *in vivo* hepatocellular response [5]. Tumor necrosis factor–α did not significantly change the secretion rates of these proteins [5]. On the contrary, cells cultured on a single collagen gel spread horizontally and albumin secretion declined rapidly [180].

The medium composition also seems of importance since it has been observed that an early peak in maximal albumin secretion rate appears in sandwich-cultured human hepatocytes in Williams' E medium, which does not persist for a long time. Dulbecco's modified Eagle medium, on the other hand, provokes a long lasting peak of albumin secretion [108]. Proline is therefore a critical component for the culture of human hepatocytes in serum free medium [108].

To date, biotransformation capacities have not yet been evaluated in these sophisticated culture systems.

Hollow fiber. Another recent development consists of gel entrapment of hepatocytes in hollow fibers [190]. For that purpose, cells are suspended in a collagen solution and inoculated into hollow fibers.

The collagen gels and a 3-dimensional cell-gel matrix are formed. Viable cells cause the gel to contract which creates enough space within the hollow fiber lumen to allow intraluminal perfusion. It was found that albumin secretion and lidocaine clearance, measured as a marker of cytochrome P450 function remained constant for 7 days in rat hepatocytes [189]. This hybrid system allows cells to be cultured at high density which is important for bioartificial liver support in the case of liver failure [154]. A potentially superior design [191], which utilized microcarrier attached hepatocytes, was recently reported for acute hepatic failure in rats. In this nonhollow-fiber system the hepatocytes were loaded within the flow stream of a 1 cm diameter column, but no more details are know about this system.

Other entrapments of hepatocytes within a 3-dimensional gel or matrix have been reported [1,47,85,131,203,219]. These have been developed as bioartificial liver supports and clinical observations have been carried out on these systems. However, not much is known about xenobiotic biotransformation capacities of these cultures.

Promising systems such as microcarrier-attached hepatocytes, spheroid aggregate hepatocytes and micro-encapsulated hepatocytes need vascularization [154] and are therefore not always suitable for use as *in vitro* systems in pharmaco-toxicological research and testing of xenobiotics. Recently, interesting systems have been described which, besides their possible role as bioartificial liver, display potential industrial applications in toxicology and drug metabolism. In one of these systems, primary rat hepatocytes are cultured as entrapped aggregates in a packed bed bioreactor [112]. In another one microcarrier-attached rat hepatocytes are cocultured with 3T3 cells [215].

Crude membrane fractions. Improvement of the stabilization of xenobiotic metabolism is observed when crude membrane fraction coating is combined with the use of culture medium supplemented with aprotinin and Se [181].

Cells adhere firmly, remain in clusters and exhibit minimal spreading. It is proposed that no single factor of the extracellular matrix membrane proteins is critical but that several components must be present in appropriate *in vivo*-like ratio's [181].

Other investigators are convinced of the fact that multiple mechanisms of hepatocyte-basement membrane interaction play a crucial role in providing specific signals for tissue development and differentiation. Mooney *et al.* [139] suggest that the mechanism of trans-membrane signaling may be independent of particular receptor binding interactions. They describe four different extracellular membrane molecules producing similar effects on cells plated at sparse densities: low extracellular matrix coating densities stimulated liver specific gene expression regardless of the molecule used. Cell spreading and growth were directly proportional to the extracellular matrix densities [139].

It is further proposed that changes in the extracellular matrix adhesivity or deformability may control hepatocyte growth and differentiation by modulating cell shape, independently of cell-cell interactions [54,139]. This seems not to be the entire reason since a cell surface protein (Liver Regulatory Protein, LRP) has been isolated from rat liver epithelial cells involved in the maintenance of hepatocyte differentiation in cocultures [40]. When antibodies against LRP are added to cocultured hepatocytes, liver specific gene activation and matrix deposition are inhibited and cytoskeleton organisation is altered. LPR does not modify the attachment of hepatocytes to different matrix components or cell-cell aggregation, suggesting that it is distinct from an extracellular matrix receptor [40].

Cell-cell interactions. Some aspects of this large field have been reviewed for rat hepatocytes by Guillouzo et al. [81] and by Donato et al. [50]. Important observations can be summarized as follows.
To mimic the microenvironment of liver cells in vivo, hepatocytes can be brought in contact with non-parenchymal cells such as sinusoidal endothelial cells [143,216], human fibroblasts [129], established fibroblastic cell lines [48,49,98], various epithelial and mesenchymal cell lines [69] or rat epithelial cells derived from primitive biliary duct cells [11].
Rat hepatocytes cultured under these conditions, especially those cocultured with rat epithelial cells [11,77] have a longer viability than hepatocytes cultured under conventional conditions, and retain to a greater extent the morphological and biochemical characteristics of adult hepatocytes in vivo, including phase I cytochrome P450-mediated and phase II biotransformations. It has been claimed that as much as 100% of the cytochrome P450 content and cytochrome P450 dependent enzymatic activities are maintained in cocultured rat hepatocytes [11,105]. More recent work with rat hepatocytes at the enzymatic, protein and mRNA level, however, points to a steady-state situation in which phase II enzymes are qualitatively maintained [152,206,207,208,209,210,213], cytochrome P450 content is partly preserved [176] and cytochrome P450 isoezymes are selectively maintained [116,152,176,206]. The mRNA's of the cytochrome P450IIB sub-family are maintained and inducible by phenobarbital and sodium valproate comparable to that observed in vivo [2,175]. Also quantitatively expressed are the genes coding for cytochrome P450 reductase, cytochrome b5 [3] and cytochrome P450IVA [3]. The extent of adult liver-specific functions expressed in cocultures of rat hepatocytes is influenced by the medium composition and fetal-like functions cannot be totally prevented [152,209]. The early production and deposition of extracellular matrix components [37,38] could play an important role both in the high transcriptional gene activity [2,3,61] and communication via gap junctions [127]. As already mentioned above a cell surface protein, important for maintenance of cell differentiation, LRP, has been isolated from epithelial cells [40].
As far as the human situation is concerned, successful cocultures of human hepatocytes with rat epithelial cells have been described [36,73].

Hepatocyte survival increased significantly in these cultures.

The addition of serum is not required but the presence of corticoids is essential, indicating that soluble factors play an important role in this model. Usually, epithelial cells are added just after attachment of the hepatocytes, however, they still can be added to 1 week-old-human hepatocyte cultures [36]. Fibronectin, an extracellular matrix component, is produced by both epithelial cells and hepatocytes, whereas collagen I, III and IV are formed only by the epithelial cells [73].

The total cytochrome P450 content is relatively stable in cocultures of human hepatocytes [78], remains inducible by phenobarbital and some isoenzymes are better maintained than in pure cultures [168,169]. Also NADPH cytochrome c reductase and epoxide hydrolase are maintained better in cocultures [168].

Factors affecting replication of hepatocytes *in vitro*. The use of growth factors in hepatocyte cultures could possibly lead to enhanced cell survival and longevity. Indeed, during the past few years several studies have strongly implicated many growth factors in stimulating DNA synthesis in cultured rat hepatocytes. The growth factors studied are epidermal growth factor (EGF) [24,97], transforming growth factor–α (TGF–α) [24,126], acidic fibroblast growth factor or heparin-binding growth factor 1 (aFGF or HBGF-I) [96], basic fibroblast growth factor (bFGF) or HBGF-II [97,130] and hepatocyte growth factor (HGF) or hepatopoietin A [4,88,113,130].

The latter is a potent mitogen for cultured rat and human hepatocytes [66,149,198]. It increases in the circulation after partial hepatectomy [128,148] but its site of synthesis and release are not yet precisely known. On the contrary, transforming growth factor–β (TGF–β) inhibits DNA synthesis both *in vivo* and *in vitro* and may act as a negative signal factor in the liver [26,125,150,179,197].

Much remains to be learnt in this field, especially concerning the expression of liver-specific functions. An interesting point is that cell density of cultured hepatocytes [88] and the presence of hormones, including insulin, glucagon, norepinephrine and vasopressin [27,41,124,178] seem to play a crucial role in the regulation process. Other factors can modulate the response of hepatocytes to growth stimuli *in vitro* such as medium factors (lactate, pyruvate, proline), the extracellular matrix [58,183], the presence of nicotinamide [89], the intralobular origin of the cells [65], the Ca^{2+} concentration [56] and other, still unknown, conditions.

Studies on the ability of hormones and growth factors to stimulate DNA

synthesis in human hepatocytes are scarce.
Ismail et al.[91] have studied the effects of EGF and TGF-α in human hepatocytes in primary culture. They found that both factors stimulate DNA synthesis at low nanomolar concentrations and that the latter was slightly more potent. TGF-β inhibited DNA synthesis at low picomolar levels and arginine-vasopressin has no effect[91].
Blanc et al.[24] confirmed the results for EGF and TGF-α and also described an important effect of human serum derived from patients with fulminant hepatitis which contains HGF.

Application of human hepatocyte cultures in pharmaco-toxicological research and testing

Since human pharmaco-toxicology is concerned with the biotransformation of xenobiotics, their eventual side effects and mode of action in man, the ideal model for investigating xenobiotic metabolism, eventual toxicity and interactions is obviously man himself. *In vivo* studies in man are limited because of ethical reasons. The development of *in vitro* methods, using organs, tissues and cells, derived from man, represents a promising alternative omitting extrapolation of data from animal to man but not from *in vitro* to *in vivo*.
Biotransformation of xenobiotics is often performed in the liver and in some cases may cause hepatic injury. Consequently, a culture system using human hepatocytes and capable of maintaining its *in vivo* xenobiotic biotransformation capacity represents the ideal model for investigating xenobiotic metabolism, liver toxicity, drug interactions and the effects of foreign compounds on cellular metabolism in man. Major advantages of this model are that the interrelationships between various types of hepatic xenobiotic biotransformations can be studied in man under well defined conditions which exclude the influence of exogenous factors and allow investigations of specific treatments. Useful information can be obtained on drug metabolic profiles, on the rate of metabolism and the metabolic fate of new drug candidates in man and if necessary in other species. Potential drug interactions may be studied. Furthermore, kinetics of drugs can be followed and small differences in metabolism of drug enantiomers can be investigated. As discussed in the previous section, maintenance *in vitro* of hepatocellular differentiation is critically dependent on exogenous soluble factors, extracellular matrix components, cell-cell interactions and factors

affecting replication of hepatocytes. Consequently, when human hepatocyte cultures are used in pharmaco-toxicological research and testing one must consider carefully the choice of the experimental conditions.

Xenobiotic biotransformation

Expression of specific genes. Cultivation of human hepatocytes is associated with a better maintenance of biotransformation capacity than is the case for rodent hepatocyte cultures.
The total cytochrome P450 concentration is better kept [23,78] but still decreases as a function of culture time. Conditions that favour long-term production of plasma proteins (extracellular matrix, cell-cell interactions) also improve the maintenance of the cytochrome P450 level and of drug-metabolizing enzymes [81]. This is particularly true for cocultures of human hepatocytes with rat epithelial cells in comparison with pure cultures [11,12,78,169].
The expression in human hepatocyte cultures of several cytochrome P450 isoenzymes has been studied by immunohistochemical techniques [168] and by Northern and Western blot analyses [141]. It was shown that human hepatocyte cultures retain the ability to induce cytochrome P450 gene expression. Indeed, cytochrome P450IIIA, IIC8,9,10, IIE1 and IA2 are expressed and remain capable of responding to some inducers [141].
It was found that cytochrome P450IIIA is induced by rifampicin but not by phenobarbital; cytochrome P450IA by 3-methylcholanthrene but not by phenobarbital or rifampicin; cytochrome P450IIC8,9,10 by phenobarbital and rifampicin but not by 3-methylcholanthrene and cytochrome P450IIE1 not by the 3 compounds tested [141]. The inducibility of these cytochrome P450 subfamilies in human hepatocyte cultures has also been studied quite intensively by other research teams [12,42,45,123,162]. They demonstrated that cytochrome P450IA1 and IA2 do not only respond to 3-methylcholanthrene but also to β–naphtoflavone and omeprazone. The cytochrome P450IIIA subfamily were found to be inducible by both rifampicin and phenobarbital. The same is true for dexamethasone, troleandomycin and several other compounds [42,45,162]. Maurice et al. [123] recently pointed to the inducing effects of clotrimazole for the cytochrome P450IIIA subfamily and the strong inhibitory effects of ketoconazole and miconazole.
The research mentioned above provides good evidence that human

hepatocyte cultures that maintain the ability to regulate cytochrome P450 expression could yield important information for clinicians [102]: new potent inhibitors and inducers can be identified, safe alternatives to drugs that interact with some cytochrome P450 dependent enzymes may be identified and potential explanations may be found for some well-known drug interactions.

Recently, Pichard et al [161] studied the effect of corticoids on the expression of different cytochrome P450 subfamilies in human hepatocytes cultured on collagen with a serum-free medium. They found that corticoids had no effect on cytochromes P450IA2, IID6 and IIE1 but dexamethasone and prednisone induced the cytochrome P450IIIA subfamily. On the contrary, prednisolone and methyl-prednisolone had no effect [161].

In a number of studies the expression of phase I enzymes, especially of cytochrome P450 dependent ones, and their inducibility by common inducers were not investigated using molecular biology techniques as is the case in the articles just mentioned but simply by measuring activities of enzymes more or less specific to certain cytochrome P450 isoenzymes. Generally speaking, high activities were present at the start of human hepatocyte cultures, but they gradually declined as a function of culture time, although the decline was less than that usually observed in rat hepatocyte cultures.

Grant et al. [70] studied the cytochrome P450 dependent mixed function oxidase by O-dealkylation of ethoxyresorufin (EROD), pentoxyresorufin (PROD) and benzyloxyresorufin (BROD), which are probes for different isoenzymes of cytochrome P450. Noteworthy is that the enzymatic activities of EROD and PROD were increased selectively by phenobarbital addition to the culture medium whereas BROD was not affected. Donato et al. [49] followed coumarin O-deethylase and aryl hydrocarbon hydroxylase activities and also observed that different inducers had different and selective effects on these monooxygenase activities.

The same observation was made by Maurice et al. [123] who examined 10 different forms of cytochromes P450 from families 1 to 4. [EROD (IA1), phenacetin O-deethylase (IA2), coumarin 7 α–hydroxylase (IIA6), benzphetamine demethylase (IIB), lauric acid 12-hydroxylase (IIC), aminopyrine demethylase (IA2-IIC), mephenytoin 4-hydroxylase (IIC8-10), mephenytoin N-demethylase (IIC8-10), debrisoquin 4-hydroxylase (IID6), aniline hydroxylase (IIE1), erythromycin demethylase (IIIA4), cyclosporin oxidase (IIIA4) and lauric acid 11-hydroxylase (IVA)]. They measured the monooxygenase activities of the enzymes just listed, with and without addition of derivatives of the imidazole family, known to be inducers of several cytochrome P450 forms in the rat [83].

For other phase I enzymes such as aldehyde dehydrogenase similar observations were made [117,118].

Until now, less attention has been paid to phase II enzymes in human hepatocyte cultures and discrepancies exist among the data published. Glutathione S-transferase (GST) activity was reported by Grant et al. [70] and Donato et al. [49] to be stable for 3 days or longer, respectively. Iqbal et al. [90] reported that the GST activity was only stable during the initial culture period but decreases afterwards. Vandenberghe et al. [211], however, measured dramatic decreases immediately. Different GST isoenzymes were expressed and the inducibility of the α class (GST A1 and A2), not of the μ class (GST M1-1), by phenobarbital, 3-methylcholanthrene and dithiolethiones, was demonstrated, using mRNA analyses. GST P1-1 (π class) was undetectable in human hepatocytes [142].

Variable results have also been found for other phase II enzymes such as UDP-glucuronyltransferase which was reported to be stable [49] or to increase [70]. Epoxide hydrolase and sulfotransferase activities, were found to decrease in human hepatocyte cultures [70].

Metabolite patterns. Another way to demonstrate the preservation of functional drug metabolising enzymes in cultured human hepatocytes is to identify the metabolites formed from various drugs and to compare these with the *in vivo* situation. A large variety of drugs, having different therapeutic actions and exhibiting *in vivo* either a simple either a complex metabolism, have been added to human hepatocyte cultures. The major metabolites or even the complete metabolite pattern has been determined.

Doxorubicin and epirubicin, both anthracycline glucoside antibiotics, were shown to be metabolized differently [7]. Glucuronidation was the major pathway of epirubicin whereas this was not the case for doxorubicin. These results were confirmed and extended by others [106]. Glucuronidation was also identified as being the only biotransformation pathway of the antiretroviral drug zidovudine [165] and was also of great importance for the cardiac drugs digoxigenin-monodigitoxoside and digoxigenin [100].

A complex metabolic profile comparable with *in vivo* data was observed for caffeine, a central nervous stimulatory drug [18]. The biotransformation rate was close to that calculated from *in vivo* data. Often the biotransformation pattern of drugs is found to compare qualitatively with the *in vivo* results but not quantitatively.

The extent of changes observed can be dependent on the drug concentration used and on the duration of the exposure time [137]. Interesting conclusions can be reached by comparison of the biotransformation patterns of the same drug by hepatocyte cultures of different species, including man. Indeed, this type of experiment shows clearly the animal species most closely related to humans in terms of drug biotransformation.

For mitoxantrone, a new anticancer drug, rabbit was shown to be the best animal species in the context just mentioned [172]. Diltiazem, a calcium channel blocker, is metabolized both by human and rabbit hepatocyte cultures through the action of the cytochrome P450IIIA subfamily [163]. For flunarizine, a selective calcium entry blocker, the biotransformation pattern in human hepatocyte cultures resembled the one observed for female rats and dogs but not that of male rat hepatocyte cultures [101]. Other examples can be given such as SC-42867 and SC-51089, both PGE_2 antagonists. SC-42867 is metabolized in human and rat hepatocytes in a comparable way, whereas this is not the case for SC-51089 [109]. Important species differences in biotransformation, (including man), have also been shown for drugs such as diazepam [31], temelastine [155], paracetamol [201], ketotifen [12], the family of doxorubicin, daunorubicin, epirubicin, esorubicin and idarubicin [106], minaprine [99], and for potential carcinogenic chemicals such as benzo(a)pyrene [138,140]. The species differences observed in hepatocyte cultures in terms of biotransformation often are a good reflection of the *in vivo* situation. This is particularly the case for caffeine [18], temelastine [155], ketotifen [12,105], pindolol and fluperlapine [79], diazepam [31] and paracetamol [201].

Finally, it must also be mentioned that a general observation made for human hepatocyte cultures is that a large individual variability on metabolism rate, induction and biotransformation pattern exists [23,73,103,142,211], however, this is not the case for all drugs examined [172]. The qualitative and quantitative differences between the cultures of different donors probably reflect individual *in vivo* differences due to genetic or environmental factors, age, coadministration of drugs and even liver disease.

Cytotoxicity of xenobiotics

Cytotoxicity end points. As is the case for cytotoxicity tests in rat hepatocytes [17] the cytotoxicity end points in human hepatocyte cultures can be divided into two distinct classes, namely liver-non-specific and liver-specific ones.

Non-specific markers include membrane integrity (trypan blue exclusion), cytosolic enzyme leakage into the medium (lactate dehydrogenase release), morphological alterations, changes in protein synthesis, glutathione content and lipid peroxidation, and covalent binding to macromolecules.

Liver-specific functions are assessed by electron microscopy, albumin and acute-phase protein production, gluconeogenesis, glycogen synthesis, ureogenesis, ATP/ADP ratio, specific cytochrome P-450 isoenzymatic activities and changes in peroxisomal β–oxidation.

The former group of parameters was used in early studies with human hepatocytes [39,73,167] whereas the latter ones have been applied more recently [22,95,103]. The evaluation of several liver-specific functions appears to be a more appropriate assay of changes in cellular integrity than the use of a single parameter [103].

Identification of cytotoxic compounds, hepatoprotectants and mechanisms of hepatotoxicity. Human hepatocyte cultures can be used to detect acute and chronic toxicity. The first attempt to study both was presented by Ratanasavanh et al. [167] using amitriptyline treatment. They were able to show cytotoxic effects 24 hours after a single dose to pure cultures and they observed time- and dose-dependent effects in cocultures kept for a longer time. Cocultured cells more closely reflect the *in vivo* situation in which drugs induce liver damage after repeated administration lasting weeks or months. Generally speaking the test compounds can be added daily for 1-3 weeks at concentrations equal to or lower than the maximum non-toxic dose defined after a 24 hrs incubation of these compounds in pure cultured human hepatocytes [167]. The determination of the cytotoxic effect of drugs in hepatocyte cultures of different species, including man, provides valuable information on existing differences in biotransformation between species and on the potential protective effect of certain molecules. Indeed, Bégué et al. [10] demonstrated that human and rat hepatocytes in culture responded, in terms of cytotoxicity, differently when exposed to aflatoxin B_1. The formation of higher amounts of a toxic epoxide metabolite in rat

hepatocytes than in human ones was the basis of this observation.
In addition, the hepatoprotective effect of (+)-cyanidanol-3, seen in rat hepatocyte cultures, was not present in human cell cultures. The same was true for malotilate, which was reported to protect rats intoxicated with CCl_4. However, this compound had no effect on either rat or human hepatocytes even after repeated treatment in vitro [35]. On the contrary, a clear hepatoprotective effect was measured for ursodeoxycholate in human hepatocyte cultures exposed to bile salts [63].
Other examples are the exposure of paracetamol and cyclophosphamide to rat and human hepatocyte cultures [103]. Both were cytotoxic in the species examined, although human cells were more sensitive to paracetamol than their rat counterparts. The same observation was made for erythromycin base [78]. Similar results were also found in vivo.
The results just mentioned are derived from research projects. It is clear that commercial screening of cytotoxic compounds and calculation of the appropriate dose-response curves and IC_{50} values could be of particular importance in the development of new therapeutic agents. Today, in modern pharmaceutical industry, screening tests to detect potential cytotoxic compounds are carried out in rat or non-human hepatocytes at an early stage of drug development. It is certainly not a common practice to perform screenings using human hepatocytes although essential information of directly practical use could be obtained. Ethical, safety, technical and logistical reasons, however, have impeded their use.
As mentioned above for the exposure to aflatoxin B_1 [10] valuable information concerning the mechanism of the hepatotoxicity can be gained out of exposure of human hepatocyte cultures to drugs. A typical example is the direct potentiation of the hepatotoxic effect of heroin and methadon by ethanol [95]. Ethanol was found to be an inducer of the cytochrome P450IIE subfamily, which was shown to be involved in the biotransformation of both opioids. Another example consists in the elucidation of the mechanism of the hepatotoxic effect of acetaminophen in human hepatocyte cultures [19]. A highly selective covalent binding occurred with proteins forming adducts which were found to be nearly similar to those observed in mouse.
Doxorubicin, daunorubicin, epirubicin, esorubicin and idarubicin have been added to rat and human hepatocyte cultures [106]. Not only differences were found in the percentages of metabolites formed and routes of biotransformation between both species but it also appeared that human cells were 2-fold less sensitive than rat hepatocytes to all

anthracyclines because of a 2-fold higher metabolisation in human cells. A close correlation between the hepatotoxic effect and biotransformation was also found for paracetamol [201]. Man seemed to be relatively resistant to the hepatotoxic effects of paracetamol in comparison with hamster and mouse due to the lower rate of conversion to the toxic metabolite N-acetyl-p-benzoquinoneimine in man. This observation was done in hepatocyte cultures as well as *in vivo* [201].

Identification of genotoxic compounds in man. Genotoxicity testing is a complex and large field which has been clearly reviewed by Garner [64]. Here, only a very small part concerned with the use of human hepatocytes has been focused on.

Hepatocyte cultures of rats are being used, already for some years, to help to assess the genotoxic potential of chemicals and drugs [29]. They are well suited for quantification of DNA fragmentation (usually measured by alkaline elution) and DNA repair (measured as unscheduled DNA synthesis detected by autoradiography) after exposure to genotoxic compounds.

In general, these assays are being considered valid models for predicting potentially genotoxic effects in human beings. Indeed, it has been shown for a wide variety of chemicals including 2-acetylaminofluorene (AAF) [200], aflatoxin B_1, CCl_4, $CHCl_3$, benzo(a)pyrene (BP), and other compounds [29] that results, in terms of DNA damage, close to those measured in human hepatocyte cultures were obtained. Similar dose-dependent inductions of DNA fragmentation and of unscheduled DNA synthesis were found in rat and human hepatocyte cultures after exposure to N-nitrosodimethylamine and methylmethanesulfonate [122] and 1,6-dinitropyrene [28], respectively.

For some molecules, however, differences in the response between rodent and human hepatocytes were noticed. Metronidazole, an antiprotozoan and antibacterial agent, yielded DNA damage in human and rat hepatocyte cultures, related to dose and length of exposure. In both cultures increases in DNA damage were observed by hypoxia and glutathione depletion and decreases by inhibition of cytochrome P450 activity. Human cells, however, were more resistant to the genotoxic activity of the drug than rat hepatocytes, highlighting the importance of species differences [119].

Snyder *et al.* [195] showed activiation of aflatoxin B_1, AAF, and aminofluorene in hepatocytes of man, hamster and rat but not of 1-aminopyrene and 1-nitropyrene in human and rat.

To see if activation of AAF proceeds *via* similar routes of metabolism in rat and human hepatocyte cultures, incubation with deacetylase inhibitors such as paraoxon and bis(p-nitrophenyl) phosphate were carried out [135]. It was found that the rat model gave similar results to one case of human hepatocytes but the effect of the deacetylase inhibitors was different with respect to subsequent alteration in DNA binding, pointing to sophisticated differences between species. In a later study by the same group [134] AAF, BP and 4-aminobiphenyl were examined in hepatocyte cultures of both species. The predominant DNA adducts formed were the same in both species but there were quantitative differences in that more carcinogenic DNA adducts were present in human cells than in those of rats.

Another example, illustrating the importance of species differences, is cimetidine, a drug for the treatment of peptic ulcer. In rat hepatocyte cultures induction of DNA fragmentation and unscheduled DNA synthesis were observed after exposure to cimetidine, whereas this was not the case in human hepatocyte cultures [121]. In other experiments, β–naphtylamine gave a positive result in rat hepatocyte cultures but in none of the human cultures examined, whereas the opposite was seen for 2,6-diaminotoluene and 5-methylchrysene [29].

Ten N-nitrosocompounds were analysed for the DNA damage and unscheduled DNA repair, they elicited when added to rat and human hepatocyte cultures. Again the same conclusion was reached, namely the responses of human cells were qualitatively similar to those of their rat counterparts, but statistically significant differences between both species were observed [120]. However, since the quantitative differences in the genotoxic effects between the cultures of both species were greater than average interspecies differences it was concluded that the rat DNA repair assay still remained a valid model.

Because of the various species differences just mentioned, it has been suggested that for some compounds the rat model might be an inappropiate predictor for the human situation [121] and whenever information on human carcinogenic hazards must be obtained, human hepatocyte cultures would provide more useful information [134].

In order to obtain results as close as possible to the *in vivo* situation, it is essential that human hepatocyte cultures maintain their *in vivo* biotransformation capacity, which is, as already discussed, sometimes a problem when long-term cultures are involved. Since genotoxic assays, however, only require a limited exposure time, short-term cultures can be used which usually do not pose the problem of dedifferentiation. Phase I and II biotransformation pathways must remain intact. As shown by Monteith et al. [137,138] BP and AAF were found to undergo not only oxidative biotransformation in primary cultures of human hepatocytes but also to be conjugated with the formation of glucuronides and sulphates [136]. This was an important observation since the possible genotoxic effect of conjugates formed (e.g. N-sulphate conjugate of AAF) is taken into account in this model.

Finally, it must be emphasized that, as is the case for the biotransformation of xenobiotics, significant interindividual variation exists with regard to genotoxic compounds complicating general conclusions when human hepatocyte cultures are being used.

Conclusion

This review presents evidence demonstrating that the use of human hepatocytes in primary monolayer culture represents a suitable alternative and/or complementary tool in pharmaco-toxicological research and testing. Human hepatocyte cultures provide the unique possibility for gaining valuable information, directly in human cells, concerning biotransformation, hepatotoxicity, cytotoxicity, genotoxicity, drug interactions and mechanism of drug action. Major problems, however, still exist because of the limited availability of human liver tissue. This problem is likely to become even more serious due to the increasing use of livers for transplantation and the growing fear of viral infections. Furthermore, important interindividual variation exists making it sometimes difficult to draw general conclusions. The use of cryopreserved human hepatocytes may solve, at least partly, this problem. Although, it is known that only a part of the thawed cells attach and survive [32,51,114,174] the attached cells retain their functional capacities [32,43,51]. Important improvements, such as culture on plastic precoated with human liver extracellular matrix have been reported [145] and probably even better results may be obtained when all the new developments mentioned above (soluble factors, extracellular matrix, cell-cell interactions and growth factors) will be taken into account. Cryopreserved and thawed human hepatocytes can thus be of great value in screening tests in the selection of compounds early during their development, in defining priorities and in identifying molecules with special properties so that *in vivo* experimentation can be optimized: in particular, human hepatocytes may be very helpful in the proper choice of the species to be studied *in vivo*. Consequently, serious efforts should now be made to ensure that human cells, such as hepatocytes, are made available under strictly controlled and ethical conditions for pharmaco-toxicological research reasons. For human transplantation reasons, cell, tissue and organ banks already function properly within the European Community (EC) but for experimental purposes no European and national legislation, no official institute, and no generally accepted ethical rules exist. It must be mentioned here that in the USA some organisations and firms already exist that deliver worldwide human derived cells, tissues and organs. One can easily imagine the following potentially ambiguous situation in which human cells obtained outside Europe are being used during the development of a new drug which will then be commercialised within the EC. Measures should be taken immediately to prevent such situations arising. In addition, different ethical attitudes exist in the various European countries making the establishment of a European tissue bank for experimental purposes a difficult task. It is therefore absolutely necessary that the EC address this problem and develop a set of standard guidelines which will be adhered to by all participating countries. It is also essential that the clinical world, medical staff, patients and their relatives, the academic and industrial worlds and the general public be made aware of these developments.

References

1. Akimoto T., Ikeda Y. and Irumi R. Fundamental studies on biological artificial liver support: liver functions of entrapped hepatocytes. Japanese Journal of Artificial Organs 1985;14:249-252.
2. Akrawi M., Rogiers V., Vandenberghe Y., Palmer C.N.A., Vercruysse A., Shephard E.A. and Phillips I.R. Maintenance and induction in co-cultured rat hepatocytes of components of the cytochrome P-450 mediated monooxygenase. Biochemical Pharmacology 1993;45:1583-1591.
3. Akrawi M., Shephard E.A., Phillips I.R., Vercruysse A. and Rogiers V. Effects of phenobarbital and valproate on the expression of cytochrome P-450 in co-cultured rat hepatocytes. Toxicology in Vitro 1993 (in press).
4. Asami O., Ihara I., Shimizu N., Shimizu S., Tomita Y., Ichihara A. and Nakamura T. Purification and characterization of hepatocyte growth factor from injured liver of carbon tetrachloride-treated rats. Journal of Biochemistry 1991;109:8-13.

5. Bader A., Borel M., Rinkes I.H., Closs E.I., Ryan M., Toner M., Cunningham J.M., Tompkins R.G. and Yarmush M.L. A stable long-term hepatocyte culture system for studies of physiologic processes: cytokine stimulation of the acute phase response in rat- and human hepatocytes. Biotechnology Progress 1992;8:219-225.
6. Ballet F., Bouma M.E., Wang S.R., Amit N., Marais J. and Infante R. Isolation, culture and characterization of adult human hepatocytes from surgical liver biopsies. Hepatology 1984;4:849-854.
7. Ballet F., Robert J., Bouma M.E., Vrignaud P. and Infante R. Metabolism of doxorubicin and epirubicin in adult human hepatocytes in culture. Pharmaceutical Research Communications 1986;18:343-347.
8. Bars R.G., Mitchell A.M., Wolf C.R. and Elcombe C.R. Induction of cytochrome P450 in cultured rat hepatocytes. Biochemical Journal 1989;262:151-158.
9. Bauer J., Lengyel G., Thung S.N., Jonas U., Gerok W. and Acs G. Human fetal hepatocytes respond to inflammatory mediators and excrete bile. Hepatology 1991;13:1131-1141.
10. Bégué J.M., Baffet G., Campion J.P. and Guillouzo A. Differential response of primary cultures of human and rat hepatocytes to aflatoxin B_1-induced cytotoxicity and protection by the hepatoprotective agent (+)-cyanidanol-3. Biology of the Cell 1988;63:327-333.
11. Bégué J., Guguen-Guillouzo C., Pasdeloup N. and Guillouzo A. Prolonged maintenance of active cytochrome P-450 in adult rat hepatocytes co-cultured with another liver cell type. Hepatology 1984;4:839-842.
12. Bégué J.M., Le Bigot J.F., Guguen-Guillouzo C., Kiechel J.R. and Guillouzo A. Cultured human adult hepatocytes: a new model for drug metabolism studies. Biochemical Pharmacology 1983;32:1643-1646.
13. Belleman P., Gebhardt R. and Mecke D. An improved method for the isolation of hepatocytes from liver slices. Analytical Biochemistry 1977;81:408-415.
14. Belzer F.O. and Southard J.H. Principles of solid-organ preservation by cold storage. Transplantation 1988;45:673-676.
15. Ben-Ze'ev A., Robinsen G.S., Bucher M.L.R. and Farmer S.R. Cell-cell and cell-matrix interaction differentially regulate the expression of hepatic and cytoskeletal genes in primary cultures of rat hepatocytes. Proceedings of the National Academy of Sciences of the USA 1988;85:2161-2165.
16. Berry M.N. and Friend D.S. High yield preparation of isolated rat liver parenchymal cells. Journal of Cell Biology 1969;43:506-520.
17. Berry M.N., Halls H.J. and Grivell M.B. Techniques for pharmacological and toxicological studies with isolated hepatocyte suspensions. Life Sciences 1992;51:1-16.
18. Berthou F., Ratanasavanh D., Riche C., Picart D., Voirin T. and Guillouzo A. Comparison of caffeine metabolism by slices, microsomes and hepatocyte cultures from adult human livers. Xenobiotica 1989;19:401-417.

19. Birge R.B., Bartolone J.B., Hart S.G.E., Nishanian E.V., Tyson C.A., Khairallah E.A. and Cohen S.D. Acetaminophen hepatotoxicity: correspondence of selective protein arylation in human and mouse liver *in vitro*, in culture and *in vivo*. Toxicology and Applied Pharmacology 1990;105:472-482.
20. Bissell D.M., Arenson D.M., Maher J.J. and Roll F.J. Support of cultured hepatocytes by laminin-rich gel. Journal of Clinical Investigation 1987;79:801-812.
21. Bissell D.M., Caron J.M., Babiss L.E. and Friedman J.M. Transcriptional regulation of the albumin gene in cultured rat hepatocytes. Role of basement membrane matrix. Molecular Biology and Medicine 1989;10:636.
22. Blaauboer B.J., van Holsteijn C.W.M., Bleumink R., Mennes W.C., van Pelt F.N.A.M., Yap S.H., van Pelt J.F., Van Iersel A.A.J., Timmerman A. and Schmid B.P. The effect of beclobric acid and clofibric acid on peroxisomal β-oxidation and peroxisome proliferation in primary cultures of rat, monkey and human hepatocytes. Biochemical Pharmacology 1990;40:521-528.
23. Blaauboer B.J., van Holsteyn I., van Graft M. and Paine A.J. The concentration of cytochrome P-450 in human hepatocyte culture. Biochemical Pharmacology 1985;34:2405-2408.
24. Blanc P., Etienne H., Daujat M., Fabre I., Zindy F., Domergue J., Astre C., Saint Aubert B., Michel H. and Maurel P. Mitotic responsiveness of cultured adult human hepatocytes to epidermal growth factor, transforming growth factor and human serum. Gastroenterology 1992;102:1340-1350.
25. Bojar H., Basler M., Fuchs F., Dreyfurst R. and Staib W. Preparation of parenchymal and non-parencymal cells from adult human liver. Morphological and biochemical characteristics. Journal of Clinical Chemistry and Clinical Biochemistry 1976;14:527-532.
26. Braun L, Mead J.E., Panzica M., Mikumo R., Bell G.I. and Fausto N. Transforming growth factor β mRNA increases during liver regeneration: a possible paracrine mechanism of growth regulation. Proceedings of the National Academy of Sciences of the USA 1988;85:1539-1543.
27. Bucher N.L.R. and Swaffield M.N. Regulation of hepatic regeneration in rats by synergistic action of insulin and glucagon. Proceedings of the National Academy of Sciences of the USA 1975;72:1157-1160.
28. Butterworth B.E., Earle L.L., Strom S., Jirtle R. and Michalopoulos G. Induction of DNA repair in human and rat hepatocytes by 1,6-dinitropyrene. Mutation Research 1983;122:73-80.
29. Butterworth B.E., Smith-Oliver T., Earle L., Lowry D.J., White R.D., Doolittle D.J., Working P.K., Cattley R.C., Jirtle R., Michalopoulos G. and Strom S. Use of primary cultures of human hepatocytes in toxicology studies. Cancer Research 1989;49:1075-1084.
30. Caron J.M. Induction of albumin gene transcription in hepatocytes by extracellular matrix protein. Molecular and Cellular Biology 1990;3:1239-1243.
31. Chenery R.J., Ayrton A., Oldham H.G., Standring P., Norman S.J., Seddon T. and Kirby R. Diazepam metabolism in cultured hepatocytes from rat, rabbit, dog, guinea pig and man. Drug Metabolism and Disposition 1987;15:312-317.

32. Chesné C., Guyomard C., Grislain L., Clerc C., Fautrel A. and Guillouzo A. Use of cryopreserved animal and human hepatocytes for cytotoxicity studies. Toxicology in Vitro 1991;5:479-482.
33. Christiansen B.S., Ingerslev J., Heickendorff L., and Petersen C.M. Human hepatocytes in culture synthesize and secrete fibronectin. Scandivavian Journal of Clinical and Laboratory Investigations 1988;48:685-690
34. Clayton D.F. and Darnell J.E. Changes in liver-specific compared to common gene transcription during primary culture of mouse hepatocytes. Molecular Cellular Biology 1983;3:1552-1561.
35. Clément B., Dumont J.M., Ratanasavanh D., Latinier M.F., Brissot P. and Guillouzo A. Effects of malotilate on human and rat hepatocytes in short-term and long-term primary culture. In: Liver Cells and Drugs (Guillouzo A., ed.) Les Editions INSERM and John Libbey Eurotext, Paris, 1988:417-421.
36. Clément B., Guguen-Guillouzo C., Campion J.P., Glaise D., Bourel M. and Guillouzo A. Long-term co-cultures of adult human hepatocytes with rat liver epithelial cells: modulation of active albumin secretion and accumulation of extracellular material. Hepatology 1984;4:373-380.
37. Clément B., Guguen-Guillouzo C., Grimaud J.A., Rissel M. and Guillouzo A. Effect of hydrocortisone on deposition of types I and IV collagen in cultured rat hepatocytes. Cellular and Molecular Biology 1988;34:449-460.
38. Clément B., Resean P.Y., Baffet G., Loréal O., Lehry D., Campion J.P. and Guillouzo A. Hepatocytes may produce laminin in fibrotic liver and primary culture. Hepatology 1988;8:794-803.
39. Cole K.E., Hsu I.C. and Trump B.F. Comparative ultrastructural effects of aflatoxin B_1 on mouse, rat and human hepatocytes in primary culture. Cancer Research 1986;46:1290-1296.
40. Corlu A., Kneip B., Lhadi C., Leray G., Glaise D., Baffet G., Bourel D. and Guguen-Guillouzo C. A plasma membrane protein involved in cell contact-mediated regulation of tissue specific genes in adult hepatocytes. Journal of Cell Biology 1991;115:505-515.
41. Cruise J.L., Houck K.A. and Michalopoulos G. Induction of DNA synthesis in cultured rat hepatocytes through stimulation of $\alpha-1$ adrenoreceptor by norepinephrine. Science 1985;227:749-751.
42. Daujat M., Pichard L., Fabre I., Pineau T., Fabre G., Bonfils C. and Maurel P. Induction protocols for cytochromes P450IIIA *in vivo* and in primary cultures of animal and human hepatocytes. Methods in Enzymology 1991;206:345-353.
43. de Sousa G., Dou M., Barbe D., Lacarelle B., Placidi M. and Rahmani R. Freshly isolated or cryopreserved human hepatocytes in primary culture: influence of drug metabolism on hepatotoxicity. Toxicology in Vitro 1991;5:483-486.
44. Demoise C.F., Galambos J.T. and Falek A. Tissue culture of adult human liver. Gastroenterology 1971;60:390-399.
45. Diaz D., Fabre I., Daujat M., Saint Laurent B., Bories P., Michel H. and Maurel P. Omeprazole is an aryl hydrocarbon-like inducer of human hepatic cytochrome P450. Gastroenterology 1990;99:737-747.

46. Dich J., Vind C. and Grumet N. Long-term cultures of hepatocytes: effects of hormones on enzyme activities and metabolic capacity. Hepatology 1988;8:39-45.
47. Dixit V., Darvasi R. and Arthur M. Restoration of liver function in Gunn rats without immunosuppression using transplanted micro-encapsulated hepatocytes. Hepatology 1990;12:1342-1349.
48. Donato M.T., Castell J.V. and Gomez-Lechon M.J. Co-cultures of hepatocytes with epithelial-like cell-lines: expression of drug-biotransformation activities by hepatocytes. Cell Biology and Toxicology 1991;7:1-14.
49. Donato M.T., Castell J.V. and Gomez-Lechon M.J. Prolonged expression of biotransformation activities of rat hepatocytes co-cultured with established cell-lines. Toxicology in Vitro 1990;4:461-466.
50. Donato M.T., Gomez-Lechon M.J. and Castell J.V. Co-cultures of hepatocytes: a biological model for long-lasting cultures. In: *In vitro* alternatives to animal pharmaco-toxicology (Castell J.V. and Gomez-Lechon M.J., eds.) Farmaindustria, Serie Cientifica, Madrid, Spain, 1992:110-127.
51. Dou M., de Sousa G., Lacarelle B., Placidi M., Lechene de la Porte P., Domingo M., Lafont H. and Rahmani R. Thawed human hepatocytes in primary culture. Cryobiology 1992;29:454-469.
52. Dreikorn K., Horsch R. and Rohl L. Forty-eight-to ninety-six hour preservation of canine kidneys by initial perfusion and hypothermic storage using Euro-Collins solution. European Urology 1980;6:221-225.
53. Dunn J.C.Y., Tompkins R.G. and Yarmush M.L. Hepatocytes in collagen sandwich: evidence for transcriptional and translational regulation. Journal of Cell Biology 1992;116:1043-1053.
54. Dunn J.C.Y., Tompkins R.G. and Yarmush M.L. Long-term *in vitro* function of adult hepatocytes in a collagen sandwich configuration. Biotechnology Progress 1991;7:237-245.
55. Dunn J.C.Y., Yarmush M.L., Koebe H.G. and Tompkins R.G. Hepatocyte function and extracellular matrix geometry: long-term culture in a sandwich configuration. FASEB Journal 1989;3:174-177.
56. Eckl P.M., Whitcomb W.R., Michalopoulos G.K. and Jirtle R.L. Effects of EGF and calcium on adult parenchymal hepatocyte proliferation. Journal of Cellular Physiology 1987;132:363-366.
57. Edwards A.M., Glistake M.L., Lucas C.M. and Wilson P.A. 7-ethoxycoumarin deethylase activity as a convenient measure of liver drug metabiolizing enzymes. Biochemical Pharmacology 1984;33:1537-1546.
58. Enat R., Jefferson D.M., Ruiz-Opazo N., Gatmaitan Z., Leinwand L.A. and Reid L.M. Hepatocyte proliferation *in vitro*; its dependence on the use of serum-free hormonally defined medium and substrata of extracellular matrix. Proceedings of the National Academy of Sciences of the USA 1984;81:1411-1415.
59. Engelmann G.L., Richardson A.G. and Fierer J.A. Maintenance and induction of cytochrome P-450 in cultured rat hepatocytes. Archives of Biochemistry and Biophysics 1985;238:359-367.

60. Fabre G., Rahmani R., Placidi M., Combalbert J., Coco J., Cano J.P., Coulange C., Ducros M. and Rampal M. Characterization of midazolam metabolism using human hepatic microsomal fractions and hepatocytes in suspension obtained by perfusing whole human livers. Biochemical Pharmacology 1988;37:4389-4397.
61. Fraslin J.M., Kneip B., Vaulont S., Glaise D., Munnich A. and Guguen-Guillouzo C. Dependence of hepatocyte specific gene expression on cell-cell interactions in primary culture. EMBO Journal 1985;4:2487-2491.
62. Fujita M., Spray D.C., Choi H., Saez J.C., Watanabe T., Rosenberg L.C., Hertzberg E.L. and Reid L.M. Glycosaminoglycans and proteoglycans induce gap junction expression and restore transcription of tissue specific mRNA's in primary liver cultures. Hepatology 1987;7:1s-9s.
63. Galle P.R., Theilmann L., Raedsch R., Otto G. and Stiehl A. Ursodeoxycholate reduces hepatotoxicity of bile salts in primary human hepatocytes. Hepatology 1990;12:486-491.
64. Garner R.C. Genotoxicity testing. In: Animals and Alternatives in Toxicology. Present status and future prospects. (Balls M., Bridges J. and Southee J., eds.) Mac Millan Press Scientific & Medical, London, 1991:91-120.
65. Gebhardt R. Different proliferative activity *in vitro* of periportal and perivenous hepatocytes. Scandinavian Journal of Gastroenterology (suppl). 1988;151:8-18.
66. Gohda E., Tsubouchi H., Nakayama H., Hirono S., Sakiyama O., Takahashi K. and Miyazaki H. Purification and partial characterization of hepatocyte growth factor from plasma of a patient with fulminant hepatic failure. Journal of Clinical Investigation 1988;81:414-419.
67. Gomez-Lechon M.J., Fabra R., Lopez P., Donato M.T., Montoya A., Larrauri A., Trullenque R. and Castell J.V. Isolation and culture of human hepatocytes from surgical liver biopsies. In: *In vitro* alternatives to animal pharmaco-toxicology (Castell J.V. and Gomez-Lechon M.J., eds.) Farmaindustria, Serie Cientifica, Madrid, 1992:129-147.
68. Gomez-Lechon M.J., Lopez P., Donato T., Montoya A., Larrauri A., Gimenez P., Trullenque R., Fabra R. and Castell J.V. Culture of human hepatocytes from small surgical liver biopsies. Biochemcial characterization and comparison with *in vivo*. In Vitro Cellular Development Biology 1990;26:67-74.
69. Goulet F., Normand C. and Morin O. Cellular interactions promote tissue-specific function, biomatrix deposition and functional communication of primary cultured hepatocytes. Hepatology 1988;8:1010-1018.
70. Grant M.H., Burke M.D., Hawksworth G., Duthie S.J., Engeset J. and Petrie J.C. Human adult hepatocytes in primary monolayer culture. Biochemical Pharmacology 1987;36:2311-2316.
71. Grant M.H., Melvin M.A.L., Shaw P., Melvin W.T. and Burke M.D. Studies on the maintenance of cytochromes P-450 and b_5, monooxygenases and cytochrome reductases in primary cultures of rat hepatocytes. FEBS Letters 1985;190:99-103.

72. Grislain L., Ratanasavanh D., Mocquard M.T., Raquillet L., Bégué J.M., Du Vignaud P., Genissel P., Guillouzo A. and Bromet N. Primary cultures of rat and human hepatocytes as a model system for the evaluation of cytotoxicity and metabolic pathways of a new drug S-3341. In: Liver Cells and Drugs (Guillouzo A. ed.) Les Editions INSERM, Paris and John Libbey Eurotext, London, 1988:357-363.
73. Guguen-Guillouzo C., Bourel M. and Guillouzo A. Human hepatocyte cultures. In: Progress in Liver Diseases vol III (Popper H. and Schassner F., eds.) Grune & Stratton, New York, 1986:33-50.
74. Guguen-Guillouzo C., Campion J.P., Brissot P., Glaise D., Launois B., Bourel M. and Guillouzo A. High yield preparation of isolated human adult hepatocytes by enzymatic perfusion of the liver. Cell Biology International Reports 1982;6:625-628.
75. Guillouzo A. and Guguen-Guillouzo C. *In vitro* approaches to hepatotoxicity studies. In: *In vitro* Methods in Toxicology (Yolles G. and Cordier A., eds.) Academic Press, London, 1992:133-160.
76. Guillouzo A., Ondea P., Le Guilly Y., Ondea M.C., Lenoir P. and Bourel M. An ultrastructural study of primary cultures of adult human liver tissue. Experimental and Molecular Pathology 1972;16:1-15.
77. Guillouzo A. Use of cultured hepatocytes for xenobiotic metabolism and cytotoxicity studies. In: Isolated and Cultured Hepatocytes (Guillouzo A. and Guguen-Guillouzo C., eds.) Les Editions Inserm, John Libbey-Eurotext, Paris, France, 1986:313-332.
78. Guillouzo A., Beaune P., Gascoin M.N., Bégué J.M., Campion J.P., Guengerich F.P. and Guguen-Guillouzo C. Maintenance of cytochrome P-450 in cultured adult human hepatocytes. Biochemical Pharmacology 1985;34:2991-2995.
79. Guillouzo A., Bégué J.M., Maurer G. and Koch P. Identification of metabolic pathways of pindolol and fluperlapine in adult human hepatocyte cultures. Xenobiotica 1988;18:131-139.
80. Guillouzo A., Grislain L, Ratanasavanh D., Mocquard M.T., Bégué J.M., Du Vignaud P., Bromet N., Genissel P. and Beau B. Use of hepatocyte cultures for preliminary metabolism and cytotoxicity studies of a new anti-hypertensive agent, oxaminozoline. Xenobiotica 1988;18:757-763.
81. Guillouzo A., Morel F., Ratanasavanh D., Chesné C. and Guguen-Guillouzo C. Long-term culture of functional hepatocytes. Toxicology in Vitro 1990;4:415-427.
82. Guzelian P.S., Li D., Schuetz E.G., Thomas P., Levin W., Mode A. and Gustafsson J.A. Sex change in cytochrome P-450 phenotype by growth hormone treatment of adult rat hepatocytes maintained in a culture system on matrigel. Proceedings of the National Academy of Sciences of the USA 1988;85:9783-9787.
83. Harmsworth W.L. and Franklin M.R. Induction of hepatic and extrahepatic cytochrome P-450 and monooxygenase activity by N-substituted imidazoles. Xenobiotica 1990;20:1053-1063.
84. Hsu I.C., Lipsky M.M., Cole K.E., Su C.H. and Trump B.F. In Vitro Cellular Developmental Biology 1985;21:154-160.

85. Hu W.S., Nyberg S.L. and Shatford R.A. Cultivation of hepatocytes in a new entrapment reactor: A potential bioartifical liver. In: Animal Cell Culture and Production of Biologicals (Sasaki R. and Ikura K., eds.) Kluwer Academic Publishers, Dordrecht, The Netherlands,1991:75-80.
86. Hümpel M., Sostarek D., Gieschen H. and Labitzky C. Studies on the biotransformation of lonazolac, bromerguride, lisuride and terguride in laboratory animals and their hepatocytes. Xenobiotica 1989;19:361-377.
87. Hunt C.M., Guzelian P.S., Molowa D.T. and Wright S.A. Regulation of rat hepatic cytochrome P450IIE1 in primary monolayer hepatocyte culture. Xenobiotica 1991;40:1621-1631.
88. Ichihara A. Mechanisms controlling growth of hepatocytes in primary culture. Digestive Diseases and Sciences 1991;36:489-493.
89. Inoue C., Yamamoto H., Nakamura T., Ichihara A. and Okamoto H. Nicotinamide prolongs survival of primary cultured hepatocytes without involving loss of hepatocyte-specific functions. Journal of Biological Chemistry 1989;264:4747-4750.
90. Iqbal S., Elcombe C.R. and Elias E. Maintenance of mixed-function oxidase and conjugation enzyme activities in hepatocyte cultures prepared from normal and diseased human liver. Journal Hepatology 1991;12:336-343.
91. Ismail T., Howl J., Wheatly M., Mc Master P., Neuberger J.M. and Strain A.J. Growth of normal human hepatocytes in primary culture: effect of hormones and growth factors on DNA synthesis. Hepatology 1991;14:1076-1082.
92. Jauregui H.O., Gann K.L. and Waxman D.J. Xenobiotic induction of P450 b4 (IIB1) and P450 c (IA1) and associated monooxygenase activities in primary cultures of adult rat hepatocytes. Xenobiotica 1991;21:1091-1106.
93. Jefferson D.M., Clayton D.F., Darnell J.E. and Reid L.M. Post-transcriptional modulation of gene expression in cultured rat hepatocytes. Molecular Cellular Biology 1984;4:1929-1934.
94. Jolles G. and Cordier A. General discussion. In: *In vitro* methods in toxicology. (Jolles G. and Cordier A., ed.) Academic Press, London, 1992:555-584.
95. Jover R., Ponsoda X., Gomez-Lechon M.J. and Castell J.V. Potentiation of heroin and methadone hepatotoxicity by ethanol: an *in vitro* study using cultured human hepatocytes. Xenobiotica 1992;22:471-478.
96. Kan M., Huang J., Mansson P.E., Yasumitsu H., Carr B. and Mc Keehan W.L. Heparin-binding growth factor type 1 (acidic fibroblast growth factor): a potential biphasic autocrine and paracrine regulator of hepatocyte regeneration. Proceedings of the National Academy of Sciences of the USA 1989;86:7432-7436.
97. Koch K.S., Lu X.P., Brenner D.A., Feu G.H., Martinez-Conde A. and Leffert H. Mitogens and hepatocyte growth control *in vivo* and *in vitro*. In Vitro Cellular Developmental Biology 1990;26:1011-1023.
98. Kuri-Harcuch W. and Mendoza-Figueroa T. Cultivation of adult rat hepatocytes on 3T3 cells: expression of various liver differentiated functions. Differentiation 1989;41:148-157.

99. Lacarelle B., Marre F., Durand A., Dair H. and Rahmani R. In vitro metabolism of minaprine in human and four animal species. Xenobiotica 1990;21:317-329.
100. Lacarelle B., Rahmani R., de Sousa G., Durand A., Placidi M. and Cano J.P. Metabolism of digoxin, digoxigenin-digitoxosides and digoxigenin in human hepatocytes and liver microsomes. Fundamental and Clinical Pharmacology 1991;5:567-582.
101. Lavrijzen K., Van Houdt J., Van Dijck D., Hendrickx J., Bockx M., Hurkmans R., Meuldermans W., Le Jeune L., Lauwers W. and Heykants J. Comparative metabolism of flunarizine in rats, dogs and man: an in vitro study with subcellular liver fractions and isolated hepatocytes. Xenobiotica 1992;22:815-836.
102. Lown K.S. and Watkins P.B. Predicting drug interactions using cultured human hepatocytes. Hepatology 1991;14:396-398.
103. Lawrence J.N. and Benford D.J. Toxicity of paracetamol and cyclophosphamide in monolayer cultures of rat and human hepatocytes. Toxicology in Vitro 1990;4:443-448.
104. Lazizi Y., Guillon J.C. and Pillot J. Long term cultivation of functionally active normal human adult hepatocytes. Developments in Biological Standardization 1983;54:75-79.
105. Le Bigot J.F., Bégué J.M., Kiechel J.R. and Guillouzo A. Species differences in the metabolism of ketotifen in rat, rabbit and man: demonstration of similar pathways in vivo and in cultured hepatocytes. Life Sciences 1987;40:883-889.
106. Le Bot M.A., Bégué J.M., Kernaleguen D., Robert J., Ratanasavanh D., Airian J., Riché C. and Guillouzo A. Different cytotoxicity and metabolism of doxorubicin, daunorubicin, epirubicin, esorubicin and idarubicin in cultured human and rat hepatocytes. Biochemical Pharmacology 1988;37:3877-3887.
107. Le Guilly Y., Lenoir P., Bourel M., Poupan R. and Guillouzo A. La culture prolongée du tissu hépatique humain adult. Pathologie Biologie 1970;18:733-741.
108. Lee J., Morgan J.R., Tompkins R.G. and Yarmush M.L. The importance of proline on long-term hepatocyte function in a collagen gel sandwich configuration: regulation of protein secretion. Biotechnology and Bioengineering 1992;40:298-305.
109. Lee K., Vandenberghe Y., Herin M., Cavalier R., Beck D., Li A., Verbeke N., Lesne M. and Roba J. Comparative metabolism of SC-42867 and SC-51089, two PGE_2 antagonists, in rat and human hepatocyte cultures 1993 (submitted).
110. Lemonnier F., Gautier M., Moatti N. and Lemonnier A. Comparative study of extracellular aminoacids in culture of human liver and fibroblastic cells. In Vitro 1976;12:460-466.
111. Lescoat G., Loreal O., Desvergne B., Pasdeloup N., Deugnier Y. and Brissot P. Effect of transferrin secretion of rat and human hepatocyte cultures. Liver 1988;8:360-365.

112. Li A.P., Barker G., Beck D., Colburn S., Monsell R. and Pellegrin C. Culturing of primary hepatocytes as entrapped aggregates in a packed bed bioreactor: a potential bioartificial liver. In Vitro Cellular Development Biology 1993;29A:249-254.
113. Lindroos P.M., Zarnegar R. and Michalopoulos G.K. Hepatocyte growth factor (hepatopoietin A) rapidly increases in plasma before DNA synthesis and liver regeneration stimulated by partial hepatectomy and carbon tetrachloride administration. Hepatology 1991;13:743-749.
114. Loretz L.J., Li A.P. and Flye M.W. Optimization of cryopreservation procedures of rat and human hepatocytes. Xenobiotica 1989;19:489-498.
115. Maekubo H., Ozaki S., Mitmaker B. and Kalant N. Preparation of human hepatocytes for primary culture. In Vitro 1982;18:483-491.
116. Maier P. Development of *in vitro* toxicity tests with cultures of freshly isolated rat hepatocytes. Experientia 1988;44:807-817.
117. Marselos M., Strom S.C. and Michalopoulos G. Enhancement of aldehyde dehydrogenase activity in human and rat hepatocyte cultures by 3-methylcholanthrene. Cell Biology and Toxicology 1986;2:257-269.
118. Marselos M., Strom S.C. and Michalopoulos G. Effect of phenobarbital and 3-methylcholanthrene on aldhyde dehydrogenase activity in cultures of Hep G2 cells and normal human hepatocytes. Chemico-Biological Interactions 1987;62:75-88.
119. Martelli A., Allavena A., Robbiano L., Mattioli F. and Brambilla G. Comparison of the sensitivity of human and rat hepatocytes to the genotoxic effects of metronidazole. Pharmacology and Toxicology 1990;66:329-334.
120. Martelli A., Robbiano L., Gazzaniga G.M. and Brambilla G. Comparative study of DNA damage and repair induced by ten N-nitroso compounds in primary cultures of human and rat hepatocytes. Cancer Research 1988;48:4144-4152.
121. Martelli A., Robbiano L., Ghia M., Giuliano L., Angelini G. and Brambilla G. A study of the potential genotoxicity of cimetidine using human hepatocyte primary cultures: discrepancy from results obtained in rat hepatocytes. Cancer Letters 1986;30:11-16.
122. Martelli A., Robbiano L., Giuliano L., Pino A., Angelini G. and Brambilla G. DNA fragmentation by N-nitrosodimethylamine and methylmethane-sulfonate in human hepatocyte primary cultures. Mutation Research 1985;144:209-211.
123. Maurice M., Pichard L., Daujat M., Fabre I., Joyeux H., Domergue J. and Maurel P. Effects of imidazole derivatives on cytochromes P450 from human hepatocytes in primary culture. FASEB Journal 1992;6:752-758.
124. Mc Gowan J.A., Strain A.J. and Bucher N.L.R. DNA synthesis in primary cultures of adult rat hepatocytes in a defined medium: effects of epidermal growth factor, insulin, glucagon and cyclic AMP. Journal of Cellular Physiology 1981;108:353-363.
125. Mc Mahon J.B., Richards W.L., del Campo A.A., Song H.H. and Thorgeirsson S.S. Differential effects of transforming growth factor β on the proliferation of normal and malignant rat liver epithelial cells in culture. Cancer Research 1986;46:4665-4671.

126. Mead J.E. and Fausto N. Transforming growth factor α may be a physiological regulator of liver regeneration by means of an autocrine mechanism. Proceedings of the National Academy of Sciences of the USA 1989;68:1558-1562.
127. Mesnil M., Fraslin J.M., Piccoli C., Yamasaki H. and Guguen-Guillouzo C. Cell contact but not junctional communication (dye coupling) with biliary epithelial cells is required for hepatocytes to maintain differentiated functions. Experimental Cell Research 1987;173:524-533.
128. Michalopoulos G., Houck K.A., Dolan M.L. and Luetteke N.C. Control of hepatocytes replication by two serum factors. Cancer Research 1984;44:4414-4419.
129. Michalopoulos G., Russel F. and Biles C. Primary cultures of hepatocytes on human fibroblasts. In Vitro 1979;15:796-806.
130. Michalopoulos G.K., Zarnegar R., Houck K. and Pediaditakis P. Hepatopoietins A and B and hepatocyte growth. Digestive Diseases and Sciences 1991;36:681-686.
131. Miura Y., Akimoto T. and Yagi K. Liver functions in hepatocytes entrapped within calcium alginate. Annals of the New York Academy of Sciences 1988;542:521-532.
132. Miyazaki K., Takaki R., Nakayama F., Yamanchi S., Koga A. and Todo S. Isolation and primary culture of adult human hepatocytes. Cell and Tissue Research 1981;218:13-21.
133. Miyazaki M., Handa Y., Oda M., Yabe T., Miyano K. and Sato J. Long-term survival of functional hepatocytes from adult rat in the presence of phenobarbital in primary culture. Experimental Cell Research 1985;159:176-190.
134. Monteith D.K. and Gupta R.C. Carcinogen-DNA adducts in cultures of rat and human hepatocytes. Cancer Letters 1992;62:87-93.
135. Monteith D.K. and Strom S.C. A comparison of the inhibition of deacetylase in primary culture of rat and human hepatocytes affecting metabolism and DNA-binding of 2-acetylaminofluorene. Cell Biology and Toxicology 1990;6:269-285.
136. Monteith D.K., Michalopoulos G. and Strom S.C. Conjugation of chemical carcinogens by primary cultures of human hepatocytes. Xenobiotica 1990;20:753-763.
137. Monteith D.K., Michalopoulos G. and Strom S.C. Metabolism of acetylaminofluorene in primary cultures of human hepatocytes: dose-response over a four-log range. Carcinogenesis 1988;9:1835-1841.
138. Monteith D.K., Novotny A., Michalopoulos G. and Strom S.C. Metabolism of benzo(a)pyrene in primary cultures of human hepatocytes: dose-response over a four-log range. Carcinogenesis 1987;8:983-988.
139. Mooney D., Hansen L., Vacanti J., Langer R., Farmer S. and Ingber R. Switching from differentiation to growth in hepatocytes: Control by extracellular matrix. Journal of Cellular Physiology 1992;151:497-505.
140. Moore C.J. and Gould M.N. Metabolism of benzo(a)pyrene by cultured human hepatocytes from multiple donors. Carcinogenesis 1984;5:1577-1582.

141. Morel F., Beaune P., Ratanasavanh D., Flinois J.P., Yang C.S., Guengerich F.P. and Guillouzo A. Expression of cytochrome P-450 enzymes in cultured human hepatocytes. European Journal of Biochemistry 1990;191:437-444.
142. Morel F., Fardel O., Meyer D.J., Langouet S., Gilmore K.S., Meunier B., Tu C.P.D., Kensler T.W, Ketterer B. and Guillouzo A. Preferential increase of glutathione transferase class & transcripts in cultured human hepatocytes by phenobarbital, 3-methylcholanthrene and dithiolethiones. Cancer Research 1993;53:231-234.
143. Morin O. and Norman C. Long-term maintenance of hepatocyte functional activity in coculture: requirements for sinusoidal endothelial cells and dexamethasone. Journal of Cellular Physiology 1986;129:103-110.
144. Moscow J.A. and Cowan K.H. Multidrug resistance. Journal of the National Cancer Institute 1992;80:14-20.
145. Moshage H.J., Rijntjes P.J.M., Hafkenscheid J.C.M., Roelofs H.M.J. and Yap S.H. Primary culture of cryopreserved adult human hepatocytes on homologous extracellular matrix and the influence of monocytic products on albumin synthesis. Journal of Hepatology 1988;7:34-44.
146. Nagao M., Oyanagi K., Tsuchiyama A., Aoyama T. and Nakao T. Studies on the expression of liver-specific functions of human fetal hepatocytes in primary culture. Tohoku Journal of Experimental Medicine 1987;152:23-29.
147. Nakagami O. and Ishida N. Morphological and functional studies of human fetal liver cells in primary monolayer culture. Tohoku Journal of Experimental Medicine 1980;132:277-287.
148. Nakamura T., Nawa K. and Ichihara A. Partial purification and characterization of hepatocyte growth factor from serum of hepatectomized rats. Biochemical and Biophysical Research Communications 1984;122:1450-1459.
149. Nakamura T., Nawa K., Ichihara A., Kaise N. and Nishino T. Purification and subunit structure of hepatocyte growth factor from rat platelets. FEBS Letters 1987;224:311-316.
150. Nakamura T., Tomita Y., Hirai R., Yamaoka K., Kaji K. and Ichihara A. Inhibitory effects of transforming growth factor β on DNA synthesis of adult rat hepatocytes in primary culture. Biochemical and Biophysical Research Communications 1985;133:1042-1050.
151. Nau H., Liddiard C. and Merker H.J. Preparation, morphology and drug metabolism of isolated hepatocyte and liver organ cultures from the human fetus. Life Science 1978;23:2361-2372.
152. Niemann C., Gauthier J.C., Richert L., Ivanov M.A., Melcion C. and Cordier A. Rat adult hepatocytes in primary pure and mixed monolayer culture. Biochemical Pharmacology 1991;42:373-379.
153. Noyes W.F. Culture of human fetal liver. Proceedings of Experimental Biological Medicine 1973;144:245-248.
154. Nyberg S.L., Shatford R.A., Hu W.S., Payne W.D. and Cerra F.B. Hepatocyte culture systems for artificial liver support: implications for critical care medicine (bioartificial liver support) Critical Care Medicine 1992;20:1157-1168.

155. Oldham H.G., Standring P., Norman S.J., Blake T.J., Beattie I., Cox P.J. and Chenery R.J. Metabolism of temelastine (SK&F 93944) in hepatocytes from rat, dog, cynomolgus monkey and man. Drug Metabolism and Disposition 1990;18:146-152.
156. Paine A.J. and Hockin L.J. The maintenance of cytochrome P450 in liver cell culture: recent studies on P450 mediated mechanisms of toxicity. Toxicology 1982;25:41
157. Paine A.J. The maintenance of cytochrome P450 in rat hepatocyte culture: some applications of liver cell cultures to the study of drug metabolism, toxicity and the induction of the cytochrome P450 system. Chemico-Biological Interactions 1990;74:1-31.
158. Paine A.J., Lesley J.W. and Legg R.F. Apparent maintenance of cytochrome P450 by nicotinamide in primary cultures of rat hepatocytes. Life Science 1979;24:2185-2192.
159. Pasco D.S. and Fagan J.B. Efficient DNA-mediated gene transfer into primary cultures of adult rat hepatocytes. DNA 1989;8:535-541.
160. Peng D.R., Pacifici G.M. and Rane A. Human fetal liver cultures: basal activities and inducibility of epoxide hydrolase and aryl hydrocarbon hydroxylase. Biochemical Pharmacology 1984;33:71-77.
161. Pichard L. Fabre I., Daujat M., Domergue J., Joyeux H. and Maurel P. Effects of corticosteroids on the expression of cytochromes P450 and on cyclosporin A oxidase activity in primary cultures of human hepatocytes. Molecular Pharmacology 1992;41:1047-1055.
162. Pichard L., Fabre I., Fabre G., Domergue J., Saint Aubert B., Mourad G. and Maurel P. Screening for inducers and inhibitors of cytochrome P450 (cyclosporin A oxidase) in primary cultures of human hepatocytes and in liver microsomes. Drug Metabolism and Disposition 1990;18:595-605.
163. Pichard L., Gillet G., Fabre I., Dalet-Beluche J., Bonfils C., Thenot J.P. and Maurel P. Identification of the rabbit and human cytochromes P450IIIA as the major enzymes involved in the N-demethylation of diltiazem. Drug Metabolism and Disposition 1990;18:711-719
164. Rahmani R., Richard B., Fabre G. and Cano J.P. Extrapolation of preclinical pharmacokinetic data to therapeutic drug use. Xenobiotica 1988;18:71-78.
165. Rajaonarison J.F., Lacarelle B., de Sousa G., Catalin J. and Rahmani R. *In vitro* glucuronidation of 3'-azido-3'-deoxy-thymidine by human liver. Role of UDP-glucuronosyltransferase 2 form. Drug Metabolism and Disposition 1991;19:809-815.
166. Ramsdell H.S. and Eaton D.L. Species susceptibility to aflatoxin B_1 carcinogenesis: comparative kinetics of microsomal biotransformation; Cancer Research 1990;50:615-620.
167. Ratanasavanh D., Baffet G., Latinier M., Rissel M. and Guillouzo A. Use of hepatocyte co-cultures in the assessment of drug toxicity from chronic exposure. Xenobiotica 1988;18:765-771.
168. Ratanasavanh D., Beaune P., Baffet G., Rissel M., Kremers P., Guengerich F.P. and Guillouzo A. Immunochemical evidence for the maintenance of cytochrome P-450 isozymes, NADPH cytochrome C reductase, and epoxide hydrolase in pure and mixed primary cultures of adult human hepatocytes. Journal of Histochemistry and Cytochemistry 1986;34:527-533.

169. Ratanasavanh D., Berthou F., Dreano Y., Mondine P., Guillouzo A. and Riche C. Methylcholanthrene but not phenobarbital enhances caffeine and theophylline metabolism in cultured adult human hepatocytes. Biochemical Pharmacology 1990;39:85-94.
170. Reese J.A. and Byard J.L. Isolation and culture of adult hepatocytes from liver biopsies. In Vitro 1981;17:935-940.
171. Reid L.M., Narita M., Fujita M., Murray Z., Liverpool C. and Rosenberg L. Matrix and hormonal regulation of differentiation in liver cultures. In: Isolated and Cultured Hepatocytes (Guillouzo A. and Guguen-Guillouzo C., eds.) Les Editions INSERM, Paris and John Libbey Eurotext, London,1986:225-258.
172. Richard B., Fabre G., de Sousa G., Fabre I., Rahmani R. and Cano J.P. Interspecies variability in mitoxantrone metabolism using primary cultures of hepatocytes isolated from rat, rabbit and humans. Biochemical Pharmacology 1991;41:255-262.
173. Rijntjes P.J.M., Moshage H.J. and Yap S.H. In vitro infection of primary cultures of cryopreserved human hepatocytes with hepatitis B virus. Virus Research 1988;10:95-110.
174. Rijntjes P.J.M., Moshage H.J., Van Gemert P.J.L., De Waal R. and Yap S.H. Cryopreservation of adult human hepatocytes. Journal of Hepatology 1986;3:7-18.
175. Rogiers V., Callaerts A., Vercruysse A., Akrawi M., Shephard E. and Phillips I. Effects of valproate in xenobiotic biotransformation in rat liver. In vivo and in vitro experiments. Pharmaceutisch Weekblad (scientific ed.) 1992;14:127-131.
176. Rogiers V., Vandenberghe Y., Callaerts A., Verleye G., Cornet M., Mertens K., Sonck W. and Vercruysse A. Phase I and phase II xenobiotic biotransformation in cultures and co-cultures of adult rat hepatocytes. Biochemical Pharmacology 1990;40:1701-1706.
177. Rogiers V., Vandenberghe Y., Callaerts A., Sonck W. and Vercruysse A. Effects of dimethylsulphoxide on phase I and phase II biotransformation in cultured rat hepatocytes. Toxicology in Vitro 1990;4:439-442.
178. Russell W.E. and Bucher N.L.R. Vasopressin modulates liver regeneration in the Brattlebora rat. Americal Journal of Physiology 1983;245:G321-G324.
179. Russell W.E., Coffey J.R., Quellette A.J. and Moses H.L. Type β transforming growth factor reversibly inhibits the early proliferative response to partial hepatectomy in the rat. Proceedings of the National Academy of Sciences of the USA 1988;85:5126-5130.
180. Ryan C.M., Carter E.A., Jenkins R.L., Sterling L.M., Yarmusch M.L., Malt R.A. and Tompkins R.G. Isolation and long-term culture of human hepatocytes. Surgery 1993;113:48-54.
181. Saad B., Schawalder H. and Maier P. Crude liver membrane fractions as substrate preserve liver specific functions in long term, serum free rat hepatocyte cultures. In Vitro Cellular and Developmental Biology 1993 (in press).
182. Sandström B. Maintenance in vitro of functionally active adult human liver. Acta Hepatogastroenterologica 1973;20:19-23.

183. Sawada N., Tomomura A., Sattler C.A., Sattler G.L., Kleinman H.K. and Pitot H.C. Extracellular matrix components influence DNA synthesis of rat hepatocytes in primary culture. Experimental Cell Research 1986;167:458-470.
184. Schuetz E.G., Li D., Omiecinski C.J., Muller-Eberhard U., Kleinman H.K., Elswick B. and Guzelian P.S. Regulation of gene expression in adult rat hepatocytes cultured on a basement membrane matrix. Journal of Cellular Physiology 1988;134:309-323.
185. Schuetz E.G., Wrighton S.A., Safe S.H. and Guzelian P.S. Regulation of cytochrome P-450p by phenobarbital and phenobarbital-like inducers in adult rat hepatocytes in primary monolayer cultures and *in vivo*. Biochemistry 1986;25:1124-1133.
186. Schuetz J.D. and Schuetz E.G. Extracellular matrix regulation of multidrug resistance in primary monolayer cultures of adult rat hepatocytes. Cell Growth and Differentiation 1993;4:31-40.
187. Scotto J.M., Sauron B., Dupy-Coin A.M. and Gautier M. Kinetics of nuclear changes during herpetic infection of human primary liver cell cultures. Journal of Submicroscopic Cytology and Pathology 1979;11:229-241.
188. Seglen P.U. Preparation of isolated rat liver cells. Methods in Cell Biology 1976;18:29-83.
189. Shatford R.A., Nyberg S.L. and Payne W.D. A hepatocyte bioreactor as a potential bio-artificial liver: demonstration of prolonged tissue-specific functions. Surgical Forum 1991;42:54-56.
190. Shatford R.A., Nyberg S.L., Meier S.J., White J.G., Payne W.D., Hu W. and Cerra F.B. Hepatocyte function in a hollow fiber bioreactor. A potential bioartificial liver. Journal of Surgery Research 1992;53:549-557.
191. Shnyra A., Bocharov A. and Bochkova N. Bioartificial liver using hepatocytes on Biosilon microcarriers. Treatment of chemically induced acute hepatic failure in rats. Artificial Organs 1991;15:189-197.
192. Sidhu J.S., Farin F.M. and Omiencinski C.J. Influence of extracelular matrix overlay on phenobarbital-mediated induction of CYP2B1, CYP2B2 and 3A1 genes in primary adult rat hepatocyte culture. Archives of Biochemistry and Biophysics 1993;301:108-113.
193. Sinclair P.R., Bement W.J., Haugen S.A., Sinclair J.F. and Guzelian P.S. Induction of cyt P450 and 5-aminolevulinate synthase activities in cultured rat hepatocytes. Cancer Research 1990;50:5219-5224.
194. Sirica A.E. and Pitot H.C. Drug metabolism and effects of carcinogens in cultured hepatic cells. Pharmacology Reviews 1980;31:205-228.
195. Snijder S., Hsu I.C. and Trump B.F. Comparison of metabolic activation of carcinogens in human, rat and hamster hepatocytes. Mutation Research 1987;182:31-39.
196. Steward A.R., Dannan G.A., Guzelian P.S. and Guengerich F.P. Changes in the concentration of seven forms of cytochrome P450 in primary cultures of adult rat hepatocytes. Molecular Pharmacology 1984;27:125-132.
197. Strain A.J., Frazer A., Hill D.J. and Milner R.D.G. Transforming growth factor β inhibits DNA synthesis in hepatocytes from normal and regenerating rat liver. Biochemical and Biophysical Research Communications 1987;145:436-442.

198. Strain A.J., Ismail T., Tsubouchi H., Hishida T., Kitamura N., Daikuhara Y. and Mc Master P. Native and recombinant human hepatocyte growth factor are highly potent promotors of DNA synthesis in both human and rat hepatocytes. Journal of Clinical Investigation 1991;87:1853-1857.
199. Strom S.C., Jirtie R.L., Jones R.S., Novicki D.L., Rosenberg M.R., Novotny A., Irons G., Mc Lain J.R. and Michalopoulos G. Isolation, culture and transplantation of human hepatocytes. Journal of the National Cancer Institute 1982;68:771-778.
200. Strom S.C., Jirtle R.L. and Michalopoulos G. Genotoxic effects of 2-acetylaminofluorene on rat and human hepatocytes. Environmental Health Perspectives 1983;49:165-170.
201. Tee L., Davies D.S., Seddon C.E. and Boobis A.R. Species differences in the hepatotoxicity of paracetamol are due to differences in the rate of conversion to its cytotoxic metabolite. Biochemical Pharmacology 1987;36:1041-1052.
202. Thomas D.B. and Yoffey J.M. Human foetal haematopoiesis in the human foetus. British Journal of Haematology 1964;10:193-197.
203. Tompkins R.G. and Carter E.A. Enzymatic function of alginate immobilized rat hepatocytes. Biotechnology and Bioengineering 1988;31:11-18.
204. Turner N.A. and Pitot H.D. Dependence of the induction of cytochrome P-450 by phenobarbital in primary cultures of adult rat hepatocytes. Biochemical Pharmacology 1989;38:2247-2251.
205. Turner N.A., Wilson M.N., Jefcoate C.R. and Pitot H.C. The expression and metabolic activity of cytochrome P-450 isoenzymes in control and phenobarbital cultures of rat hepatocytes. Archives of Biochemistry and Biophysics 1988;263:204-215.
206. Utesch D., Platt K.L. and Oesch F. Xenobiotic metabolizing enzyme activities in mono- and cocultures of rat-liver parenchymal cell with rat liver non-parenchymal epithelial cells or mouse embryo fibroblasts. Abstract in: Third International ISSX meeting 1991: Drug metabolism: molecules, models and man, 24-28 June. Amsterdam, The Netherlands 1991:310.
207. Vandenberghe Y., Glaise D., Meyer D., Guillouzo A. and Ketterer B. Glutathione transferase isoenzymes in cultured rat hepatocytes. Biochemical Pharmacology 1988;37:2482-2485.
208. Vandenberghe Y., Morel F., Foriers A., Ketterer B., Vercruysse A., Guillouzo A. and Rogiers V. Effect of phenobarbital on the expression of glutathione S-transferase isoenzymes in cultured rat hepatocytres. FEBS Letters 1989;251:59-64.
209. Vandenberghe Y., Morel F., Pemble S., Taylor J.B., Rogiers V., Ratanasavanh D., Vercruysse A., Ketterer B. and Guillouzo A. Changes in expression of mRNA coding for glutathione S-transferase subunits 1-2 and 7 in cultured rat hepatocytes. Molecular Pharmacology 1990;37:372-376.
210. Vandenberghe Y., Ratanasavanh D., Glaise D. and Guillouzo A. Influence of medium composition and culture conditions on glutathione S-transferase activity in adult rat hepatocytes during culture. In Vitro Cellular Developmental Biology 1988;24:281-288.
211. Vandenberghe Y., Rogiers V. and Guillouzo A. Glutathione S-transferase activity in cultured human hepatocytes. Cell Biology International Reports 1988;12:959-967.

212. Vandenberghe Y., Tee L., Morel F., Rogiers V., Guillouzo A. and Yeoh G. Regulation of glutathione S-transferase gene expression by phenobarbital in cultured adult rat hepatocytes. FEBS Letters 1991;284:103-108.
213. Vons C., Pegorier J.P., Girard J., Kohl C., Ivanov M.A., and Franco D. Regulation of fatty-acid metabolism by pancreatic hormones in cultured human hepatocytes. Hepatology 1991;13:1126-1130.
214. Vons C., Pegorier J.P., Ivanov M.A., Girard J., Melcion C., Cordier A. and Franco D. Comparison of cultured human hepatocytes isolated from surgical biopsies or cold-stored organ donor livers. Toxicology in Vitro 1990;4:432-434.
215. Voss J.U. and Seibert H. Microcarrier-attached rat hepatocytes as a xenobiotic metabolizing system in cocultures. Cell Biology and Toxicology 1991;7:387-399.
216. Wanson J.C. and Mosselmans R. Co-culture of adult rat hepatocytes and sinusoidal cells: a new experimental model for the study of ultrastructural and functional properties of liver cells. In: Communications of Liver Cells (Popper H., Bianchi F. and Gudat F., eds.) MTP Press, Ltd, Lancaster, England 1980:2329-2389.
217. Waxman D.J., Morrissey J.J., Naik S. and Jauregui H.O. Phenobarbital induction of cytochrome P450. High level long responsiveness of primary rat hepatocyte cultures to drug induction and glucocorticoid dependence of the phenobarbital response. Biochemical Journal 1990;271:113-119.
218. Wiebkin P., Dees J.H., Mathis J.M. and Prough R.A. Drug metabolism by isolated fetal human hepatocytes in suspension and primary culture. Drug Metabolism and Disposition 1985;13:163-168.
219. Yanagi K., Ookawa K. and Mizuno S. Performance of a new hybrid artificial liver support system using hepatocytes entrapped within a hydrogel. ASAIO Journal 1989;35:570-572.
220. Caron J.M. and Bissell D.M. Extracellular matrix induces albumin gene expression in cultured rat hepatocytes. Hepatology 1989;10:636-642.

7
Potential of freshly isolated and cryopreserved human hepatocytes in drug research and development

R. Rahmani, G. de Sousa, F. Marre, F. Nicolas and M. Placidi

INSERM U 278, Faculté de Pharmacie
27, Bd Jean Moulin, 13385 Marseille Cedex 05 (France).

Introduction

The liver plays a major role in handling foreign chemicals and is also the most active mammalian tissue with respect to xenobiotic metabolism. As hepatocytes isolated from various species were shown to retain most of the functions of the intact liver, this model has been extensively and increasingly applied over the last decade in various pharmaceutical research areas, including pharmacology, pharmacokinetics and toxicology. Applications include the evaluation of drug efficacy, metabolic fate and hepatotoxicity [1-3].

The majority of studies performed with hepatocyte systems have 'however' utilized preparations of cells from animals, mostly rodents. Hence, because both qualitative and quantitative interspecies variabilities are likely to occur in the hepatic fate and effect of drugs, extrapolating data obtained with animal cells to the human situation remains hazardous. This drawback, together with the ethical considerations in performing human experimentation *in vivo*, makes the development of human *in vitro* systems critical in the evaluation of human health risks prior to clinical trials. Indeed, early information concerning the metabolic pattern of a novel drug in human hepatocytes could be highly relevant in choosing the optimal species for preclinical pharmaco-toxicological evaluation and in optimizing the information obtained from early clinical studies.

However, before applying these tools in prospective studies on drug transport, biotransformation and toxicity, one must ensure that in vitro models are reliable in elucidating and/or predicting drug metabolic pathways (including drug interactions), and interspecies as well as interindividual variabilities as compared to in vivo data. In that context, our laboratory has, over the last few years, developed efficient procedures for isolating large amounts of human hepatocytes which can be used freshly isolated in suspension, in primary culture or for the preparation of subcellular fractions (microsomes, membranes) [4-6]. Moreover, specifically designed cryopreservation protocols have made long-term storage of these hepatocytes possible under conditions maintaining their metabolic functions [6,7]. Various potential applications of these in vitro systems in drug discovery and development are presented.

Methodology

Preparation and incubation conditions of hepatocytes

Freshly isolated hepatocytes in suspension: The isolation of animal and human hepatocytes, the incubation procedure, drug transport and metabolic evaluation were as previously described [5-9]. Freshly isolated hepatocytes were incubated in a final concentration of 1 to 5.10^6 cells/ml at 37°C in Waymouth medium (pH 7.4 ; 95% O_2 - 5% CO_2). The radiolabelled drug was added in the incubation medium to initiate transport and metabolic experiments. Fractions of the extra- and/or intracellular medium were analyzed using various High-Performance-Liquid-Chromatography (HPLC) methodologies specific to each drug.

Primary cultures of hepatocytes: Hepatocytes were resuspended in F12 Coon's modification/DMEM medium containing 10% fetal calf serum (FCS), insulin, glucagon, L-thyroxine, transferrine, linoleic acid and antibiotics. Cells (2.5×10^6) were plated on Petri dishes (60 mm diameter); after incubation (4 or 8 h) with cells adhering to the plastic, medium was renewed and supplemented with 10^{-6} M dexamethasone. Metabolic and toxicologic studies were performed as previously described [4,10,11].

Hepatocyte cryopreservation and thawing

Human hepatocytes were resuspended in HAM F12 medium supplemented with 10% dimethylsulphoxide and 20% FCS. Cell freezing was performed with a NICOOL ST 20 apparatus which can be programmed to optimize temperature drop. Hepatocytes were stored at - 196°C. After thawing in a water bath at 37°C, the cells were purified by a rapid centrifugation in a culture medium containing Percoll [7].

Liver microsomes

Microsomes prepared from various species [12,14] (rat, rabbit, baboon, dog and human) were incubated at 37°C and drug metabolic reactions initiated by adding NADPH (1 mM).

Results and discussion

In vitro *interspecies and interindividual variability of Minaprine biotransformation: comparison with* in vivo *studies*

Minaprine is a psychotropic agent with antidepressant properties and is effective in the treatment of various types of depressive disorders [15-19]. This drug was selected as a good candidate for our validation strategy since its biotransformation has been extensively studied *in vivo* in man and various animal species [20,21]. These studies have shown: 1/ diverse and complex metabolic pathways (hydroxylation, oxidation, N-dealkylation, N-oxidation, reductive ring cleavage, etc.) (Fig. 1); 2/ significant interspecies variability ; and 3/ in patients, large intersubject variations in Minaprine plasma levels and a significant relationship between debrisoquine phenotype and Minaprine/ 4-hydroxyminaprine metabolic ratios.

We therefore investigated Minaprine metabolism *in vitro*, using freshly isolated hepatocytes and liver microsomes from different species (rat, rabbit, dog, baboon, and human) [22,23]. *In vivo* and *in vitro* data were then compared to evaluate the reliability of these *in vitro* models in assessing drug metabolic pathways, and interspecies and interindividual variabilities, as well as in identifying the cytochrome P450 responsible for Minaprine polymorphic hydroxylation.

Our results showed that the major metabolic route (4-hydroxylation of

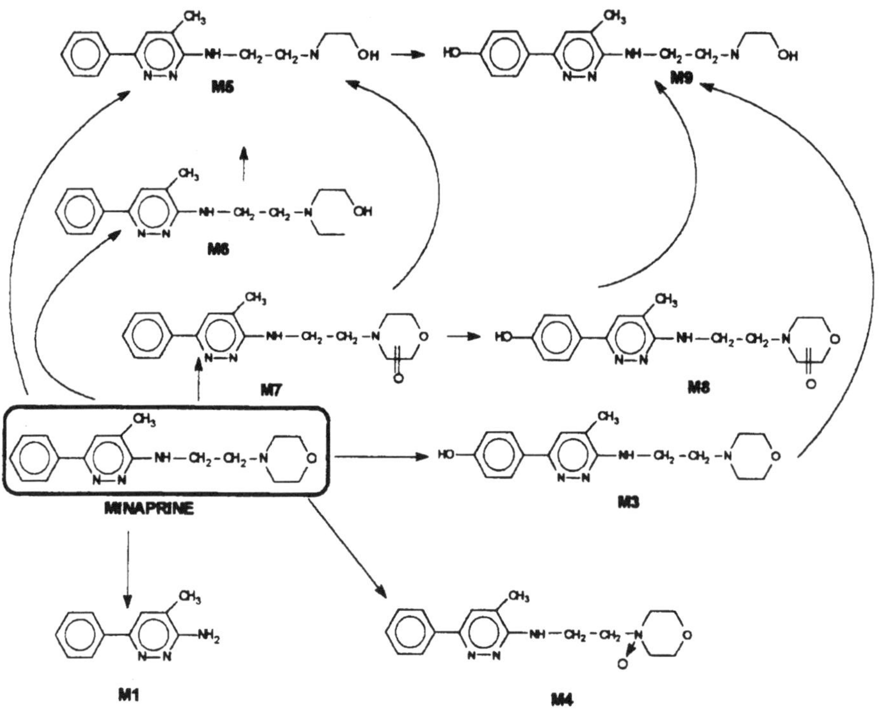

Figure 1 :
Metabolic pathways of Minaprine [20,22].
M1=3-amino-4-methyl-6-phenyl-pyridazine,
M3=4-hydroxyminarpine,
M4=Minaprine N-oxyde,
M5=3-[2-(hydroxyethylamino)ethylamino]-4-methyl-6-phenyl-pyridazine.

the aromatic ring - M_3) is the same *in vivo* and *in vitro*. Other *in vivo* biotransformation pathways, were also confirmed in hepatocytes. Indeed, a good correlation between *in vitro* and *in vivo* findings was established for the major chloroform-extractable metabolites of Minaprine in the rat (Table I). Minaprine exhibits rapid biotransformation *in vitro*, which may explain its short *in vivo* plasma half-life ($t_{1/2}$ = 2.5 h).

Furthermore, the interspecies variability of metabolism *in vivo* was reproduced by *in vitro* models ; the major difference concerned the formation of the Minaprine N-oxide derivative (M_4). In the dog, large amounts of this compound were present, whereas in the other species only trace amounts were observed. The overall metabolic pattern of this drug appeared to be less complex in man than in rat, dog and monkey,

	M	M1	M3	M4	M5
In vitro (%)	5.7	7.8	55.5	8.3	22.6
In vivo (%)	1.7	5.5	66.1	5.3	21.3

Table I :
Comparison of *in vivo* and *in vitro* metabolism of Minaprine in rat[20,22]
In vitro data represent the relative proportions of each chloroform-extractable metabolite in the extracellular medium 2 h after exposure of rat hepatocytes in suspension to [^{14}C]Minaprine (50 µM). *In vivo* data correspond to extractable metabolites excreted in the 0-48 h urine fraction[20].
M = Minaprine, M_1 (see Figure 1) ; M_3 = 4-hydroxyminaprine ;
M_4 = Minaprine N-oxide ; M_5 (see Figure 1)

since only one metabolite (M_3) was being produced in high amounts by human hepatocytes. A similar interspecies variability of Minaprine was demonstrated *in vivo*, leading to the same conclusions, i.e., that the dog is not suitable as a surrogate species for man in these pharmacological and toxicological evaluations of Minaprine [22].
Finally, the marked interindividual variability in Minaprine metabolism, already reported *in vivo* in patients, was also found *in vitro* using human hepatocytes in suspension from six different human liver samples (HL26-29, HL32-33) (Table II). For instance, whereas HL 29 hepatocytes metabolized Minaprine poorly, HL 26 and HL 33 hepatocytes extensively converted Minaprine to M_3 and then to its glucuronide. In addition, small amounts of the metabolite M_5 and the lactam derivative were formed by some hepatocyte samples. Traces of M_4 were found whereas M_1 was not detectable.
Complementary studies with human hepatic microsomal fractions allowed us to establish that the cytochrome P450 isoenzyme involved in the 4-hydroxylation of Minaprine and responsible for *in vivo* Minaprine polymorphic hydroxylation belongs to the CYP2D subfamily and is probably the human liver CYP2D6 [23]. Identifying the isoenzymes specifically involved in the biotransformation of a given drug is of utmost importance not only from a theoretical point of view but also in predicting potential drug interactions.
In conclusion, these studies on Minaprine confirm the reliability of *in vitro* models for the assessment of drug metabolism in man and animal

HUMAN LIVER	EXTRACELLULAR CONCENTRATION (µM)		
	M3-GLU	M3	MINAPRINE
HL 26	0.69	7.06	0.07
HL 27	0.46	1.43	3.85
HL 28	0.34	6.40	0.49
HL 29	ND	0.46	6.67
HL 32	0.48	1.21	3.87
HL 33	0.86	5.99	0.11

Table II :
Variability of Minaprine metabolism in human hepatocytes in suspension [22]
Human hepatocytes in suspension (2.5×10^6 cells/ml) were incubated for 1 h with a 10 µM initial concentration of [^{14}C]Minaprine. Extracellular media were further analyzed by HPLC.
ND=Not detected ; M_3-GLU=glucuronide of 4-hydroxyminaprine ; M_3= 4-hydroxyminaprine

species in vivo, as has been shown previously by other authors [1-3]. During the preclinical development of new compounds, such in vitro systems can be powerful tools in selecting the animal species most closely related to humans in terms of metabolic patterns. These models also may make it possible to detect any potential genetic polymorphisms in the metabolism of a drug.

Benzodiazepine metabolism in human and animal hepatocytes; role in the duration of pharmacological activity

Because of their pharmacological properties, i.e. anxiolytic, sedative, anti-convulsant and hypnotic, benzodiazepines represent one of the major advances in medicine. The pharmacokinetics of these drugs differ in terms of elimination half-life ($t_{1/2}$), plasma clearance (Cl), and distribution volume as well as metabolic routes and rates [24, 25]. These drugs have been tentatively classified according to an experimental parameter, the QR (or Quotient for Recovery, which represents the maximum circulating concentration over the 12 h plasma concentration ratio). The higher the QR for a benzodiazepine, the more hypnotic the drug [26]. Midazolam (MDZ) and Diazepam (DZP) belong to this important class of drugs. MDZ exhibits rapid hypnotic action ($t_{1/2}$ = 1-3 h ; QR = 100), and DZP shows both hypnotic and anxiolytic effects ($t_{1/2}$ = 20-60 h ; QR = 3.2) (Table III).

We sought to determine whether these *in vivo* features could be

	QR	QRapp
DIAZEPAM	3.2	3.6
MIDAZOLAM	100	70-200
MDZ/DZP QR Ratio	31	20-55

Table III :
Comparison of *the in vivo* recovery quotient (QR) and the *in vitro* apparent QR (QRapp) for Diazepam and Midazolam[26,27].

retrospectively predicted by *in vitro* models [4,8,27]. The cellular kinetics and metabolism of HDZ and DZP were investigated in human hepatocytes and *in vitro* apparent QR (QRapp) was estimated. QRapp was defined as initial unchanged drug extracellular concentration over that which existed after 90 min. HPLC analysis allowed us to identify and quantify the various metabolites formed by human cells. The appearance kinetics of the various biotransformation products are illustrated in Fig. 2 for DZP and MDZ. The phase I cytochrome P450-mediated derivatives corresponded to oxazepam (OX), temazepam (TEM) and nordiazepam (NOR) for DZP, and 1-hydroxy, 4-hydroxy and 1-4 dihydroxy-midazolam for MDZ. Phase II compounds corresponded to the glucuronides of the hydroxylated metabolites for each drug.

DZP was slowly metabolized to these different products and, after a 2 h exposure, the unchanged drug remained the main product in the extracellular compartment. In contrast, MDZ was rapidly metabolized and at the end of the 2 h exposure, conjugated metabolites represented 90% of the extracellular drug. This particularly highlights on the difference in affinity of both benzodiazepines for the cytochrome P450 enzymatic complex. Hence, after exposure to equimolar concentrations of both benzodiazepines, 50% of DZP was still present in the extracellular

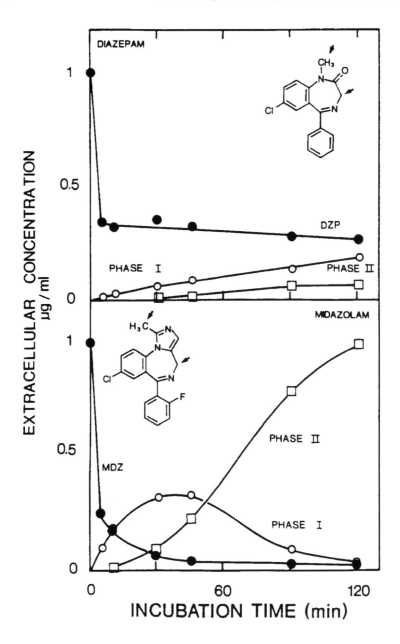

Figure 2 :
Extracellular kinetics of unchanged drug and of various metabolites after exposure of freshly isolated human hepatocytes to DZP or MDZ.
Substrate concentrations of DZP and MDZ were 1 μg/ml.
Arrows represent the main potential sites of drug biotransformation.

compartment after 2 h, whereas only 15% of unchanged MDZ remained in the extracellular compartment after 30 min (Fig. 2).
The QRapp of MDZ and DZP, calculated as described above, were 70-200 and 3.6 respectively (Table III), which is in agreement with previously

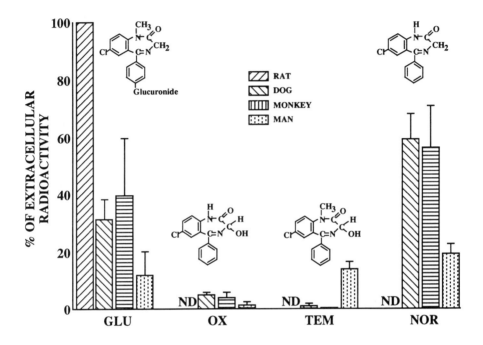

Figure 3:
Drug metabolism profiles of DZP in primary cultures of hepatocytes isolated from rat, dog, monkey and man.
Glu=hydroxy-DZP-glucuronide, OX=Oxazepam, TEM=Temazepam, NOR=Nordiazepam, ND=Not detected. Substrate concentration of DZP was 10 µM. Incubation time period was 24 h.

reported data *in vivo* [26]. The rapid metabolism of MDZ and its further catabolism to the pharmacologically less active 1-hydroxy-midazolam glucuronide may explain the short duration of the pharmacodynamic effects observed after administration in patients. Both the relatively rapid onset and the short duration of action of MDZ, as compared to DZP, could be associated with their metabolic clearance.
DZP and MDZ were also used as substrates in drug metabolism studies in order to characterize the differences in the metabolite profiles obtained in hepatocytes isolated from four species: Sprague-Dawley rat,

cynomolgus monkey, beagle dog and man. The metabolite patterns obtained by HPLC analysis of the culture medium indicated that substantial differences exist, corresponding to known species differences in the metabolite profile of both drugs *in vivo* [28-32]. For DZP, the hepatocytes of all species were found to produce NOR, TEM and OX; NOR was the principal metabolite in dog and monkey, TEM and NOR were the main metabolites in human hepatocytes (Fig. 3). Glucuronides were also produced in all species; indeed, they represented the most preponderant terminal metabolites in the rat. These results are in accordance with previous reports on the *in vitro* metabolism of DZP [2]. For MDZ, the interspecies variability also appeared highly significant, but only quantitatively since all the species produced, in various amounts, the same phase I and phase II metabolites as reported *in vivo* [31,32].

These findings substantiate the usefulness of hepatocytes in elucidating or predicting, at the preclinical stage of drug development, the pharmacokinetic behaviour of drugs within the same chemical family. For benzodiazepines, they could be used in assessing the duration of action of future analogs during early development stages. Moreover, the results support the value of this model in drug metabolism studies and especially in studies concerned with species differences in biotransformation.

Anticancer drug transport and metabolism in human hepatocytes: relationships between in vitro data, clinical pharmacokinetics and toxicity

Both, pharmacokinetics and drug metabolism are now recognized as being major determinants of the pharmacodynamics of cytotoxic anticancer agents [27,33]. Metabolic studies are included at all stages of anticancer drug development. By understanding the impact of metabolism on both drug activity and toxicity, the development of new compounds may be stimulated and a better insight into the mechanism involved may be provided.

Vincaalkaloids: Vincaalkaloids (V.A.), including vinblastine (VLB), vincristine (VCR), vindesine (VDS) and navelbine (NVB), are anticancer drugs widely used both as single agents and in combination with other drugs in chemotherapy [34]. Although these molecules are structurally related, marked differences have been observed in their antitumor

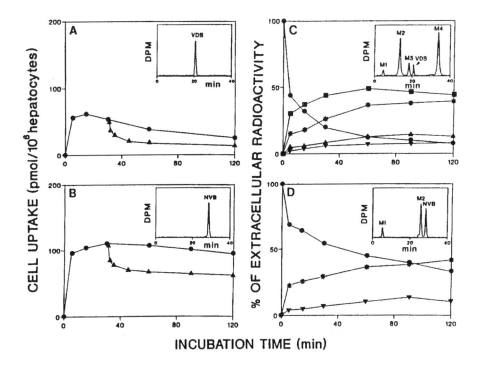

Figure 4:

<u>Left panels</u>: Uptake (●) and release (▲) kinetics of Vindesine (A) and Navelbine (B) in freshly isolated human hepatocytes in suspension.

<u>Right panels</u>: Extracellular kinetics of the disappearance of parent Vincaalkaloids (●) and the appearance of their respective metabolites (C:Vindesine; D:Navelbine) (M1,▼, M2,✻, M3,▲, M4,■).

<u>Inserts</u>: HPLC profiles (120 min portions) in intracellular (A, B) and extracellular media (C, D). Substrate concentration of Vincaalkaloids was 0.5 µM.

activity, toxicity and pharmacokinetic behaviour. Moreover, the clinical pharmacokinetic parameters of V.A. show large inter- and intra-individual variabilities, probably resulting from individual differences in hepatic drug disposition. *In vivo* and *in vitro* studies in humans and animals have been conducted for several years in our laboratory with the aim of reaching a better understanding of the large interindividual and interdrug variabilities of V.A. and the consequences with regards to toxicity and efficacy [9,27,35-41]. Their metabolic fate is nearly completely unknown and inhibits not only their rational therapeutic use but also the development of new analogues with a better therapeutic index.

Studies were carried out to evaluate the uptake, release and metabolism of the four currently used V.A. by using freshly isolated human hepatocytes in suspension. During incubation, V.A were intensely biotransformed. For example, VDS was metabolized into more (M_4) and less (M_1, M_2, M_3) polar metabolites than the unchanged drug (Fig. 4C); whereas for NVB, only polar metabolites (M_1, M_2) were produced (Fig. 4D). The absence of hydrophobic metabolites in NVB biotransformation might be at the origin of its much lower toxicity as compared with other V.A.. The highly lipophilic metabolites may readily bind to the peripheral nervous system and result in the neurotoxicity commonly found in patients receiving this family of anticancer drugs [34]. Despite their extremely high lipophilicities, these metabolites are almost completely excreted by the cells without binding to intracellular and/or membraneous hydrophobic components. Indeed, HPLC analysis revealed only unchanged drug in the intracellular compartment (Fig. 4A, 4B inserts). A similar observation was made when the drugs (VDS and NVB) were transferred to a drug - free medium. The extent of cell uptake appeared to parallel the lipophilicity of the compounds: NVB, which is more lipophilic than VDS, was more rapidly accumulated by the cells and to a greater extent than VDS. This observation may at least in part explain the higher distribution volume (Vd) of NVB (Vd = 28.6 ± 11.7 l/kg) compared with VDS (Vd = 8.8 ± 5 l/kg), as estimated after I.V. bolus injection in patients.

Especially noteworthy was the observation that the uptake rates of the drugs VCR, VDS, VLB and NVB by human hepatocytes showed an excellent correlation with their serum clearances as previously reported in patients [34,38] (r = 0.9995, p<0.001) (Table IV). This finding is compatible with the high *in vivo* hepatic extraction and is likely to be at the origin of the vincaalkaloid pharmacokinetic characteristics reported *in vivo*.

Human hepatocytes also provide the opportunity to advance the idea that the large interindividual variation observed for V.A. pharmacokinetics in cancer patients is linked with the extensive differences in drug metabolic capacities among the population. Indeed, with a library of human livers, a variability factor of 10 was observed between the lowest and the highest metabolic rates of V.A.. This variability was further explained by identifiying the human liver CYP3A involved in the biotransformation of VDS and VLB; the isoenzyme level, measured by Western-blot, also varied considerably between individuals [41].

Finally, the combination of cellular and subcellular microsomal models enables the prediction of eventual drug interactions in clinical practice

	PLASMA CLEARANCE [34-38] (l/h/kg)	UPTAKE RATE MEAN ± SD (pmol/min/10^6 cells)
VCR	0.101	0.279 ± 0.155
VDS	0.250	0.343 ± 0.193
VLB	0.740	0.568 ± 0.259
NVB	1.260	0.834 ± 0.069

Table IV :
Comparison of *in vivo* clearance and *in vitro* uptake of Vincaalkaloids

between V.A. and a number of anticancer drugs currently associated with the V.A. Indeed, of the compounds tested, epipodophyllotoxins (Etoposide, Teneposide), Doxorubicine, and Lomustine are potent inhibitors of VDS and VLB biotransformation [41]. These agents may interfere with the V.A., thereby altering their metabolic processes and hence also their pharmacotoxicological activity. These findings have both fundamental and clinical implications and have to be taken into account in the safety evaluation and design of combined cancer chemotherapy regimens.

In conclusion, these data are of great importance as well as for a better understanding of the structure-activity relationships in this class of anticancer drugs as for a reliable extrapolation of *in vitro* results to the *in vivo* situation. They have made it possible to validate human *in vitro* models and have pointed to the importance of applying them as soon as possible during the development of new anticancer drugs. This approach may also identify potential ways of overcoming anticancer drug resistance, which is the major drawback in cancer chemotherapy.

Mitoxantrone: Mitoxantrone (MT) is a recent anticancer drug currently used for the treatment of metastatic breast cancer and acute leukemias [42,43]. It is an anthracenedione drug which can be compared to Doxorubicine, but its toxic side effects, particulary cardiotoxicity, are much less pronounced. All the chemical and experimental studies showed a large interindividual and interspecies variability in pharmacokinetic parameters. Moreover, by comparing two groups of patients, a group with hepatic impairment and a control group without, some authors concluded that MT administration has to be carefully monitored in the former group to avoid hematological toxicity associated with high MT plasma levels [44,45].

Numerous studies were performed to determine the main hepatic pathways for drug elimination, but little attention was paid to the importance of biotransformation. Furthermore the results of these studies are difficult to compare since they were obtained in various animal models on different biological fluids [42]. Although the urine excretion of the two main metabolites of MT (i.e. mono- and dicarboxylic acid derivatives) after I.V. injection in cancer patients [46-48] was studied, little additional information was available on humans.

The metabolism of MT was hence studied in primary cultures of hepatocytes from rat, rabbit and man [4,10,27]. Biotransformation occurred in all the species; extracellular unchanged MT levels represented around 50%, 25% and 20% of total radiolabel at 48 h, respectively. The data showed that MT was slowly but extensively metabolized to various derivatives which rapidly effluxed into the extracellular compartment. Minor interspecies variability was demonstrated in the overall biotransformation rate of the drug but large variability in the metabolic pattern was found. In the rat, only trace amounts of the mono- and dicarboxylic acid metabolites were present, the main derivatives being two polar compounds (Fig. 5). In man, only minor metabolites and mainly the mono- and di-carboxylic acid derivatives were detected. Moreover, the monocarboxylic derivate was predominant in the rabbit wheras the dicarboxylic was predominant in humans (Fig. 5). The rabbit therefore appears to be the animal species most closely related to humans in terms of MT metabolism. Furthermore, only small interindividual differences (n = 4) were observed in the biotransformation of MT by human hepatocytes.

Finally, the comparative hepatotoxicity of MT and its two main metabolites was assessed to determine the influence of drug metabolism on the occurrence of side effects [11]. Cytotoxicity tests, evaluated as impairment of 3-(4,5-dimethylthiazol-2-yl)-diphenyl tetrazolium bromide (MTT) biotransformation and neutral red (NR) incorporation [49], demonstrated the importance of adding carboxylic acid (one or two groups) in decreasing the toxicity (Fig. 6). Indeed, whatever the test used and the exposure-time, metabolites were always found to be less toxic than the parent compound (Table V).

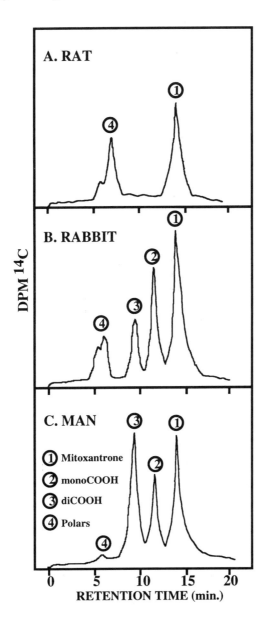

Figure 5:
HPLC analysis of [14]C Mitoxantrone and its metabolites in the extracellular medium after exposure of primary cultures of hepatocytes isolated from rat, rabbit and man [10].
Substrate concentration of Mitoxantrone was 5 µM.
Incubation time period was 12 h.

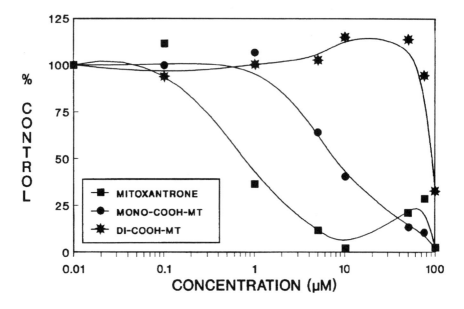

Figure 6:
In vitro cytotoxicity of Mitoxantone and its two main metabolites, as determined by MTT reduction in human hepatocytes after 48 h exposure.

These findings on MT underscore another interesting aspect of cultured hepatocytes, in particular human ones: one can measure metabolism and toxicity simultaneously. By using specific metabolic inhibitors and by studying the toxicity of individual metabolites, one can further study the role of xenobiotic metabolism in toxicity.

Conclusion

The results shown here for psychotropic and anticancer agents together with the data obtained in our laboratory for other therapeutic families (immunosuppressive agents [27], digitalics [50], antiviral drugs [51]...) allow us to make a number of general conclusions concerning the potential of these *in vitro* tools in facilitating drug discovery and development processes, and on *in vivo/in vitro* relationships in general. Used in combination with the most advanced analytical techniques, these hepatic models provide a very rapid and efficient means of: 1/ determining the animal species that metabolically most ressembles man; 2/ assessing

	NR test		MTT test	
	24 h	48 h	24 h	48 h
MT	7.4	2	6.8	0.39
Monocarboxylic MT	80.0	7.8	90.0	9.80
Dicarbocylic MT	90.0	80.0	95,0	95.0

Table V :
IC_{50} values (µM) obtained after 24 and 48 h of exposure of human hepatocytes to MT and its two main metabolites[11]

the duration of drug action, particularly those drugs exhibiting different metabolic clearances; 3/ explaining the structure pharmacokinetics properties within a same therapeutic family ; 4/ elucidating the metabolic origin of interindividual variability in drug response and toxicity; and 5/ predicting drug interactions. The application of such systems to drug design may greatly enhance the rational design of safe and effective drugs allowing savings in cost, time, test materials as well as minimizing the use of animals.

The use of human hepatocytes offers considerable advantages which cannot be obtained with animals *in vivo*: namely the availbility of human data before the performance of clinical trials. However, a major problem exists with regard to obtaining human hepatocytes on a regular basis; because of the increasing development and success of organ transplantation, adequate amounts of fresh normal liver portions are becoming rare. This has led to vigorous attempts to find suitable methods for human hepatocyte storage until they can be conveniently used for further *in vitro* studies. The only conceivable method of acheiving long term storage of these cells and their regular supply appears to be cryopreservation.

We concentrated on procedures for cryopreserving hepatocytes with the knowledge that large numbers are needed for studies on the metabolism and toxicity of xenobiotics [7]. The results show that reproducible freeze/thaw protocols can be used to store human hepatocytes for several years. After thawing, a large fraction of the cells are still able to survive and retain membrane integrity and protein synthesis functions, as well as the major phase I and phase II metabolic activities [6,7,11]. Indeed, benzodiazepines, digoxin and zidovudine, which used as diagnostic substrates for the characterization of human hepatocytes, were equally biotransformed in fresh and cryopreserved cells. However, multicenter studies with a large set of parameters representative of the main hepatic functions should be conducted to optimize and more extensively validate this promising approach.

Hepatocyte storage procedures should contribute significantly to the efficient use of human and higher mammalian species hepatocytes as models for the study of relationships between structure, metabolism, pharmacokinetics and toxicokinetics, thereby providing a more rational selection criteria for the safety assessment of candidate drugs.

References

1. Guillouzo A. and Guguen-Guillouzo A. Isolated and Cultured hepatocytes. Editions INSERM, Paris and John Libbey Eurotext, London, 1986.
2. Chenery R.J. The utility of hepatocytes in drug metabolism studies. In: Progress in drug metabolism (Gibson G.G., ed.), Taylor and Francis, London, 1988:217-265.
3. Guillouzo A. Liver Cells and Drugs, Editions INSERM, Paris and John Libbey Eurotext, London, 1988.
4. Cano J.P., Rahmani R., Fabre G., Richard B., Lacarelle B., Bore P., Bertault-Peres P., de Sousa G., Fabre I., Placidi M., Coulange C., Ducros M. and Rampal M. Human hepatocytes as an alternative model to the use of animal in experiments. In: Liver cells and Drugs (Guillouzo A., ed.), Editions INSERM, Paris and John Libbey Eurotext, London, 1988;164:301-307.
5. Cano J.P., Rahmani R., Lacarelle B., Fabre G., Bore P., Richard B., de Sousa G., Bertault-Peres P., Sengewald I. and Placidi M. Evaluation of hepatic transport and metabolism of drugs, using cellular and subcellular animal and human models. In: Recent Trends in Clinical Pharmacology (Strauch G. and Morselli P.L., eds.), INSERM, PARIS, 1988;168:33-58.
6. Rahmani R., de Sousa G., Lacarelle B., Rahmani-Jourdheuil D., Placidi M. and Catalin J. Use of human hepatic cellular and subcellular models for assessing drug transport, biotransformation and toxicity. In: Man and the laboratory animal: perspectives for 1992, (Fondation Merieux, ed.), Lyon, 1990:539-543.
7. Dou M., de Sousa G., Lacarelle B., Placidi M., Lechene De La Porte P., Domingo M., Lafont H. and Rahmani R. Thawed human hepatocytes in primary culture. Cryobiology 1992;29:454-469.
8. Fabre G., Rahmani R., Placidi M., Combalbert J., Covo J., Cano J.P., Coulange C., Ducros M. and Rampal M. Characterization of Midazolam using human hepatic microsomal fractions and hepatocytes in suspension obtained by perfusing whole human livers. Biochemical Pharmacology 1988;37:4389-4397.

9. Zhou X.J., Martin M., Placidi M., Cano J.P. and Rahmani R. In vivo and in vitro pharmacokinetics and metabolism of Vincaalkaloids in rats - Part II: Vinblastine and Vincristine. European Journal of Drug Metabolism and Pharmacokinetics 1990;15:323-332.
10. Richard B., Fabre G., de Sousa G., Fabre I., Rahmani R. and Cano J.P. Interspecies and inter-individual variabilities in Mitoxantrone metabolism using primary-culture of hepatocytes from rat, rabbit and human. Biochemical Pharmacology 1991;41:255-262.
11. de Sousa G., Dou M., Barbe D., Lacarelle B., Placidi M. and Rahmani R. Freshly isolated or cryopreserved human hepatocytes in primary-culture : influence of drug metabolism on hepatotoxicity. Toxicology in Vitro 1991;5:483-486.
12. Van Der Hoven T.A. and Coon M.J. Preparation and properties of partially purified cytochrome P450 and reduced nicotinamide adenine dinucleotide phosphate P450 reduced from rabbit liver microsomes. Journal of Biological Chemistry 1974;249:6302-6310.
13. Lacarelle B., Marre F., Blanc-Gauthier T., Zhou X.J., Placidi M., Catalin J. and Rahmani R. Use of human and animal liver microsomes in drug metabolic studies. European Journal of Drug Metabolism and Pharmacokinetics 1992;3:458-465.
14. Lacarelle B., Rajaonarison J.F., Gauthier T., Placidi M., Catalin J. and Rahmani R. Use of a human liver microsome bank in drug glucuronidation studies. Toxicology in Vitro 1991;5:559-562.
15. Bohacek N., Ravic M. and Biziere K. A double-blind comparison of Minaprine and Imipramine in the treatment of depressed patients. Journal of Clinical Psychopharmacology 1986;6:320-321.
16. Jouvent R., Lancrenon S., Patay M., Biziere K. and Widlocher D. A controlled study of Minaprine versus placebo in inhibited depressed outpatients. In: Minaprine, a New Psychotropie Drug Active in Affective Disorders (Dugay K. and Mandel P., eds.), Montpellier, Sanofi Recherche, 1984:33-40.
17. Mikus P., Biziere K. and Bentel U. A controlled study of Minaprine and Nomifensine in outpatients with masked depression. Clinical Trials Journal 1985;22:477-488.
18. Radmayr E., Biziere K. and Bentel U. Minaprine and Maprotiline in endogenous depression. A double-blind controlled study. Clinical Trials Journal 1986;23:100-109.
19. Passeri M., Cucinotta D., De Mello M. and Biziere K. Comparison of Minaprine and placebo in the treatment of Alzheimer's disease and multi-infarct dementia. International Journal of Geriatric Psychiatry 1987;2:97-103.
20. Davi H., Dupont P., Jeanniot J.P., Roncucci R. and Cautrells W. The biotransformation of ^{14}C Minaprine in man and five animal species. Xenobiotica 1981;11:735-747.
21. Fong M.H., Abbiati A., Benfenati E. and Caccia S. Quantitative analysis of Minaprine and some of its metabolites with application to kinetic studies in rats. Journal of Chromatography 1983;259:141-149.

22. Lacarelle B., Marre F., Durand A., Davi H. and Rahmani R. Metabolism of Minaprine in human and animal hepatocytes and liver microsomes. Prediction of metabolism in vivo. Xenobiotica 1991;21:317-329.
23. Marre F., Fabre G., Lacarelle B., Bourrie M., Catalin J., Berger Y., Rahmani R. and Cano J.P. Involvement of the cytochrome P450IID subfamily in Minaprine 4-hydroxylation by human hepatic microsomes. Drug Metabolism and Disposition 1992; 20:316-321.
24. Amrein R. and Leishman B. The importance of pharmacokinetic data for clinical practice. In: Benzodiazepines Today and Tomorrow. (Priest RG., Vianna Filho U., Amrein R. and Skreta M., eds.), Lancaster, 1980:61-75.
25. Amrein R., Eckert M., Haefeli H. and Leishman B. Pharmacokinetic and clinical considerations in the choice of an hypnotic. British Journal of Clinical Pharmacology 1983;16:5-10.
26. Gerecke M. Chemical structure and properties of Midazolam compared with other benzodiazepines. British Journal of Clinical Pharmacology 1983;16:11-16.
27. Rahmani R., Richard B., Fabre G. and Cano J.P. Extrapolation of preclinical pharmacokinetic data to therapeutic patterns. Xenobiotica 1988;18:71-88.
28. Klotz U., Antonin K.H. and Bieck P.R. Pharmacokinetics and plasma binding of Diazepam in man, dog, rabbit, guinea pig and rat. Journal of Pharmacology and Experimental Therapeutics 1976;199:67-73.
29. Van der Kleijn E., Possum J.M., Muskens E.T.J.M. and Rijntjes N.V.M. Pharmacokinetics of Diazepam in dogs, mice and humans. Acta Pharmacologica and Toxicologica 1971;3:109-127.
30. Boxenbaum H. Comparative pharmacokinetics of benzodiazepines in dog and man. Journal of Pharmacokinetics and Biopharmaceutics 1982;10:411-425.
31. Crevat-Pisano P., Dragna S., Granthil C., Coassolo P., Cano J.P. and Francois G. Plasma concentrations and pharmacokinetics of Midazolam during anesthesia. Journal of Pharmaceutical Pharmacology 1986;38:578-582.
32. Vree T.B, Baars A.M., Booij L.H.D. and Driessen J.J. Silmultaneous determination and pharmacokinetics of Midazolam and its metabolites in plasma and urine of man and dog by means of HPLC. Arzneimittel Forschung Drug Research 1981;31:2215-2219.
33. Gesher A. and Neweel D.R. The role of pharmacokinetic and metabolism studies in anticancer drug discovery and development. In: Progress in drug metabolism (Gibson G.G., ed.), Taylor and Francis, London-Washington DC, 1992:263-294.
34. Zhou X.J. and Rahmani R. Preclinical and clinical pharmacology of Vincaalkaloids. Drugs 1992;44:1-16.
35. Rahmani R., Barbet J., Martin M. and Cano J.P. Radioimmunoassay and preliminary pharmacokinetic studies of 5'-noranhydrovinblastine (Navelbine). Cancer Research 1984;44:5609-5613.
36. Rahmani R., Martin M., Favre R., Cano J.P. and Barbet J. Clinical pharmacokinetics of Vindesine: repeated treatments by intravenous bolus injections. European Journal of Cancer and Clinical Oncology 1984;20:1409-1417.

37. Rahmani R., Gueritte F., Martin M., Just S., Cano J.P. and Barbet J. Comparative pharmacokinetics of antitumor Vinca-alkaloids : intravenous bolus injections of Navelbine and related alkaloids to cancer patients and rats. Cancer Chemotherapy and Pharmacology 1986;16:223-228.
38. Rahmani R., Bruno R., Iliadis A., Fabre R., Just S., Barbet J. and Cano J.P. Pharmacokinetics of the antitumor drug Navelbine (5'-noranhydrovinblastine) in cancer patient. Cancer Research 1987;47:5796-5799.
39. Rahmani R., Henry J.C., Bore P., Lafont H. and Cano J.P. The fate of Vindesine on isolated perfused rat liver. Journal of Cellular Pharmacology 1990;2:119-126.
40. Zhou X.J., Bore P., Monjanel S., Sahnoun Z., Favre R., Durand A. and Rahmani R. Pharmacokinetics of Navelbine (5'-noranhydrovinblastine) after oral administration in cancer patients. Cancer Chemotherapy and Pharmacology 1991;29:66-70.
41. Zhou X.J., Zhou-Pan X.R., Gauthier T., Placidi M., Maurel P. and Rahmani R. Human liver microsomal cytochrome P4503A isoenzymes mediated vindesine biotransformation: metabolic drug interactions. Biochemical Pharmacology 1993;45:853-861.
42. Smith I.E. Mitoxantrone (Novantrone): A review of experimental and early clinical studies. Cancer Treatment Review 1983;10:103-115.
43. Shenkenberg T.D. and Von Hoff. Mitoxantrone: a new anticancer drug with significant activity. Annals of Internal Medecine 1986;105:67-81.
44. Savaraj N., Lu K., Valdiviesco M. and Loo T.L. Pharmacology of Mitoxantrone in cancer patients. Cancer Chemotherapy and Pharmacology 1985;45:1879-1884.
45. Chlebowski R.T., Tong M. and Woodward D.L. Mitoxantrone administration in patients with hepatic dysfunction. In: Advances in Cancer Chemotherapy, The Current Status of Novantrone (Coltment C.A. Jr., ed.), Washington DC, 1985:23-28.
46. Ehninger G., Proksh B., Heinzel G. and Woodward D.L. Clinical pharmacology of Mitoxantrone. Cancer Treatment Reports 1986;70:1373-1378.
47. Chiccarelli F.S., Morrison J.A., Cosulich D.B., Perkinson N.A., Ridge D.N., Sum F.W., Murdock K.C., Woodward D.L. and Arnold E.T. Identification of human urinary Mitoxantrone metabolites. Cancer Research 1986;46:4858-4861.
48. Payet B., Arnoux P., Catalin J. and Cano J.P. Direct determination of Mitoxantrone and its mono- and dicarboxylic acid metabolites in plasma and urine by high-performance liquid chromatography. Journal of Chromatography 1988;424:337-345.
49. Fautrel A., Chesne C., Guillouzo A., de Sousa G., Placidi M., Rahmani R., Braut F., Pichon J., Hoellinger H., Vintezou P., Diarte I., Melcion C., Cordier A., Lorenzon G., Benicourt M., Vannier B., Fournex P., Peloux AF., Bichet N., Gary D., Cano J.P. and Lounes R. A multicentre study of acute *in vitro* cytotoxicity in rat liver cells. Toxicology in Vitro 1991; 5:543-547.
50. Lacarelle B., Rahmani R., de Sousa G., Durand A., Placidi M. and Cano J.P. Metabolism of Digoxin, digoxigenin-digitoxosides and digoxigenin in human hepatocytes and liver microsomes. Fundamental and Clinical Pharmacology 1991;5:567-582.

51. Rajaonarison J.F., Lacarelle B., de Sousa G., Catalin J. and Rahmani R. *In vitro* glucuronidation of 3'-azido-3'-deoxythymidine by human liver : role of UDP-glucuronosyl transferase 2 isoform. Drug Metabolism and Disposition 1991;19:809-815.

8

Human models for the *in vitro* assessment of neurotoxicity

C.K. Atterwill and W.M. Purcell

The CellTox Centre, Division of Biosciences, University of Hertfordshire, College Lane, Hatfield, Herts, AL10 9AB (UK)

General introduction

Having seen considerable development of animal cell culture systems for use in neurotoxicity testing, particularly for central nervous system (CNS) hazard assessment and toxicity, it is now expected that there will be some focus on the use of human cell systems with particular reference to the risk assessment process in Research and Development (R & D). In this chapter, emphasis will be placed upon cell culture systems for evaluating the effects of repeated exposure to xenobiotics in live, intact cells, rather than on the use of the many subcellular *ex vivo* preparations (such as synaptosomes, brain slices, etc) used in the past. Many extensive and up to date reviews exist on these preparations and their use in pharmacology, toxicology and drug development, e.g. for studying drug-receptor interactions and screening.

In addition to the common ethical considerations placed on the source and use of human tissues for neurotoxicological purposes, additional health and safety factors apply to tissue of neural origin. The transmission of various 'slow viruses', e.g. Creutzfeldt-Jakob disease, is of considerable importance, especially since the neuropathology of many neurodegenerative disorders is still unknown.

In the first sections, the general principles applying to models for neurotoxicological testing will be described, the advantages and disadvantages, and future prospects. The categories of cell culture models using animal tissues equally apply to human models (see Table I) and, therefore, examples of developments in these categories will be described from the recently published literature. Lastly, some emphasis will be placed on the status of a tiered *in vitro* model currently under preliminary validation in our laboratories using predominantly non-human materials. The methods for the preparation of these cell culture systems will be similar for both types of tissue and hopefully the tiered model will integrate relevant human cell models in future validation phases. With respect to this last possibility, some of our work on a human mast cell model for studying aspects of neurotoxicity and neuroimmunotoxicity in relation to neurotrophic factors will be covered in some detail.

Background

There is increasing awareness of the need to protect and enhance the quality of human life and to better protect the environment against the effects of human activities of all kinds.

This is reflected in many current developments, not least in new, proposed or revised legislation, for example, on agricultural chemicals and consumer products, on new drugs, on the assessment of existing industrial chemicals in use before current legislation came into force, and disposal of waste materials.

These initiatives could result in more toxicity testing in animals, but at the same time, there are also legal requirements, and public expectation, that laboratory animal use should progressively be reduced, refined and replaced. Hence it is important that non-animal, (i.e. alternative) methods become available, particularly when their introduction and use can be justified on scientific grounds, as well as in the interests of animal welfare.

The evolution of alternative methods is a gradual process, which must involve proper development within the laboratories of origin, thorough interlaboratory validation for scientific reproducibility and reliability, and independent assessment of relevance and suitability for use in 'real-world' situations.

Due to the recent importance and recognition of neurotoxicity testing as an important issue in xenobiotic safety assessment procedures, new and extended *in vivo* testing procedures have been proposed, for

Type	Further detail	Advantages & disadvantages
Dispersed cell lines (includes 'Micromass' type)	<u>Primary dispersed</u> Monolayer - Mixed or enriched in neurones, astrocytes, oligogendrocytes <u>Secondary dispersed</u> Derived from above or cell lines, out-growths from explants	Good reproducibility and large quantities. Can perform single cell electrophysiology. Differentiation occurs but can dedifferentiate over time. Often not organotypic
Tumorigenic cell lines	Monolayer - neuroblastoma, Schwannoma & glioma	Large quantities of uncontaminated cell types but dedifferentiated
Organotypic explants	'Lying drop' type. Different CNS regions	Good cytoarchitectural preservation for morphological studies. Not all CNS areas possible yet. Fairly specialised technique.
Whole organ explants	PNS autonomic ganglia	Can culture more 'mature' cells. Limited quantities.
Whole embryo culture	Usually rat	Very specialised technique; intact foetal metabolism & near normal brain development. Resource intensive and only narrow development period defined.
Rotation - mediated aggregation cultures	Organotypic 'suspension' cultures	Organotypic cell - association and neurochemical characteristics. Highly reproducible; morphological assessment possible; can culture larger quantities of tissue. Uses many foetuses.

Table I :

Nervous system culture types

example, under the new Environmental Protection Agency (USEPA) guidelines. Of equal importance is the development of *in vitro* alternative tests, which have long been valued for their contribution into mechanistic neurotoxicology.

The newness of this exciting field, and the number of possible combinations of different *in vitro* neurobiological systems (developed over the years by prestige neurobiology groups) now makes it possible to initiate and evolve a useful alternative testing model for potential neurotoxins as described above without the biases and problems encountered in many other fields of alternative toxicity testing.

In vitro *techniques in relation to general neurotoxicology*

Alternative methods in neurotoxicology. The objective of all toxicological development work is to prevent or minimise suffering, both animal and human, by eliminating unsuitably toxic agents from widespread use. Neurotoxicity presents a particular problem from the human point of view, because detection of the complex and diverse actions of neurotoxicants frequently requires the sensitivity and complexity of whole animal systems. The concept of safe threshold levels is particularly difficult in central nervous system (CNS) toxicity, owing to the potential for cumulative damage over long periods in irreplaceable neuronal tissue. This also has implications for the consequences of seemingly reversible pharmacological effects, which may have an irreversible action if elicited during CNS development (e.g. lead effects on synaptogenesis). Furthermore, although neurotoxic effects have the general advantage of low spontaneous incidence (c.f. cancer), they can often be very difficult to detect and quantify.

Another difficulty occurs when neurotoxicity is not associated with cell death (which many alternative *in vitro* techniques are designed to detect), but is manifest as some form of disturbance or loss of specialised cellular functions. This represents a particular problem for *in vitro* studies. Consideration should also be given to the fact that neurotoxicity may involve interactions among different CNS cell types or may require metabolism of the toxicants (within the CNS, by the liver or elsewhere). Many neurotoxic agents also show marked cellular and regional specificity of action within the nervous system [29,53]. In some cases, there may also be additional species and/or age-dependent specificity. These variations increase the difficulty of detecting such effects by using alternative systems. The limitations of the number and type of human *in vitro* 'live' cell systems available for neural work add to this difficulty.

The elimination of potential neurotoxins early in commercial, developmental screening by judicious use of *in vitro* methods, and the use of efficient and sensitive assessment methods during subsequent *in vivo* testing, are the main routes for progress. The potential cellular targets using *in vitro* models for neurotoxicity screening (in addition to factors common to all cells, such as genotoxicity) include:

1) interaction with specific neurotransmitter systems and their receptors, storage organelles, release processes, uptake transport carriers and metabolising enzymes;

2) interaction with the specialised cytoskeleton e.g. neurofilaments, microtubules;

3) interaction with specialised ion channels and second messenger systems.

With reference to the above criteria, we are currently evaluating a primary non-neuronal *in vitro* cell model, namely mast cells derived from human and rodent tissues, for possible inclusion in Phase III of our tiered model for neurotoxicity testing. The association of mast cells with nerves [46,84], their interrelationship with neurotrophic factors [2,48,61] and neuropeptides [19,49,51] is well documented and further details concerning this neuroimmune axis are being explored in our laboratories and others [62,67]. Mast cells manufacture and secrete biogenic amines [56] and possess active uptake mechanisms and metabolising enzymes for a range of amines [57]. The secretory response and post-secretory events outlined in mast cells also share many of the characteristics of neurotransmitter systems [58,59]. Hence, such a non-neuronal model may be a suitable target for studies evaluating the neurotoxic potential of a range of xenobiotics acting on the central and peripheral nervous system.

Progress in neurotoxicological applied research. In general, existing toxicological legislation provides a mandatory framework for the identification of potential hazards associated with the use of a particular chemical product. More specifically, legislators in the USA and Europe are becoming concerned over the need to identify chemicals with target organ specificity, such as those which have diverse effects on the nervous system, i.e. neurotoxicants. Neurotoxicants are defined as chemical compounds which can elicit dose-dependent, sustained changes in structure and/or function of the nervous system. Within the functional effects, there may be associated behavioural disturbances, i.e. neurobehavioural effects [4,75]. Even with such a broad definition, the actual number of chemicals known or suspected of being neurotoxic is relatively small [4,17,70] From such a small database, it is difficult to predict the neurotoxicological potential of a novel, or previously untested chemical, unless there is great structural similarity with the neurotoxic moiety of a known neurotoxin, as may be the case with some of the alkylketone solvents, organophosphorus biocides and excitotoxins [38,70].

It is apparent that some form of structured screening programme is needed. Neurotoxicological screening guidelines do exist for industrial chemicals (Federal Register, 1985) and those for agrochemicals are under active discussion. The principles and practices involved in screening for neurotoxicity have been reviewed by Gad [22]. At present they all involve *in vivo* procedures (see Appendix).

Considerable progress has been made in developing *in vitro/ex vivo* alternatives in neurotoxicity testing since the original 'Fund for Replacement of Animals in Medical Experiments' (FRAME) 1983 report. In that report, it was stressed that no single 'all-embracing' test for neurotoxicity was conceivable in the future, because of the complexities of the nervous system in terms of structure, function and response. This view remains largely unchanged but a viable place now exists in an *in vivo/in vitro* testing strategy. This is worth remembering in the context of the differing structures, functions and responses of the central, peripheral and neuroendocrine neural systems, where often one system is chosen, for technical or ethical reasons, to predict the response of another. For example, our proposed use of mast cells in mechanistic toxicity studies of potential neurotoxicants for human risk assessment purposes.

Because of the complexity of the nervous system in vertebrates, it is also still generally accepted that it is unrealistic to try and develop a single, all-embracing *in vivo* 'neurotoxicity' test [86]. Accordingly, *in vivo* neurotoxicity assessment has evolved into the development of a package or battery of complementary procedures, i.e. neurophysiological, neuropathological and neurobehavioural evaluations combined in various ways to constitute a test battery in a laboratory animal model system. The test battery combination has to be able: 1) to differentiate chemicals which are neurotoxic from those which cause some other form of toxicity; 2) to classify the type and severity of neurotoxicant-induced damage, and 3) to provide a no observed effect level (NOEL) for those chemicals which require regulatory submission and have to undergo an appropriate hazard evaluation procedure. These data are best for detecting neurological and neurobehavioural abnormalities. Confirmation that a chemical is neurotoxic can be approached via appropriate neuropathology. A Step II test would be undertaken to classify and measure the severity of the neurotoxicant and, possibly, the effects on some aspect of specialised behaviour (e.g. on learning and memory).

Looking at this type of successful screen for *in vivo* neurotoxicological assessment, it is clear that there is considerable scope also for the application of an *in vitro* 'package' for use in a stepwise fashion. This would add to the information gained in Steps I-III of the procedure described above, and could perhaps reduce the number of *in vivo* tests required for the full evaluation of a potential neurotoxicant. It is difficult to conceive at present how, for example, an *in vitro* test (or battery of tests) could be used 'blind' at Step I. However, a properly validated *in vitro* screen may eventually serve such a purpose for a series of chemically- or pharmacologically-related compounds known to be neurotoxic. Such a stepwise screen could also be evaluated for its ability to predict neurotoxicants from among a series of totally unrelated xenobiotics.

In context, the 1991 neurotoxicity subsection of the report of the FRAME toxicity committee recommended that:

1) A range of *in vitro* neurotoxicity models should be evaluated for their suitability for inclusion in a tiered *in vitro* testing scheme for neurotoxicity, which should include organotypic cultures. The use of co-culture models incorporating xenobiotic metabolising systems should also be included in this scheme.

2) Using techniques chosen from this set, a stepwise *in vitro* neurotoxicity test battery or batteries, such as that presented in Fig. 1, should be developed. In order to validate the test battery, a list of reference chemicals should be selected. The list should include both centrally-acting and peripherally-acting neurotoxicants, especially those which possess regional specificity. Whenever possible, a neurotoxicant should be screened alongside a suitable non-neurotoxic analogue.

3) It is important to build in flexibility, so that any battery can be adapted to fit the particular needs of the pharmaceutical, chemical

and agrochemical industries. This should include an awareness of the environmental aspects of screening. For example, a stepwise screen employing mammalian model systems will clearly have priority for evaluating neurotoxic hazards to man and other mammals, whereas lower vertebrate and invertebrate systems may be useful where environmental neurotoxicity is also a consideration.

Chemically-induced changes in the nervous system which result in some degree of diffuse or regionally specific neuronal cell death, are clearly more important than those which lie in the uncertain interface between a neurotoxic response and the upper limits of the neuropharmacological range of effects. This is because the repair mechanisms in the brain and spinal cord are ineffective in bringing about complete resolution of structural damage: during the process of neurogenesis in the adult, fully differentiated CNS is largely confined to the olfactory epithelium [15]. In contrast, damage in the peripheral nervous system (PNS) can be repaired to a greater or lesser degree [24]. *In vitro* neurotoxicological techniques may thus have an additional application in studying the repair processes of either system following neurotoxic 'insult'.

A place for *in vitro* neurotoxicological tests. In recent years, *in vitro* alternatives to animal toxicity testing have been the subject of a number of working parties and symposia [24,26] including those in the area of neurotoxicity [13,30,68,80].

In addition to the established role of *in vitro* neurotoxicological methods in the investigation of mechanisms of neurotoxicity, a recurring theme is the use of these methods as some form of primary screen or prescreen. Key requirements to fulfil this expectation are that: 1) the method proposed must have a sound scientific basis (i.e. be equivalent to Step I of the *in vivo* screening; 2) recognition of a realistic neurotoxicological endpoint relevant to potential human responses must be possible; 3) the method must be thoroughly validated using a number of neurotoxicants which target different regions of the nervous system, and 4) the validated system must be shown to have a high predictive value. At the present time, no single *in vitro* neurotoxicity test or package of tests has been adequately evaluated and validated [25]. Also, when developing *in vitro* neurological models, different strategies must be adopted for the PNS and CNS.

In the 1983 FRAME report, emphasis was placed on the development of

In vitro neurotoxicity testing and human models

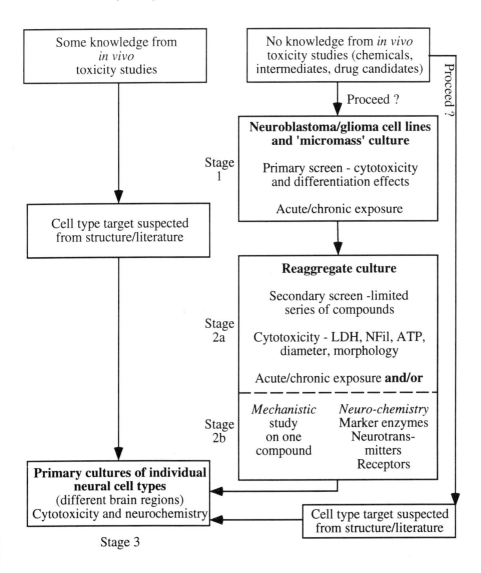

Figure 1:
A 'stepwise' scheme for *in vitro* neurotoxicity testing

suitable organotypic *in vitro* tissue culture models of the nervous system. Since then, much progress has been made, both in mechanistic neurotoxicology and in devising potential prescreening strategies for use in industry. These mostly involve culture systems derived from the mammalian CNS, with use of invertebrate and lower vertebrate models. The development of suitable human models are important areas for future research.

Recent progress, regulatory acceptance and future advances. Up to the time of the first FRAME report, i.e. in the late 1970s, most emphasis was placed on the use of *ex vivo/in vitro* models in neurotoxicological investigation. Examples included synaptosomes, brain slices and freshly-isolated neurones and glia, and these still serve as a useful adjunct in mechanistic toxicology, even where the more sophisticated culture systems described below have taken the lead. The increasing interest in both *in vitro* invertebrate and mammalian tissue culture models is re-emphasised in the proceedings of recent meetings of the Industrial *In vitro* Toxicology Society in the UK [13] and the recent book on the topic edited by Goldstein & Shahar [26]. The general interest in investigative neurotoxicology is also indicated by the growth of the International Neurotoxicology Association (INA).

Heightened regulatory awareness in the field has led to 'tighter' proposals in the form of EPA/TOSCA guidelines for both defining and maximising the information required from *in vivo* neurotoxicity tests in different species and in defining those tests which can be 'built into' standard/routine toxicity testing protocols. For example, in the case of the organophosphate insecticides, *in vivo* neuropharmacological measurements in the chicken are combined with information from *ex vivo* measurements of brain neurotoxic esterase (NTE) activity. More recently (see below) the FRAME toxicity committee has made specific and pragmatic proposals relating to the development of alternative neurotoxicity tests.

Classification of neurotoxicants

In vitro neural systems can be predictive for neurotoxicity, exceptions being cases where, for example in the CNS, xenobiotics act primarily by directly affecting blood-brain-barrier 'integrity'. In general, because of the anatomical and functional complexity of the nervous system, culture systems have been largely used in mechanistic studies where the neurochemical changes underlying *in vivo* and behavioural phenomena are further investigated *in vitro*. There are currently six acceptable classifications for neurotoxicants according to cell type and nervous system area primarily affected [87]. It is clear then, that when interpreting *in vitro* data from mechanistic investigations or developing *in vitro* models as neurotoxicological 'prescreens', much attention must be paid to both the validation of the proposed test system and to the behavioural, pathological and neurochemical correlates of neurotoxicity in the whole animal model.

Choice of end points

The wide range of *in vitro* systems presently employed in neurobiological studies is available for use in neurotoxicological investigations although often, as in the former, the choice of system is usually an arbitrary one. Careful consideration must first be given to the chosen indicators of toxicity which can include cellular viability/death, indicators of mitochondrial and lysozomal activity, lipoperoxidation and generation of reactive species, generic cell functions (such as respiration, ion transport, protein and DNA turnover), differentiated cell functions (e.g. axonal transport, synaptogenesis, myelination, enzyme activities, neurotransmitter function), and lastly, toxicant characteristics (such as accumulation, release and metabolism by the neural cells). The development of early and cell-specific indicators of the reaction of neuronal cells and astroglial cells to neurotoxicant through e.g. neurone-specific enolase (NSE) [74] and glial fibrillary acidic protein (GFAP) [44] changes respectively are of great interest.

Problems with in vivo/in vitro extrapolations in neurotoxicity testing

There are many examples of problems when predicting *in vivo* neurotoxicity from *in vitro* data [26]. For example, in the case of carbon disulphide, CNS toxicity may occur after high dose exposure whereas peripheral neuropathy occurs following long-term, low-dose exposure. This highlights the problem of using a single *in vitro* model derived from either the CNS or PNS to predict an *in vivo* neurotoxic effect. As for many other target organ toxicities metabolic factors are always extremely important. In the case of the well known dopaminergic neurotoxin, 1-Methyl-4-phenyl-1,2,3,6-tetrahydropyridine (MPTP) the presence of glial cells are necessary in a culture system in order to produce the neurotoxic metabolite 1-Methyl-4-phenylpyridinium ion (MPP+) [88] from the parent compound. Different species vary considerably in their sensitivity to MPTP. Transport and metabolism in neural cells is of importance but of equal importance is peripheral metabolism by P450-linked enzymes (which also exist intraneurally) in the cases of e.g. carbon tetrachloride [20] and fenfluramine [66]. Another factor for consideration is that cells in neural cultures perform little neurophysiological 'work' under standard culture conditions. Consequently, procedures including excitation of nerve cells should be included in the *in vitro* test model.

Culture models available

There are many *in vitro* culture systems now available (Table I) including neural, tumour-derived cell lines, organotypic explant or reaggregation cultures, and primary monolayer cultures of individual neural cell types: neurones, astrocytes and oligodendrocytes. These are supplemented by various *ex vivo/in vitro* systems, e.g. brain slices and synaptosomes and models for study the axonal transport of proteins and e.g. relationships with peripheral axonopathies [69]. Insight has been gained in understanding organophosphate-induced delayed neuropathy (OPIDN) through the hen brain assay of neuropathy target esterase. A number of human neuroblastoma and glioma cell lines are now available and have been used to a small degree in neurotoxicological investigations. For example, the human IMR32 cell line has been used to study aspects of MPP+ and kainic acid neurotoxicity [74] and the human glioma lines (86 HG-39, 87 HG-31, etc) to examine lead and calcium effects [71]. Some cell lines express specific properties, (for example SH-5Y-5Y-cholinergic; NB69-dopaminergic) and have been used to study e.g. levodopa neurotoxic effects [43]. Primary monolayer cultures of human neural tissue have also been prepared recently from cryopreserved stocks to investigate β-amyloid-related neurotoxicological mechanisms. In some cases, HeLa cell membranes from cells transfected with glutamate receptor genes and expressing the receptor proteins have been used to delineate excitotoxicant membrane binding [16]. Furthermore, two human neuroblastoma cell lines expressing recombinant nerve growth factor receptors have been developed [64], which may be a useful model in which to assess xenobiotics which exert their neurotoxic effect via interaction with nerve growth factor (NGF) or its receptors. From the culture models much success has been achieved using the organotypic explant culture type [85] for example when studying excitatory amino acid - B-N-oxalylamino-L-alanine (BOAA) & B-N-methylamino-L-alanine (BMAA) -induced neurotoxicity. Organotypic brain reaggregation cultures have been successfully used in our own laboratories to study various cholinotoxic mechanisms and there is now one report of a neurotoxicological investigation with this type of culture on the anti-HIV drug trichosthanthin [55].

Brain reaggregate cultures. Rotation-mediated aggregating cultures constructed from single cell suspensions of foetal brain have provided much valuable information regarding the neurobiological and neuropharmacological aspects of the developing brain [7]. The cells within these organotypic cultures change from a population of undifferentiated neuroepithelial cells to an integrated population of differentiated neurones, astrocytes and oligodendroglia organised in a spherical structure of 200-500 mm in diameter [7,23] Dendritic and axonal growth, and synaptogenesis peak at 21-30 days *in vitro*, myelination occurs and cell division is restricted, and aspects of neural development in the cultures are as dependent upon thyroid hormone (L-T_3) as they are *in vivo* [14].

Developmental neurotoxicants in vitro

There is now an increasing number of neurotoxicants with correlations between the functional 'perturbations' produced in developing organotypic brain reaggregate cultures *in vitro* and their known *in vivo* effects. These include methylmercury, cycloheximide and colchicine [32], 6-hydroxydopamine (6-OHDA) and the tricyclic antidepressants [39], and ascorbic acid [77]. With respect to cholinergic neurones the list includes kainic acid [77], the organophosphorus compounds [81] and in our own laboratory, ethylcholine mustard aziridinium (ECMA) and aluminium [10,50].

No formal distinction has been made in these studies between developmental and non-developmental neurotoxins as most *in vitro* culture models employ tissue derived from foetal nervous systems and data are often extrapolated to predict 'adult' neurotoxic potential. Certain models, however, such as the brain reaggregates do allow a fine comparison of exposure at different developmental stages because of their 'longevity'. Furthermore, experimentally differentiated neural cell lines can be used to predict toxicity on mature nerve cells. This information for the adult response can be supplemented for human risk-

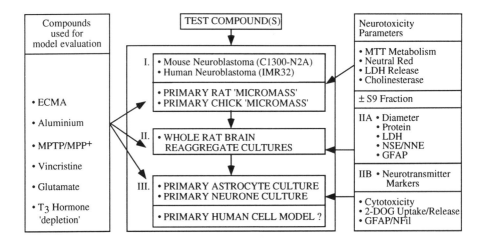

Figure 2 :
Detailed current status/plans for neurotoxicity tier testing *in vitro*.

assessment with data from e.g. neurotoxicant-exposed human cells, such as mast cells [33,61,62].

A 'tiered' neurotoxicity test in vitro?

A 'tiered' or stepwise *in vitro* CNS neurotoxicity testing procedure was recently proposed by Atterwill [8] where the first stage screen involved neurotoxicant exposure in neural cell lines or in the brain 'micromass' culture model. This will be followed by second-phase testing in a proven organotypic system such as the whole-brain reaggregate cultures for investigation of time-course, specificity and mechanism of neurotoxicity. A third phase would then allow more detailed information on mechanism, hazard and risk to be obtained using cell-type specific neural type cultures, alternative cellular systems such as mast cells, and human cell models. Such a scheme is depicted in simple terms in Fig. 1 & Fig. 2. A variety of neurotoxins have been tested in our laboratory using some of the models described in order to assess the feasibility of such a tiered testing screen (see Fig. 2). We have addressed issues such as the acceptability of the proposed endpoints to be determined as indicators of neurotoxicity, the necessity of time-course investigations, and the necessity for species comparisons. It is also important to evaluate the inter-relationships between general cytotoxicity and specific target organ toxicity to the nervous system, and in this respect the validation study described below has incorporated measurement of general cytotoxicity in non-neural cells into the scheme. The cholinotoxin ECMA (ethylcholine mustard aziridinium), the vinca alkaloid, vincristine, MPTP and its toxic metabolite MPP+, aluminium chloride and some glutamate receptor antagonists have now been tested in order to validate the use of the various proposed culture models described for Phase I of the tiered-test model. The data from some of these investigations and the methods employed for cell cultures and assays in Phase I are summarised in two previous publications and a final tiered testing scheme proposed to be fully evaluated in a blind trial under the auspices of FRAME (Fund for Replacement of Animals in Medical Experimentation) and an European Commission (EC) Commissioned Study [11,12]. Although no formal validation work has yet been carried out on the brain reaggregate models in Phase II, some work has been initiated with Phase III models including a primary astrocyte culture for the detection of gliotoxicity and an isolated, *in vitro* rat and human mast cell model for investigating aspects of human neurotoxicity with respect to neurotrophic factor interactions and aspects of monoamine function. In this chapter we will, therefore, describe the methods for the preparation of these cells and the applications and implications considered to date.

Mast cells as a model of neurone function for specialised aspects of neurotoxicity testing

Introduction

Mast cells have long been associated with immediate hypersensitivity reactions, concerning the interaction of allergens with cell-fixed IgE. However, it is clear that mast cells functionally respond to an enormous range of compounds via specific receptors clearly delimited from the IgE system. Of particular interest is the concept of a neuroimmune axis, in that mast cells are histologically associated with neurones and release an array of preformed and newly synthesised mediators upon challenge with neurotrophic factors, such as NGF, and neuropeptides, including substance P, neurotensin, CGRP and neuropeptide Y [19,21,48,51,61,62]. Furthermore, mast cells are implicated in the aetiology of a range of neuroinflammatory conditions, including multiple sclerosis and neurofibromas [18,65]. Overall, mast cells share many of the characteristics of central and peripheral neurones, in terms of receptors for compounds derived from neurones and glial cells, synthetic pathways for biogenic amines, such as histamine and 5-hydroxytryptamine, active uptake systems and metabolising enzymes [57,58,59]. Indeed, tricyclic antidepressants and monoamine oxidases have been shown to exert parallel effects in mast cell systems [57].

At the CellTox Centre, we are currently evaluating the potential of mast cells derived from human placental tissue and rodent tissues for inclusion as primary cell models in our tiered *in vitro* neurotoxicity screen (Phase III). Work to date has concentrated upon the interaction of NGF with mast cells, since these cells possess a high-affinity, *trk*A, receptor for NGF [54]. These studies will be expanded to elucidate the role of other neurotrophic factors in the development of neurotoxicity and those compounds which disrupt histaminergic and serotonergic transmitter pathways.

Since NGF is essential to the development and survival of populations of nerve cells in the peripheral and central nervous system [72,82], potential neurotoxicants may interact with this trophic factor and/or its receptor to produce apparent toxicity. The biological effects of NGF are initiated by binding with a specific cell receptor, which exists in two distinct forms: a high-affinity receptor, *trk*A, located primarily on neuronal cells and a low-affinity receptor, p75, located on a range of cell types and suggested to be involved in the regulation of normal cell growth [28,37,73]. At present it is not clear whether NGF needs to interact with both the *trk*A and p75 receptor to exhibit high-affinity binding or simply the *trk*A receptor alone [28,63]. It is known that rat peritoneal mast cells (RPMC) secrete histamine upon challenge with NGF [33,48] via the *trk*A receptor [54], and we have already demonstrated that certain alkylating and cholinergic neurotoxins, such as ECMA, interact with NGF and that this is measurable in the mast cell model [33].

It is worthy of note that mast cells interact with NGF at several levels and findings concerning this neuroimmune axis are intriguing. NGF induces histamine release from rat peritoneal mast cells [33,48] and synergises with other agonists in this respect [76]. NGF is involved in the differentiation of mast cells in embryo rat brain and NGF-primed spleen cells injected into the lateral ventricles of developing rat brain differentiated into mast cells [1]. Furthermore, NGF induces a systemic increase and phenotypic change in rat tissue mast cells [42], promotes the survival of rat mast cells in culture [31] and neurofibromas have been associated with systemic mastocytosis [65]. It has also been suggested that the clinical signs of toxicity observed upon subacute and subchronic dosing of mice with human recombinant NGF may reflect a direct action of mast cells, thereby releasing potent inflammatory mediators [67]. This later observation suggests a role for mast cells in immunotoxicity testing concerning neurotrophic factors. Overall, NGF therefore appears to have potent biological activities in addition to its neurotrophic effects.

We recently characterised a novel source of human mast cells, the placenta, in terms of their characteristic morphology, staining reactions and histamine secretion upon challenge with IgE- and non-IgE directed ligands [52,60,61,83]. Since it is known that human placental tissue contains a significant amount of NGF [27] and expresses the low-affinity receptor [37], we investigated whether human placental mast cells (HPMC) possess a functional receptor for NGF, measured by means of histamine secretion upon challenge with the ligand.

The ability to use a human cell model for *in vitro* screening and mechanistic toxicity testing of neurotrophic therapeutics and xenobiotics which may exert their neurotoxic effects by interaction with neurotrophic factors and/or their receptors would be a significant advantage in specialised areas of neurotoxicity and immunotoxicity.

Methods

Mast cells may be dispersed from human and animal tissues by means of a simple collagenase digestion technique, in a serum-supplemented media [60], and purified by means of counter current elutriation and density gradient centrifugation [3]. The isolation procedure does not significantly affect the biochemical or pharmacological profile of the collected cells [60]. Enzymic dispersal protocols need to be established for each tissue type, and methodologies have been published for a range of human tissues, including skin, lung and placenta [3,34,36,60,79]. In addition, mast cells may be collected by lavage of pleural or peritoneal spaces, e.g. RPMC, BAL fluid [35,56,78].

Collection of human placental mast cells. Human placentas, collected under ethical approval from the delivery suite at the East Hertfordshire Health Authority, were transported to our laboratories in large plastic boxes containing minimum essential medium Eagle (pH 7.2; MEM, Sigma) within 30 minutes of normal delivery or Caesarian section.

Placentae were washed free of excess blood in isotonic saline (0.9%, 4°C) and several cotyledons dissected out and rinsed in iced saline.

Placental cotyledons were further cleaned by frequent changes in MEM, supplemented with 2% human serum (MEM+), dissected into blocks of approximately 1.0g and the wet weight recorded. Each tissue block was chopped into small pieces (approx 1mm^3) in 5cm^3 of MEM+, a further 15cm^3 of MEM+ added and the samples incubated (15 min, 37°C) in a shaking water bath. Following centrifugation (200g, 5 min, 4°C) the supernatant was decanted and the tissue resuspended in 15cm^3 of prewarmed (37°C) digestion buffer (NaCl 137 mM, glucose 5.6mM, KCl 2.7 mM, $MgCl_2$ 0.5mM, NaH_2PO_4 0.4mM, DNase I 60mgl^{-1} (Sigma), human albumin 1.0g l^{-1} (Sigma), penicillin 1000 units l^{-1} (Sigma), streptomycin 1.0mg l^{-1} (Sigma); pH 7.2) and enzymatically dispersed (37°C, 90 min) with collagenase enzyme (1.5 mg cm^{-3}; Type 1A from *Clostridium histolyticum*; Sigma) in a shaking water bath. The concentration of collagenase used to disperse placental tissue was optimised at 1.5mg cm^{-3} following previous experiments in which the concentration of enzyme was altered in the range of 0 - 5.0mg cm^{-3}, and the number of dispersed mast cells (toluidine blue staining, 0.05%w/v), free nucleated cells and the viability (trypan blue dye exclusion) of the resultant cell suspension measured [60].

After digestion, the cell suspension was mechanically disrupted by 5 passages through a 5cm^{-3} plastic syringe and filtered through two layers of surgical gauze moistened with MEM+. Cells were washed (200g, 5 min, 4°C) once in MEM+ and twice in challenge buffer (NaCl 137 mM, HEPES 20mM, glucose 5.6mM, KCl 2.7mM, $CaCl_2$ 1.0 mM, $MgCl_2$ 0.5 mM, NaH_2OPO_4 0.4 mM; pH 7.2) and finally resuspended in challenge buffer to a volume required in the experiment.

Challenge of human placental mast cells. HPMC were exposed to varying concentrations of NGF, and the responsiveness of the cells measured as a function of histamine release. The secretory nature of the response was determined by experiments concerning the rate of the reaction, calcium dependency, effect of metabolic inhibitors and extremes of pH and temperature.

In simple release experiments, aliquots of HPMC were pre-incubated (5 min, 37°C) with phosphatidylserine (PS, 10.0µg cm^{-3}; Sigma) prior to challenge (15 min, 37°C) with NGF (0.001 - 10.0 µg cm^{-3}; Sigma 7S). The effect of calcium ions upon the reaction was investigated by omission of calcium ions from the buffer, or introduction of varying concentrations of ions during the preincubation stage with PS. Chelators, such as ethylene-diamine-tetraacetic acid (EDTA) and ethylene-glycol-bis-(beta-aminoethyl ether)-N-N'-tetraacetic acid (EGTA), were not added to the system since these compounds exert secondary effects upon mast cell function [47]. In experiments to determine the secretory nature of the response, glucose was omitted from the incubation media and cells pre-incubated (20 min, 37°C) with either 2-deoxyglucose (5 mM; Sigma) or antimycin A (1 µM; Sigma) prior to challenge with NGF in the presence of PS.

The reaction was halted after 15 minutes (37°C), or at specific time points to determine the rate of the reaction, by quenching with an excess of iced buffer (pH 7.2). Cells were centrifuged (200g, 5 mins, 4°C) and supernatants collected and assayed for the presence of histamine using the fluorometric OPT-condensate assays [6,60]. Basal histamine release was assessed in parallel processed samples, in the absence of NGF. Total amine content of the cells was determined after sonication (50 watts, 30 sec) and centrifugation (1340g, 10 mins, 4°C). Histamine release, corrected for basal output, was expressed as a percentage of total cellular histamine content.

Results

Effect of NGF upon histamine release from HPMC. NGF induced histamine release from HPMC in a concentration dependent manner, with an EC50 of 0.1µg cm^{-3} and maximal secretion of 22.3 ± 3.4% of total histamine content at 3.0µg cm^{-3} (Fig. 3). The secretory response had a half-life of approximately 2 minutes and required 10 minutes for completion of the secretory process.

Secretory nature of NGF-induced histamine release from HPMC. NGF-induced histamine from HPMC was dependent upon the presence of extracellular calcium ions (≥ 1.0 mM). Minimal histamine output was observed in the absence of added calcium ions (2.7 ± 1.3%) and in the presence of 0.1mM calcium (2.8 ± 1.1%).

Histamine release from HPMC induced by NGF was non-cytotoxic (Fig. 4) and was reduced by omission of glucose from the incubation medium (from 13.7 ± 2.3% to 6.1 ± 2.8%) and totally blocked by preincubation (20 min, 37°C) of the cells in the absence of glucose and with the metabolic inhibitors 2-deoxyglucose (5mM; 1.1 ± 0.6%) and antimycin A (1µM; 0.4 ± 0.4%).

Histamine release from HPMC induced by NGF was pH-dependent, being maximal at pH 7.2 and reduced under more acidic (pH 6.0, 4.6 ± 0.9%) and alkaline conditions (pH 8.5, 8.3 ± 1.7%). The reaction was temperature-dependent, being maximal at 37°C and reduced by extremes of temperature (21°C, 4.3 ± 2.5%; 45°C, 3.1 ± 1.2%).

Discussion

HPMC were shown to functionally respond to physiological levels of NGF in terms of a secretory response, measured in terms of histamine release. Indeed, on a molar basis, NGF is one of the most potent secretagogues so far studied. It is worthy of note, that while the EC50 established in HPMC is the same as RPMC, the maximal output of histamine from human cells is significantly less (approximately 25% compared with 70% in rat mast cells [33,48]); this is another example of

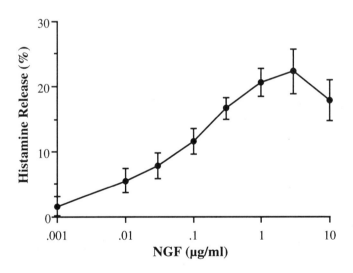

Figure 3:
Secretion of histamine from human placental mast cells in response to nerve growth factor (NGF).
Results are the mean ± SEM of duplicate observations (n=3).

mast cell heterogeneity and reinforces the importance of experiments conducted using human cells. Furthermore, this may indicate a role for NGF as a modulator of histamine release from human mast cells, since this has been established in rat mast cells [76].

While the nature of the receptor responsible for the actions of NGF on HPMC still remains to be elucidated, NGF was shown to induce secretion of histamine in a non-cytotoxic, calcium-dependent process; these results accord with studies in rat mast cells [48].

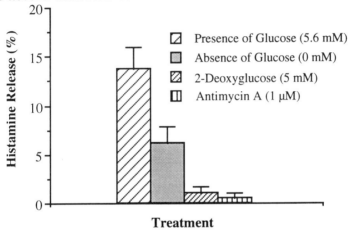

Figure 4 :
Secretory nature of histamine release from human placental mast cells in response to nerve growth factor (NGF; 0.1 µg/ml).
Results are the mean ± SEM of duplicate observations (n=3).

HPMC are suggested to provide an ideal primary *in vitro* cell model in which to assess the anaphylactoid properties of neurotrophic therapeutics. Since HPMC share many of the pharmacological properties of human skin mast cells [60], and are more readily available in quantity, these cells may be a more suitable source for toxicology studies concerning human mast cells. It has already been suggested [67] that neurotrophic therapeutics may exert immunotoxic effects in terms of inducing an anaphylactoid response; HPMC may be an ideal system in which to further study such effects and elucidate the mechanisms involved.

Furthermore, the ability to monitor the effects of xenobiotics which may exert their neurotoxic effects via interaction with NGF and/or its receptors in a human cell model, in which a functional response may be simply measured, represents a significant advantage over currently available *in vivo* models. Use of a non-neuronal model in a neurotoxicity model may appear surprising, however, mast cells display many of the functions of central and peripheral neurones, in terms of biogenic amine content, release and uptake systems and are responsive to a range of neuropeptides, such as substance P, and are often seen in close association with nerves.

Overall, the concept of a neuroimmune axis concerning mast cells and factors derived from neurones or glia validate the use of mast cells, derived from human and rodent sources, as additional models in human toxicity testing for risk assessment purposes. HPMC are suggested to provide:

1. human cells for risk extrapolation and possible inclusion in a tiered *in vitro* model for neurotoxicity testing;

2. a 'mechanistic' tool for examining the action of neurotoxins in human cells on, for example, NGF receptors;

3. a model for studying compounds affecting neural responses in human nervous tissue;

4. a model for testing potential neurotrophic therapeutics for mast cell-mediated anaphylactoid immunotoxic effects.

General Discussion & Conclusions

It is refreshing and pleasing to note at this point in time that other major bodies are recognising both the importance of neurotoxicity testing in risk-assessment and the potential usefulness of *in vitro* systems in this process. The National Research Council of the USA, Board of Environmental Studies & Toxicology, Committee on Neurotoxicology and models for assessing risk recently published (1992) their set of recommendations. Several of these recommendations have a direct bearing on the use of alternative test systems and are as follows (extracts taken from 1992 report). Recommendations (c) and (d) are worthy of special note in relation to this chapter.

(a) The committee recommends that a rational, cost-effective neurotoxicity testing strategy be developed and adopted.

(b) That studies to define mechanisms of neurotoxicity in as much detail as possible be encouraged, as well as studies to identify hazards.

(c) That putative biologic markers in animal species be evaluated and validated in *in vivo* and *in vitro* systems. The committee further recommends that biologic markers be regularly incorporated into epidemiologic and clinical studies of neurologic disease, particularly prospective studies.

(d) That existing *in vitro* test methods be exploited more extensively than at present to identify and analyze the mechanisms of neurotoxic action at cellular levels.

(e) That to improve the assessment of the human risks associated with exposure to possible neurotoxic agents, risk-assessment methods that capture the complexities of the neurologic response, including dose-time-response, logic response relationships, multiple outcomes, and integrated organ systems be developed.

One of the primary aims of the present work is to utilise relevant markers for specific neural cell types in the CNS and PNS as indicators of neurotoxicity and/or neuricidal events. With this objective in mind the Phase 1 screening models (see section below) will be used to assess for general effects using the neutral red and MTT assays whereas the Phase 2 organotypic reaggregate cultures will employ these plus more specific neural markers for neurotoxicity and neuricidal activity. In this context neuron-specific enolase (NSE) the major enolase isoenzyme found in differentiated neurones and non-neuronal enolase (NNE) the major form in mature glia and non-differentiated neurones [40,41,74] will be determined as well as neurofilament protein (NFil) and glial fibrillary acidic protein (GFAP) [44] and possibly neurotoxic esterase (NTE) activity, for the detection of those neurotoxicants causing OPIDN. With the increasing importance on the role of free radicals and oxidative stress in neurotoxicity [45] it is also considered important to investigate relevant indices for the early detection of such phenomena and to include these where appropriate.

A 'tiered' testing scheme has now been proposed utilising the original proposals of Atterwill [8,9] and preliminary validation information gained as reported in Atterwill et al [11,12]. In addition, we have new information on the potential use of a human mast cell model in Phase III of a tiered model to contribute to aspect of neurotoxicological and neuro-immunotoxicological risk assessment.

Details and validation logistics of the *in vitro* neurotoxicity tier-testing model

With all the caveats relating to extrapolation from *in vitro* models to an *in vivo* neurotoxicological risk-assessment package, an *in vitro* tier-testing model (Fig. 2) has been developed as described in the earlier sections for use as a potential prescreen for neurotoxicity of xenobiotics (pharmaceutical agents and chemicals) as a possible adjunct to *in vivo* testing strategies, and in the long-term as a potential replacement for *in vivo* testing. The use of a human cell model in this context has been addressed and described. This model is being validated under the auspices of FRAME and the EC by an interlaboratory trial co-ordinated by the CellTox Centre. The Centres involved are the Division of Biological Sciences at the University of Salford for performing aspects of the Phase III evaluation work and the Department of Human Morphology at Nottingham University for testing acute lethal potency of the validation chemicals in animal and human cell lines. Other European centres involved in the collaboration are the Department of Neurochemistry & Neurotoxicology at the University of Stockholm, Sweden, the University of Neuherberg, Germany and L'Oreal, Paris, France. All culture procedures, assays and data collection procedures have agreed written protocols. A total of forty chemicals, including different classes of known neurotoxicants plus non-toxic analogues and non-toxic general compounds will be included to be tested 'blind' in two groups of twenty compounds. It is anticipated that full results and details from this study will be known in 1994 when the data obtained from the different systems and centres will be compared with known *in vivo* data and decisions made on the usefulness and progression of this tiered model, and the future of such a test in applied *in vitro* neurotoxicology.

Acknowledgements

We are very grateful to FRAME and the EC for the research funding to establish and validate this model. Our thanks also to Dr E. Walum (University of Stockholm) and K. Atkinson (FRAME) for their help in compiling the test chemical list. Our thanks also to all the current CellTox staff involved in aspects of this work, including Dr S. Williams, Dr R. Fox and Mrs J. Davenport-Jones.

References

1. Aloe L. and De Simone R. NGF primed spleen cells injected in brain of developing rats differentiate into mast cells. International Journal of Developmental Neuroscience 1989;7:565-573.
2. Aloe L and, Levi-Montalcini R. Mast cell increase in tissues of neonatal rats injected with the nerve growth factor. Brain Research 1977;133:358-369.
3. Amon U., Ramachers U., Boggjer J. and Wolff H.H. A technique for purification of mast cells. Agents and Actions (In press).
4. Anger W.K. and Johnson B.L. Chemicals affecting behaviour. In: Neurotoxicity of Industrial and Commercial Chemicals (O'Donoghue J.L., ed.) CRC Press, Boca Raton, USA, 1985.
5. Anon. Report of the FRAME Toxicity Committee. Nottingham: FRAME, 1983.
6. Anton A.H. and Sayre D.F. A modified fluorimetric procedure for tissue histamine and its distribution in various animals. Journal of Pharmacology and Experimental Therapeutics 1969;166:285-292.
7. Atterwill C.K. Brain reaggregate cultures in neurotoxicological investigations. In: In Vitro Methods in Toxicology (Atterwill C.K. and Steele C.E., eds.), Cambridge, Cambridge University Press, 1987:133-164.
8. Atterwill C.K. Brain Reaggregate Cultures in Neurotoxicological investigations: adaptional and neuroregenerative processes following lesions. Journal of Molecular Toxicology (in press).
9. Atterwill C.K. Brain reaggregate cultures in neurotoxicological investigations: studies with cholinergic neurotoxins. ATLA 1989;6:221-230.
10. Atterwill C.K. and Collins P. Investigation of aluminium neurotoxicity using rat brain reaggregate cultures. British Journal of Pharmacology 1988;94:441p.
11. Atterwill C.K., Davenport-Jones J., Goonetilleke S., Johnston H., Purcell W.M., Thomas S.M., West M. and Williams S. New models for the *in vitro* assessment of neurotoxicity in the nervous system and the preliminary validation stages of a tiered test mode. Toxicology In Vitro (in press).
12. Atterwill C.K., Johnston H. and Thomas S.M. Models for the *in vitro* assessment of neurotoxicity in the nervous system in relation to xenobiotic and neurotrophic-factor mediated events. Neurotoxicology 1992;13:39-35.
13. Atterwill C.K. and Walum E. Neurotoxicology *in vitro*: model systems and practical applications. Toxicology in Vitro 1989;3:159-161.
14. Atterwill C.K., Kingsbury A.E. and Balazs A. Effect of thyroid hormone on neural development *in vitro*. In: Drugs and Hormones in Brain Development (Schlumpf M. and Lichtensteiger W., eds.) Karger Press, Basel, Switzerland, 1983:50-61.
15. Balls M., Riddell R. and Worden A.N. (eds.). Animals and Alternatives in Toxicity Testing. London: Academic Press, 1982.

16. Bettler B., Egebjerg J., Sharma G., Pecht G., Borgmerger I.-H., Mou C., Stevents C.F. and Heinemann S. Cloning of a putative glutamate receptor: a low affinity kainate-binding subunit. Neuron 1992;8:257-265.
17. Blum K. and Kanz L. Neurotoxicology. Marcel Dekker Inc., New York & Basel, 1985:676.
18. Bracci-Laudiero L., Aloe L., Levi-Montalcini R., Buttinelli C., Schilter D., Gillensen S. and Otten U. Multiple sclerosis patients express increased levels of β-nerve growth factor in cerebrospinal fluid. Neuroscience Letters 1992;147: 9-12.
19. Church M.K., Lowman M.A., Rees P.H. and Benyon R.C. Mast cells, neuropeptides and inflammation. Agents and Actions 1989;27: 8-16.
20. Clemedson C., Odland L. and Walum E. Differential effect of carbon tetrachloride in the cell membrane of neurons and astrocytes. Neurotoxicology and Teratology 1990;12:597-602.
21. Foreman J.C. Substance P and calcitonin gene-related peptide: effects on mast cells in human skin. International Archives of Allergy and Applied Immunology 1987;82:366-371.
22. Gad S.C. (ed.) Screening for neurotoxicity: principles and practices. Journal of the American College of Toxicology 1969;8:1-239.
23. Garber B.B. and Moscona A.A. Reconstruction of brain tissue from brain suspensions. Aggregation patterns of cells dissociated from different regions of the developing brain. Developmental Biology 1972;27:217-234.
24. Goldberg A.M. (ed.) Alternative Methods in Toxicology, Vol 3, A Progress Report from the Johns Hopkins Center for Alternatives to Animal Testing. New York: Mary Ann Leibert, 1985.
25. Goldberg A.M. (ed.) Alternative Methods in Toxicology, Vol 5, Approaches to Validation. New York: Mary Ann Leibert, 1987.
26. Goldstein A.M. and Shahar A. Model Systems in Neurotoxicology. Alternative approaches to Animal Testing. Alan R Liss Inc, 1987.
27. Goldstein L.D., Reynolds C.P. and Perez-Polo J.R. Isolation of human nerve growth factor from placental tissue. Neurochemical Research 1978;3:175-183.
28. Hempstead B.L., Martin-Zanca D., Kaplan D.R., Parada L.F. and Chao M.V. High-affinity NGF binding requires coexpression of the *trk* proto-oncogene and the low-affinity NGF receptor. Nature 1991;350:678-682.
29. Hirano A. and Henn J.F. The central nervous system as a target in toxic-metabolic states. In Experimental and Clinical Neurotoxicology (Spencer S. and Schaumburg H.H., eds.) Williams and Wilkins, Baltimore, USA, 1980:24-35.
30. Hooisma J. Tissue culture and neurotoxicology. Neurobehavioural Toxicology and Teratology 1982;4:617-622.
31. Horigome K., Lampe P.A. and Johnson E.M. Effects of NGF on rat peritoneal mast cells: survival promotion and immediate early gene induction. Society for Neuroscience (Abstract) 1992;950:401.16.
32. Jacobs A.L., Maniscalco W.M. and Finkelstein J.N. Effects of methylmercuric chloride, cycloheximide and colchicine on the reaggregation of dissociated mouse cerebellar cells. Toxicology and Applied Pharmacology 1986;86:362-371.

33. Johnston H.B. and Atterwill C.K. Nerve Growth Factor (NGF) receptors on mast cells. Effects of the cholinergic neurotoxin ethylcholine mustard aziridinium ion (ECMA). Neurotoxicology 1992;13:155-161.
34. Lawrence I.D., Warner J.A., Cohan V.L., Hubbard W.C., Kagey-Sobotka A. and Lichenstein L.M. Purification and characterisation of human skin mast cells. Journal of Immunology 1987;139:3062-3069.
35. Leung K.B.P., Flint K.C., Brostoff J., Hudspith B.N., Johnson N.M.I. and Pearce F.L. Some properties of mast cells obtained by human bronchoalveolar lavage. Agents and Actions 1986;18:110-112.
36. Lowman M.A., Rees P.H., Benyon R.C. and Church M.K. Human mast cell heterogeneity: histamine release from mast cells dispersed from skin, lung, adenoids, tonsils and colon in response to IgE-dependent and nonimmunologic stimuli. Journal of Allergy and Clinical Immunology 1988;81:590-597.
37. MacGrogan D., Saint-Andre J.P. and Dicou E. Expression of nerve growth factor and nerve growth factor receptor genes in human tissues and in prostatic adenocarcinoma cell lines. Journal of Neurochemistry 1992;59:1381-1391.
38. McGeer E.G. and McGeer D.L. Neurotoxin-induced animal models of human diseases. In: Neurotoxicology (Blum K. & Manzo L., eds.) Marcel Dekker, New York & Basel, 1985.
39. Majocha R.E., Pearse R.N., Baldersarini R.J., Delong G.R. and Walton K.G. The noradrenergic system in cultured aggregates of fetal rat brain cells: Morphology of the aggregates and pharmacological indices of noradrenergic neurones. Brain Research 1981;230:235-252.
40. Marangos P.J., Parma A.M. and Goodwin F.K. Functional properties of neuronal and glial isoenzymes of brain enolase. Journal of Neurochemistry 1978;31:727-732.
41. Marangos P.J., Schmechel D.E., Parma A.M. and Goodwin F.K. Developmental profile of neuron-specific (NSE) and non-neuronal (NNE) enolase. Brain Research 1986;190:185-193.
42. Marshall J.S., Stead R.H., McSharry C., Nielsen L. and Bienenstock J. The role of mast cell degranulation products in mast cell hyperplasia. I. Mechanisms of action of nerve growth factor. Journal of Immunology 1990;144:1886-1892.
43. Mena M.A., Pardo B., Casarejos M.J., Fahn S. and Yebenes J.G. Neurotoxicity of levodopa on catecholamine-rich neurons. Movement Disorders 1992;7:23-37.
44. O'Callaghan J.P. and Jensen C.K. Enhanced expression of glial fibrillary acidic protein and the cupric silver degeneration reaction can be used as sensitive and early indicators of neurotoxicity. In: Current Issues in Neurotoxicology (Mutti A. et al., eds.) InTox Press Inc., 1992:113-122.
45. Oliver C.N., Starke-Reed P.E., Liu G.J., Carney J.M. and Floyd R.A. Oxidative damage to brain proteins, loss of glutamine synthetase activity, and production and free radicals during ischemia/reperfusion-induced injury to gerbil brain. Proceedings of the National Academy of Sciences of the USA 1990;87:5144-5147.

46. Olsson Y. Mast cells in peripheral nerve. Acta Neurologica Scandinavica 1971;47:357-368.
47. Pearce F.L. Calcium and histamine release from mast cells. Progress in Medicinal Chemistry 1982;19:59-109.
48. Pearce F.L. and Thompson H.L. Some characteristics of histamine secretion from rat peritoneal mast cells stimulated with nerve growth factor. Journal of Physiology 1986;372:379-393.
49. Pearce F.L., Kassessinoff T.L. and Kiu W.L. Characteristics of histamine secretion induced by neuropeptides: implications for the relevance of peptide-mast cell interactions in allergies and inflammation. International Archives of Allergy and Applied Immunology 1989;88:129-131.
50. Pillar A.M., Prince A.K. and Atterwill C.K. The effect of the cholinergic neurotoxin ECMA on neuronal function in brain reaggregate cultures. Archives of Toxicology, Suppl 1987;11:243-246.
51. Piotrowski W., Devoy M.A.B., Jordan C.C. and Foreman J.C. The substance P receptor on rat mast cells and in human skin. Agents and Actions 1984;14:420-424.
52. Postyalko A., Kelly J.L. and Purcell W.M. Histochemical and immunohistochemical characterisation of human placental mast cells. Journal of Histochemistry and Cytochemistry (submitted).
53. Price D.L. and Griffin J.W. Neurons and ensheathing cells as targets of disease processes. In: Experimental and Clinical Neurotoxicology (Spencer S. and Schaumburg H.H., eds.) Williams and Wilkins, Baltimore, USA, 1980:2-23.
54. Pryor J.C., Horigome K. and Johnston E.M. Mast cells express *trk* but not low affinity nerve growth factor receptor. Soc Neurosci Abs 1992;950:401-17.
55. Pulliam L., Herndier B.G. and McGrath M.S. Purified trichosthanthin (GLQ223) exacerbation of indirect HIV-associated neurotoxicity *in vitro*. AIDS 1991;5:1237-1242.
56. Purcell W.M., Cohen D.L. and Hanahoe T.H.P. Comparison of histamine and 5-hydroxytryptamine content and secretion in rat mast cells isolated from different anatomical locations. International Archives of Allergy and Applied Immunology 1989;90:382-386.
57. Purcell W.M., Cohen D.L. and Hanahoe T.H.P. Contribution of post-secretory mechanisms to the observed pattern of histamine and 5-hydroxytryptamine secretion, from rat peritoneal mast cells in response to compound 48/80. International Archives of Allergy and Applied Immunology 1989;90:387-394.
58. Purcell W.M. and Hanahoe T.H.P. Differential release of histamine and 5-hydroxytryptamine from rat mast cells; the contribution of amine uptake to the apparent pattern of secretion. Agents and Actions 1990;30:38-40.
59. Purcell W.M. and Hanahoe T.H.P. The activity of amitriptyline as a differential inhibitor of amine secretion from rat peritoneal mast cells: the contribution of amine uptake. Agents and Actions 1990;30:41-43.
60. Purcell W.M. and Hanahoe T.H.P. A novel source of mast cells: the human placenta. Agents and Actions 1991;33:8-12.

61. Purcell W.M. and Atterwill C.K. Human placental mast cells *in vitro* possess a functional receptor for nerve growth factor. Human and Experimental Toxicology (in press).
62. Purcell W.M. and Atterwill C.K. Human mast cells as an *in vitro* model system in aspects of neuro-immunotoxicity testing. Human and Experimental Toxicology (in press).
63. Ragsdale C. and Woodgett J. trking neurotrophic receptors. Nature 1991;350:660-661.
64. Reddy U.R., Ventatakrishnan G., Roy A.K., Chen J., Hardy M., Mavilio F., Rovero G., Pleasure D. and Ross A.H. Characterisation of two neuroblastoma cell lines expressing recombinant nerve growth factor receptors. Journal of Neurochemistry 1991;56:67-74.
65. Riccardi V.M. Tuberous sclerosis and neurofibromatosis. The potential role of trauma and mast cells in the pathogenesis of neurofibromas. Elsevier, 1990:167-190.
66. Ricuarte G.A., Molliver M.E., Martello M.G. and Katz J.L. Dexfenfluramine neurotoxicity in brains of non-human primates. Lancet 1991;338:1487-1488.
67. Rogers B.C., Hardy L., Thomsen K., Nixon A. and Green J.D. Reduction in dosing frequency increases the toxicity of human recombinant nerve growth factor (rhNGF) in mice. Society of Toxicology of the USA 1993;13:397.
68. Schrier B. Nervous system cultures as toxicologic test systems. In Nervous System Toxicology (Mitchell C.L., ed.) Raven Press, New York, 1982:337-348.
69. Schwartz J.H. Synthesis and trafficking of neuronal proteins. In: Principles of Neural Science. IIIrd edition. (Kandel E. *et al.*, eds.) Elsevier 1991;4:49-65.
70. Spencer P.S. and Schaumberg H.H. Experimental and Clinical Neurotoxicology. Williams & Wilkins, Baltimore, USA, 1980.
71. Stark M., Wolff J.E.A. and Korbmacher A. Modulation of glial cell differentiation by exposure to lead and cadmium. Neurotoxicology and Neuroenterology 1992;14:247-252.
72. Thoenen H., Bandtlow C. and Heumann R. The physiological function of nerve growth factor in the central nervous system: comparison with the periphery. Reviews of Physiology Biochemistry and Pharmacology 1987;109:145-178.
73. Thoenen H. The changing scene of neurotrophic factors. Trends in Neurosciences 1991;14:165-170.
74. Thomas S.M., Hartley C.L. and Mason H.J. Effects of neurotoxins on neurone-specific enolase and lactate dehydrogenase activity and leakage in neuroblastoma cells. Toxicology In Vitro 1991;5:439-442.
75. Tilson H.A. Screening for neurotoxicity principles and practices: introduction. Journal of the American College of Toxicology 1989;8:13-18.
76. Tomioka M., Stead R.H., Nielsen L., Coughlin M.D. and Bienenstock J. Nerve growth factor enhances antigen and other secretagogue-induced histamine release from rat peritoneal mast cells in the absence of phosphatidylserine. Journal of Allergy and Clinical Immunology 1988;82:599-607.

77. Trapp B.P. and Richelson E. Usefulness for neurotoxicology of rotation mediated aggregating cell cultures. In: Experimental and Clinical Neurotoxicology (Spencer P.S. and Schaumberg H.H., eds.) Williams and Wilkins, Baltimore/London, 1980:803-819.
78. Valdez Y.E. and Lehnert B.E. A procedure for instilling agents into the pleural space compartment of the rat without co-administration into the lung compartment. Animal Techniques 1988;39:1-8.
79. Van Overveld F.J. Some aspects of mast cell subtypes from human lung tissue. Fisons Cara Service, 1988.
80. Vernadakis A., Davies D.L. and Gremok F. Neural culture: a tool to study cellular neurotoxicity. In: Neurotoxicology (Blum K. and Manzo L., eds.), Marcel Dekker Inc., New York & Basel, 1985.
81. Wehner J.M., Smolen A., Ness-Smolen T. and Murphy C. Recovery of acetylcholinesterase activity after acute organophosphate treatment of CNS reaggregate cultures. Fundamental and Applied Toxicology 1985;5:1104-1109.
82. Whittemore S.R. and Seiger A. The expression, localization and functional significance of β-nerve growth factor in the central nervous system. Brain Research 1987;12:439-464.
83. Wilson A.J., Kelly J.L. and Purcell W.M. Electron microscopy studies of human placental mast cells. Journal of Clinical Pathology (submitted).
84. Woesner-Menzel L., Schultz B., Vakilzadeh F. and Czarnezki B.M. Electron microscopical evidence for a direct contact nerve fibers and mast cells. Acta Dermato-Venereologica 1981;61:465-469.
85. Yonezawa T., Bernstein M.B. and Peterson E.R. Organotypic cultures of nerve tissue as a model system for neurotoxicity investigation and screening. In: Experimental and Clinical Neurotoxicology. (Spencer P.S. and Schaumburg H.H., eds.) Williams and Wilkins, Baltimore/London, 1980:788-802.
86. Dewar A. Neurotoxicity. In: Animals and Alternatives in Toxicity Testing. (Balls M., Riddell R. and Worden A.N., eds.) McMillan, New York, 1982:359-386.
87. Norton S. Toxic responses of the central nervous system. In: Cassarrat and Doulls Toxicology, 3rd edition. (Klaasen C.D., Amdur M.D. and Doull J., eds.) MacMillan, New York, 1986:359-386.
88. Barnes B.M., Cheng C.H.K., Costall B., Jenner P.G. and Naylor R.J. The toxicity of MPTP and MPP+ in rat neuronal and glial cell cultures. British Journal of Pharmacology 1989;96:332P.

9
Interference of sesquiterpenoid unsaturated dialdehydes with neuronal transduction studied in human neuroblastoma cells

A. Forsby*,**, M.I. Andres*,*** and E. Walum*

*Stockholm University, Department of Neurochemistry and Neurotoxicology, 106 91 Stockholm (Sweden)
**Lund University, Department of Animal Physiology, Helgonavägen 3b, 223 62 Lund (Sweden)
***National Institute of Toxicology, P.O Box 863, 41080 Seville (Spain)

Introduction

During the past years, we have been studying effects of pungent sesquiterpenes on neuronal transduction. The studies have been performed on human neuroblastoma SH-SY5Y cells, which possess properties of sympathetic ganglion cells [1]. The traditional cellular model for investigating noxious substances, is primary cultures of rat dorsal root ganglia (DRG). However, the disadvantages of using primary cultures are many. For example, the cultures are never homogeneous, the yield of isolated cells is low, and it is difficult to perform reliable biochemical measurements. There is a great interest in developing alternatives to primary animal cultures and to find models for pharmacotoxicological studies on human cells. We therefore used the SH-SY5Y cell line to investigate effects of sesquiterpenoid unsaturated dialdehydes on neuronal transduction mechanisms.

The human neuroblastoma SH-SY5Y cell line

The SK-N-SH neuroblastoma cell line was established in culture by Dr. June Biedler in 1970, from a bone marrow biopsy of a 4-year old girl. It comprised two morphologically distinct cell types, one neuroblastic and one epithelial-like [2]. SK-N-SH cells were later subcloned into several sublines, of which SH-SY5Y is one. SH-SY5Y has been characterised by means of neurospecific properties; adrenergic neurotransmitter enzymes and neuron-specific enolase are expressed and it has a low resting membrane potential. The cells also express opioid, muscarinic and nerve growth factor receptors. However, the SH-SY5Y cell line can be further differentiated along different neuronal linages [3]. The differentiation includes growth of neuronal processes, increased excitability of the plasma membrane, specific induction of neurotransmitter enzymes and neurotransmitter receptors, and formation of functional synaptic contacts with appropriate target cells [4]. The differentiation can be chemically induced by retinoic acid (RA), 12-O-tetradecanoylphorbol-13-acetate (TPA), nerve growth factor or dibuturyl cyclic AMP [5].

Yu and Sadée [6] found that of several differentiation agents tested, RA was the most potent enhancer of the negative coupling of μ opioid receptors to adenylate cyclase. RA was also found to enhance the ability of prostaglandin E_1 to raise cyclic AMP levels, whereas other neurotransmitter systems were much less affected. Furthermore, RA has been shown to increase the number of muscarinic binding sites, and to increase both acetylcholine esterase and choline acetyltransferase activities [4]. These latter observations indicate that RA may cause the redifferentiation of SH-SY5Y cells from mainly adrenergic to a more cholinergic phenotype. RA also induces a shift in the enolase profile towards more neuron-specific enolase, and after RA treatment, ornithine decarboxylase can be induced by fetal calf serum [3]. The SH-SY5Y cell line is frequently used as a model for studies of proto-oncogene expression in relation to RA- and TPA-induced neuronal differentiation and growth control.

SH-SY5Y cells have been used in a number of different applications. Studies on receptor binding, second messenger levels, differentiation and gene expression, are some examples. In our laboratory, general cytotoxicity analyses have been performed on undifferentiated SH-SY5Y cells in comparison with cells, differentiated by RA [7]. Inhibition of

RA-induced differentiation, as judged by morphological observations, has also been investigated, as well as manganese-uptake *via* transferrin receptors [8]. The effects of sesquiterpenes on neuronal signal transduction, i.e. SH-SY5Y cell membrane permeability, intracellular free Ca^{2+} concentrations, inositol phosphate mobilization and neurotransmitter release, will later be discussed in detail.

In our laboratory, stock cultures of SH-SY5Y cells are grown as monolayers in 75 cm^2 tissue culture flasks (Costar) in 15 ml Eagles minimal essential medium with Earle's salts (EMEM), supplemented with (to final concentrations) 1% non essential amino acids, 2 mM L-glutamine, 100 μg streptomycin/ml, 100 U penicillin/ml and 10% fetal calf serum. The cells are detached once a week with trypsin (0.05%) and ethylenediamine tetraacetic acid (EDTA, 0.02%) in a calcium- and magnesium-free phosphate buffered salt solution. The detached cells are suspended in complete growth medium, counted in a Coulter counter, diluted and re-inoculated at a cell density of 10,000 cells/cm^2. The medium is changed once between each subculturing and the cells are kept in a humidified, 4% CO_2 atmosphere at 37 ºC.

Sesquiterpenoid Unsaturated Dialdehydes

Sesquiterpenes containing an unsaturated dialdehyde group are naturally occurring compounds which can be isolated from various organisms such as higher plants [9,10], fungi [11,12], and molluscs [13]. Most of the unsaturated dialdehydes are very hot tasting and possess a powerful antifeedant activity towards insects [14,15] and higher animals [16]. It is therefore believed that these compounds take part in natural defence systems. In addition to the antifeedant activity and their hot taste, many of the sesquiterpenes have also been reported to possess cytotoxic, antimicrobial and mutagenic activities [17,18,19]. This presentation is focused on the investigations of the two pungent sesquiterpenes, polygodial and isovelleral, and the non-pungent epipolygodial (Fig. 1). Polygodial was first isolated from the plant *Polygonum hydropiper*, but as some other sesquiterpenoids, it is also a product from the East African trees, *Warburgia ugandensis* and *W. stuhlmanii*, that is used as food spices and in folk medicine [14]. Isovelleral and other hot tasting substances are formed in a sophisticated lactifier system of the pungent Lactarii mushrooms when they are attacked by fungivores [11]. Although it primarily is the unsaturated dialdehyde functionality that is responsible for the biological activities of the compounds [14,15,19],

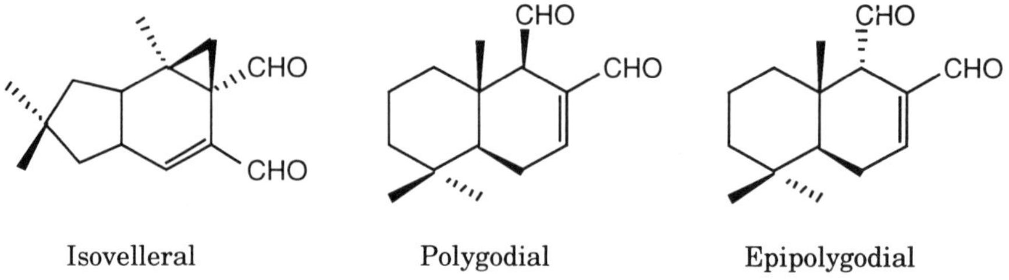

Figure 1 :
The structures of the sesquiterpenes polygodial, epipolygodial and isovelleral.

their biological activities often vary considerably in spite of the apparent structural similarities between the compounds. Efforts to survey such variations have been made by Quantitative Structure-Activity Relationships-studies (QSAR) [20,21], which have shown that certain chemical and structural characteristics are strongly correlated with biological activities of the unsaturated dialdehydes. Efforts have also been made to find a molecular mechanism to the sensory stimulation of the pungent terpenes. Covalent binding of the dialdehyde functionality with primary amines [22,23] and sulfhydryl groups [24] in 'hot taste receptors' have been suggested. However, such receptors have not yet been characterized and therefore, the molecular mechanism for the sensory stimulation of the pungent sesquiterpenes is still unknown.

Membrane Toxicity

The cell membrane appears to be an important cellular target for at least some of the sesquiterpenoid unsaturated dialdehydes, as demonstrated in yeast cells [25] and in the mouse cell line ELD [20]. The pungency as well as the antifeedant activity of the unsaturated dialdehydes indicate that they stimulate sensory neurons, and a different effect of the compounds on neuronal cells as compared to yeast cells and the non-neuronal mouse cells could therefore be anticipated. The effects of six sesquiterpenoid unsaturated dialdehydes on the membrane permeability in SH-SY5Y cells were investigated. In addition, these effects were compared with the pungency of the compounds as well as their membrane toxicity in other cells. A search for structure-activity relationships was carried out by correlating the ability of the compounds to increase the membrane permeability in neuronal cells with 22 chemical and structural descriptors, by the multivariate PLS method (Partial Least Square in latent variables). The method of PLS is based on principal component analysis and correlates large numbers of descriptors with variables. PLS presents principal components which simultaneously explain as much of the variance in both the descriptors and the variables as possible. For a more detailed description of the method, see ref. 26.

The glucose analogue 2-deoxyglucose (2-dGl) is taken up by the cells *via* glucose carriers and phosphorylated by hexokinase. The product, 2-deoxyglucose-6-phosphate, is not further converted, nor can it leave the cell *via* the plasma membrane, and is therefore accumulated in the cytoplasm [27]. The effects of the sesquiterpenes on the cell membrane permeability were studied by measuring the kinetic efflux of radioactivity from cells preloaded with tritiated 2-dGl. The experimental procedure and calculations of the relative efflux, have previously been described in detail [28]. The concentrations that gave 5 and 20 percent efflux compared to the control cells (EC_5 and EC_{20}) were calculated. The ability of the compounds to increase the cell membrane permeability, expressed as pEC_5 and pEC_{20} (EC-values in mol/l), were correlated with the chemical descriptors discussed below by multivariate PLS analysis.

The theoretical descriptors were chosen to characterize the unsaturated dialdehyde functionality and have previously been described in detail [28]. The following descriptors were included in the PLS correlation: molecular weight, dihedral angles, intraatomic distances between the two aldehyde carbons, the energy differences between the lowest unoccupied molecular orbital (LUMO) and the highest occupied molecular orbital (HOMO), and the next lowest unoccupied molecular orbital (NLUMO) and the HOMO, atomic charges, X, Y and Z components of the dipole moment when the structure is fixed in a coordinate system, the total dipole moment, and the experimental log P-value.

Structure-Activity Relationships

The six sesquiterpenes had quite different effects on the cell membrane permeability. The most active compounds, polygodial, isovelleral and warburganal, increased the 2-dGl-6-P efflux at low concentrations with the EC_{20} values 2.5, 3.9, and 9.0 µM, respectively, after 20 minutes of incubation. The structural isomers of isovelleral and polygodial, iso-isovelleral and epipolygodial, were much less active (EC_{20} values 28 and

180 µM, respectively), whereas EC_{20} for merulidial could not be determined. Rather, merulidial seemed to have a stabilizing effect on the cell membrane by decreasing the 2-dGl-6-P efflux, compared to control. The results indicate that the sesquiterpenes that increased the membrane permeability the most, are also the most pungent ones. However, these results are rather similar to sesquiterpene-induced membrane leakage in ELD cells and there is nothing that suggests that these compounds give any specific effects on neuronal cell membranes.

The results of the QSAR analysis of the five active compounds showed that a small distance between the two aldehyde carbons, a large dipole moment, a relatively low LUMO-HOMO energy difference, and a relatively low charge on the oxygen atom in the unsaturated dialdehyde group were important for the membrane toxic activity. The results also indicated that a high lipophilicity (log P) was correlated with a high activity. These molecular properties suggest that the induction of membrane permeability depends on the tendency of the sesquiterpenes to accumulate in the cell membrane, with the lipophilic part dissolved in the lipid bilayer and the reactive dialdehyde groups sticking out from the inside or outside of the membrane.

Calcium Fluxes

The membrane toxicity study indicated a relationship between the pungency of the sesquiterpenes and their ability to increase the cell membrane permeability in SH-SY5Y cells. However, the findings were not unique for neuronal cells and we therefore conclude that the sesquiterpenes do not primarily exert their pungency by simply causing unspecific permeability changes in sensory neurons. To evaluate a possible neuronal transduction mechanism coupled to sensory stimulation, we have studied effects of polygodial, isovelleral and epipolygodial on intracellular free calcium concentrations, $[Ca^{2+}]_i$, in the human neuroblastoma cells.

Free $[Ca^{2+}]_i$ was determined by the fura-2 method, first described by Grynkiewicz et al. [29]. Fluorescence is emitted when free Ca^{2+} binds to fura-2 and is thereby directly proportional to the $[Ca^{2+}]_i$. The effects on $[Ca^{2+}]_i$ were measured in a large population of monolayer-cultured cells in a multicell set-up, to get an average value. Polygodial-induced effects were also studied in single cells by video microscopy image analyses. The changes in $[Ca^{2+}]_i$ were registered continuously during 10 minutes in all experiments and the sesquiterpenes were investigated in concentrations subtoxic to the SH-SY5Y cell membrane. The methods, including ratio calibration and calculation of $[Ca^{2+}]_i$, have previously been described in detail [30].

The two pungent sesquiterpenes, polygodial and isovelleral, induced an increased $[Ca^{2+}]_i$ at very low concentrations (0.43 µM and 2.2 µM, respectively), but the non-pungent epipolygodial, was practically inactive and induced only a weak Ca^{2+} increase at high concentrations (43 µM). Kinetic analysis of the average Ca^{2+}-increase induced by polygodial and isovelleral revealed, that after a short lag phase of 30-60 seconds, an initial constant and rapid increase in the $[Ca^{2+}]_i$ occurred. The rate of increase then declined after 5 minutes. The rate of the initial rapid Ca^{2+}-influx was concentration dependent. The results indicate that there may be a relationship between the Ca^{2+}-increase and the pungency (i.e. stimulation of sensory neurons) of the dialdehyde sesquiterpenes.

Experiments in extracellular solution with EGTA-chelated Ca^{2+}, showed that the initial rise in $[Ca^{2+}]_i$ occurred after incubation with polygodial and isovelleral, although the rate and maximum level was reduced as compared to experiments performed in the presence of extracellular Ca^{2+}. These findings suggest that a Ca^{2+}-release from intra-cellular stores takes place. Thus, the terpenes may induce inositol 1,4,5-trisphosphate (IP$_3$) mobilization (possibly via an activation of phospholipase C, PLC).

The image analysis of single cells incubated with polygodial, showed that the rapid increase in the $[Ca^{2+}]_i$, registered in the multi-cell experiments, was represented by an initial rise in the $[Ca^{2+}]_i$ which, in most of the cells, was reversed back to the normal cytoplasmatic Ca^{2+} concentration. In addition to the initial peak, oscillations in the $[Ca^{2+}]_i$ took place in some cells after prolonged incubation with polygodial. The fluctuations in $[Ca^{2+}]_i$, may also be a result of an initial IP$_3$ stimulation and eventually activation of Ca^{2+}-activated Ca^{2+}-channels [31]. Cells completely unresponsive to polygodial were also present in the cultures. One may attribute this phenomenon to the fact that cells in a culture are in different phases of the cell cycle and thus, the properties of the cell membranes differ between cells due to differences in their protein and lipid composition.

Inositol Phosphate Mobilization

The investigation on sesquiterpene-induced fluxes in $[Ca^{2+}]_i$, indicated a relationship between the pungency of the compounds and their ability to increase $[Ca^{2+}]_i$. The effect on $[Ca^{2+}]_i$ was observed under physiological concentrations of extracellular Ca^{2+}, as well as under extracellular Ca^{2+}-free conditions, which suggests a release from intracellular Ca^{2+} stores. Such release of Ca^{2+} is known to be initiated by IP_3 and we have therefore investigated the effect of polygodial, isovelleral and epipolygodial, on inositol phosphate (IP) mobilization. Polygodial's effect on carbachol-induced IP mobilization was also studied as well as the effect of polygodial on the carbachol-induced increase of $[Ca^{2+}]_i$.

The IP measurements were performed, with some modifications, according to the technique of Berridge et al.[32]. SH-SY5Y cells for the IP experiments were plated in 24 well plates at a density of 250 000 cells/well and cultured for 24 hours before the ^{3}H-*myo*-inositol loading. The cultures were exposed to the dialdehydes or carbachol for 30 minutes. IP_3 was measured indirectly as accumulated inositol 1-phosphate, IP_1, and inositol 1,4-bisphosphate, IP_2. The experimental procedures have previously been described in detail [33].

The effects of the three sesquiterpenes on IP mobilization were unexpected. According to our hypothesis, both pungent compounds polygodial and isovelleral, should activate IP mobilization, but the non-pungent epipolygodial should have no effect. This presumption was based on the finding that polygodial and isovelleral release Ca^{2+} from intracellular Ca^{2+} compartments [30] and on the assumption that the Ca^{2+}-release should be IP_3 dependent. However, isovelleral did not have any significant effect on the IP mobilization. On the other hand, polygodial increased, at the highest concentration tested (4.3 µM), the IP_1 and IP_2 content by about 140% and 180% respectively as compared to the control. Epipolygodial in 171 µM, increased the IP_1 and IP_2 content by 100% and 60%, respectively. These results show that there is no relationship between an IP mobilization and the nociceptive potential (cf. Introduction) of the three sesquiterpenes. Furthermore, IP mobilization does not seem to be a prerequisite for the isovelleral induced intracellular Ca^{2+} release. The different effects of isovelleral and polygodial on the IP mobilization, indicated that the polygodial-induced increase of the IP levels, was not a result of a general cell membrane disruption and release of membrane associated phosphoinositides. This could have been the case since we have previously shown that isovelleral and polygodial increase the general cell membrane permeability and have a damaging effect on the SH-SY5Y cell membrane at the incubation times used in the IP assay [28]. We therefore assume that polygodial specifically interacts with some steps in the IP pathway, possibly activates PLC. The epipolygodial-activated IP mobilization in SH-SY5Y cells may be attributed to its molecular homology to polygodial.

It has been claimed that intracellular calcium oscillations and feedback interactions between IP_3 and Ca^{2+} could account for a periodic activation of PLC[31]. As mentioned in a previous section, we have found that polygodial induces transient calcium oscillations in SH-SY5Y cells. To investigate the role of a of Ca^{2+}-induced PLC activation in the SH-SY5Y cells, we studied the effect of carbachol and polygodial on IP mobilization in Ca^{2+}-free extracellular solution (EGTA-chelated Ca^{2+} in KRH buffer). We found that the IP_1 formations were inhibited by 78% for carbachol and 74% for polygodial. These results indicate, that a feedback activation of PLC was followed by an increase in $[Ca^{2+}]_i$ under physiological extracellular conditions. Contrary to polygodial, the increase of $[Ca^{2+}]_i$ induced by isovelleral, did not have any stimulatory effect on the PLC activity as judged by the lack of an IP mobilization. The reason may be that isovelleral inhibits some steps in the IP pathway or, perhaps more likely, that a Ca^{2+}-independent, primary induction of PLC is necessary for IP mobilization [34]. Polygodial, but not isovelleral, would then be capable of such an initial induction of PLC.

Polygodial's effect on carbachol induced receptor signal transduction was investigated with emphasis on IP mobilization and Ca^{2+} influx. The results showed that 4.3 µM polygodial inhibited the carbachol-stimulated IP_1 formation by 77%, despite the fact that polygodial by it self had a stimulatory effect on IP formation. Ten minutes of pre-incubation with polygodial, had a significant inhibitory effect on the carbachol-induced increase of the $[Ca^{2+}]_i$ in the neuroblastoma cells. Previous studies on receptor binding, showed that the affinity for the muscarinic acetyl choline receptor (mACh-r) ligand ^{3}H-quinuclidinyl benzilate, to rat striatal membranes was not affected by polygodial or any other sesquiterpenoid unsaturated dialdehyde [35]. Consequently, polygodial does not interact with the agonist binding site of the mACh-r, but rather interferes with the receptor / G protein / PLC coupling, or has a direct effect on IP-mobilizing enzyme activities.

Neurotransmitter release

Ca^{2+}-influx is a profound requirement for the release of transmitter substances since Ca^{2+} trigger the mechanism of exocytosis. We have shown that polygodial is able to increase the $[Ca^{2+}]_i$ in the neuroblastoma cells without affecting the general cell membrane permeability. We were therefore interested to investigate the possibility that polygodial might be able to induce transmitter release from the SH-SY5Y cells.

Scott et al. have shown that the SH-SY5Y cell line expresses depolarization-evoked release of noradrenaline (NA) following treatment of TPA for several days to induce differentiation [36]. However, Murphy et al. demonstrated that undifferentiated SH-SY5Y cells exhibited potassium- and carbachol-evoked, calcium-dependent release of NA [37]. We chose to use a modified version of the undifferentiated model according to Murphy, for the studies of polygodial-induced NA-release. Cells for experiments were monolayers, cultured for 6 or 7 days. After the ^{3}H-NA loading, the release of radioactivity into the extracellular solution, was registered during 3 minutes of incubation. Cells incubated with buffer which contained the polygodial solvent (0.1% ethanol) served as a control, whereas carbachol and KCl were used to verify the method.

The results indicate that low concentrations of polygodial, i.e. 0.43 µM to 2.1 µM, increase the transmitter release from SH-SY5Y cells in a concentration dependent way. The relative release reached a maximum of 14% at 2.1 µM. At concentrations higher than 2.1 µM but lower than 15 µM, an increased NA-release was still apparent. It is our believe, that polygodial in low concentrations, is able to activate the physiological mechanism of neurotransmitter release as a result of increased $[Ca^{2+}]_i$. At 15 µM, no effect was registered, whereas 21 µM showed an increase of the released ^{3}H-NA by 7.3%. However, 21 µM of polygodial has been shown to be toxic to the SH-SY5Y cell membrane, and the effect on transmitter release can be attributed to a general disruption of cell- and vesicle-membranes, and a leakage of incorporated ^{3}H-NA as a result.

Conclusions

From our results (summarized in Table I) it appears that the pungent compounds also possess the highest membrane toxic activity and cause the greatest Ca^{2+}-influx in the human neuroblastoma cells. On the other hand, sesquiterpene-induced IP-mobilization does not seem to be a prerequisite for the sensory stimulation. The finding that polygodial and isovelleral have a different effect on the IP turnover mechanism, indicates that the two compounds interact with different cellular constituents, although both of the compounds possess the unsaturated dialdehyde functionality.

The biological mechanism behind the antifeedant activity and hot taste of the sesquiterpenes, is not known. It has been suggested that polygodial binds covalently to taste receptors, by interactions with -SH or -NH$_2$ groups of the receptors [14,23]. The differences in the activity between polygodial and epipolygodial have been assigned to the positions of the two aldehyde groups. Polygodial possesses a β-aldehyde group at C-9, whereas the corresponding aldehyde group of epipolygodial is in alpha configuration. The β-aldehyde configuration of polygodial would facilitate the binding to the receptors.

It is, however, quite possible that the pungent terpenes interact with cell membrane proteins other than taste receptors. The agonists histamine, glutamate and carbachol were screened in terms of Ca^{2+}-influx to investigate the presence of other functional receptors in the SH-SY5Y cell line. Carbachol was found to be the only agonist which could induce an increase in [Ca^{2+}]$_i$. However, binding studies on muscarinic acetyl

	Polygodial	Isovelleral	Epipolygodial
Membrane toxicity	+++	+++	+
Ca2+-influx	+++	+++	+
IP-mobilization	++	0	+
NA-release	+++	++[a]	b

Table I :
Summary of the effects of polygodial, isovelleral and epipolygodial on neuronal transduction mechanisms. Three pluses indicate the highest biological activity.
a = Preliminary results; b= not determined.

choline receptors in membranes isolated from the rat striatum, showed that the binding affinity of ^{3}H-quinuclidinyl benzilate was not affected by polygodial, isovelleral or epipolygodial [35]. Nevertheless, polygodial was able to inhibit the carbachol initiated increase in $[Ca^{2+}]_i$. Preliminary results from experiments performed in the presence of the L-type Ca^{2+} channel blocker PN200-110, and from experiments performed under extracellular Na$^+$-free conditions (NaCl replaced with choline chloride), indicated that the increase in the $[Ca^{2+}]_i$ was not dependent on a previous Na$^+$-influx to the cytoplasm. Consequently, the neuronal response elicited by the sesquiterpenes may not result from an initial depolarization of the cells. According to these results, we assume that the increased $[Ca^{2+}]_i$, induced by the pungent sesquiterpenes in the SH-SY5Y cells, was mediated by chemical interactions between the unsaturated dialdehyde group of the terpene molecule and cell membrane proteins (e.g. neurotransmitter receptors, G-proteins, PLC), either through a specific activation, or through alterations in the structural environment of the functional proteins. It has been stated that the disturbances in cell membrane permeability caused by the sesquiterpenes are related to their accumulation in the cell membrane, where they orient themselves with the dialdehyde group exposed on the inner or outer side of the membrane, and react chemically with proteins associated with the membrane [20,27]. The reaction of the two aldehyde groups with a primary amine group to form a pyrrole derivate, could be one possible mechanism responsible for the effects of polygodial on neuronal signal transduction.

Our findings indicate that neuronal transduction does not necessarily have to be receptor mediated. Rather, the Ca^{2+}-influx, induced by the pungent sesquiterpenes, may be initiated by non-agonistic interactions between the compounds and membrane-associated proteins. The polygodial-induced ^{3}H-NA release is an indication of the physiological significance of the increased $[Ca^{2+}]_i$. Preliminary studies on isovelleral-induced transmitter release revealed that also this compound is able to induce ^{3}H-NA release, although some what higher concentrations were needed. Possible mechanisms of sesquiterpene mediated increased intracellular Ca^{2+} concentration and the known consequences of the Ca^{2+} elevation are presented in Fig. 2.

In this presentation, we have shown that the human neuroblastoma cell line SH-SY5Y, may be used as a model in studies of neuronal signal transduction mechanisms and the induction of nociceptive responses. It is our intention to continue the investigations on the primary

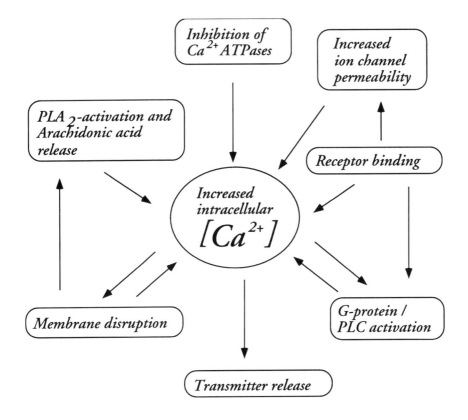

Figure 2:
Possible mechanisms of sesquiterpene mediated increased intracellular Ca^{2+} concentration and the known consequences of the Ca^2-elevation.

interactions between the sesquiterpenes and cell membrane proteins. The mechanism behind the Ca^{2+}-fluxes has to be explored further.

Acknowledgements

The investigations were supported by Hierta Retzius' Foundation, The Lars Hierta Foundation, The Swedish Fund for Research Without Animal Experiments and the National Swedish Board for Laboratory Animals.

References

1. Biedler J.L., Roffler-Tarlov S., Schachner M. and Freedman L.S. Multiple neurotransmitter synthesis by human neuroblastoma cell lines and clones. Cancer Research 1978;38:3751-3757.
2. Biedler J.L., Melson L. and Spengler B.A. Morphology and growth, tumorigenicity and cytogenetics of human neuroblastoma cells in continuous culture. Cancer Research 1973;33:2643-2652.
3. Pålman S., Mamaeva S., Meyerson G., Mattson M.E.K., Bjelfman C., Örtoft E. and Hammerling U. Human neuroblastoma cells in culture: A model for neuronal cell differentiation and function. Acta Physiologica Scandinavica 140, suppl. 592:25-37.
4. Adem A., Mattson M.E.K., Norberg A. and Pålman S. Muscarinic receptors in human SH-SY5Y neuroblastoma cell line: Regulation by phorbol ester- and retinoic acid-induced differentiation. Developmental Brain Research 1987;33:235-247.
5. Yu W.C., Hochhaus G., Fu-Hsiung C., Richards M.L., Bourne H.R. and Sadée W. Differentiation of human neuroblastoma cells: Marked potentiation of prostaglandin E-stimulated accumulation of cyclic AMP by retinoic acid. Journal of Neurochemistry 1988;51:1892-1899.
6. Yu, W.C. and Sadée W. Efficacy and tolerance of narcotic analgesics at the mu opioid receptor in human neuroblastoma cells. Journal of Pharmacology and Experimental Therapeutics 1988;55:350-355.
7. Walum E., Wang L., Jones K., Nordin M., Clemedson C. and Varnbo I. Cellular neuronal development In vitro-neurobiological and neurotoxicological studies in cultured model systems. In: The brain in bits and pieces. In vitro techniques in neurobiology, neuropharmacology and neurotoxicology (Zbinden G., ed.) M.T.C. Verlag, Zollikon, Switzerland, 1992:115-135.
8. Suárez N. and Eriksson H. Receptor mediated endocytosis of a manganese complex of transferrin into neuroblastoma (SH-SY5Y) cells in culture. Journal of Neurochemistry 1993;61 (in press).
9. Kubo I., Lee Y-W., Pettei M., Pilkiewicz F. and Nakanishi K. Potent armyworm antifeedants from the east African Warburgia plants, J.C.S. Chemical Communications 1976;1013-1014.
10. Fukuyama Y., Sato T., Asakawa Y. and Takemoto T. A potent cytotoxic warburganal and related drimane-type sesquiterpenoids from Polygonum hydropiper. Phytochemistry 1982;12:2895-2898.
11. Camazine S. and Lupo A.T., Labile toxic compounds of the Lactarii: The role of the laticiferous hyphae as a storage depot for precursors of pungent dialdehydes. Mycologia 1984;2:355-358.
12. Sterner O., Bergman R., Kihlberg J. and Wickberg B. The sesquiterpenes of Lactarius vellereus and their role in a proposed chemical defense system. Journal of Natural Products 1985;2:279-288.
13. Cimino G., De Rosa S., De Stefano S., Sodano G. and Villani G. Dorid nudibranch elaborates its own chemical defence. Science 1983;219:1237-1238.
14. Kubo I. and Ganjian I. Insect antifeedant terpenes, hot tasting to humans. Experientia 1981;31:1063-1064.

15. Caprioli V., Cimino G., Colle R., Gavagnin M., Sodano G. and Spinella A. Insect antifeedant activity and hot taste for humans of selected natural and synthetic 1,4-dialdehydes. Journal of Natural Products 1987;2:146-151.
16. Camazine S.M., Resch J.F., Eisner T. and Meinwald J. Mushroom chemical defence: Pungent sesquiterpenoid dialdehyde antifeedant to opossum. Journal of Chemical Ecology 1983;10:1439-1447.
17. Forsby A., Andersson M., Lewan L. and Sterner O. The cytotoxicity of 22 sesquiterpenoid unsaturated dialdehydes, as determined by the neutral red absorption assay and by protein determination. Toxicology in Vitro 1991;5:9-14.
18. Anke H., Sterner O. and Steglich W. Structure-activity relationships for unsaturated dialdehydes. 3. Mutagenic, antimicrobial, cytotoxic, and phytotoxic activities of merulidial derivatives. Journal of Antibiotics 1989;42:738-744.
19. Sterner O., Carter R.E. and Nilsson L.M. Structure-activity relationships for unsaturated dialdehydes 1. The mutagenic activity of 18 compounds in the Salmonella/microsome assay. Mutation Research 1987;188:169-174.
20. Andersson M., Bocchio F., Sterner O., Forsby A. and Lewan L. Structure-activity relationships for unsaturated dialdehydes 7. The membrane toxicity of 15 sesquiterpenoids measured as the induction of ATP leakage in ELD cells. The correlation of the activity with structural descriptors by the multivariate PLS method. Toxicology in Vitro 1993;7:1-6.
21. Nilsson L.M., Carter R.E., Sterner O. and Liljefors T. Structure-activity relationships for unsaturated dialdehydes 2. A PLS correlation of theoretical descriptors for six compounds with mutagenic activity in the Ames Salmonella assay. Quantitative Structure-Activity Relationships 1988;7:84-91.
22. D'Ischia M., Prota G. and Sodano G. Reaction of polygodial with primary amines: An alternative explanation to the antifeedant activity. Tetrahedron Letters 1982;23:3295-3298.
23. Cimino G., Sodano G. and Spinella A. Correlation of the reactivity of 1,4-dialdehydes with methylamine in biomimetic conditions to their hot taste: Covalent binding to primary amines as a molecular mechanism in hot taste receptors. Tetrahedron 1987;43:5401-5410.
24. Taniguchi M., Adachi T., Haraguchi H., Oi S. and Kubo I. Physiological activity of warburganal and its reactivity with sulfhydryl groups. Journal of Biochemistry 1983;94:149-154.
25. Kubo I. Polygodial, an antifungal potentiator. Journal of Natural Products 1988;51:22-29.
26. Dunn W.J., Wold S., Edlund U., Hellberg S. and Gasteiger J. Multivariate structure-activity relationships between data from a battery of biological tests and an ensemble of structure descriptors: The PLS method. Quantitative Structure-Activity Relationships 1984;3:131-137.
27. Smith D.E. and Gorski J. Estrogene control of uterine glucose metabolism. An analysis based on the transport and phosphorylation of 2-deoxyglucose. Journal of Biological Chemistry 1968;243:4169-4174.
28. Forsby A., Walum E. and Sterner O. The effect of six sesquiterpenoid unsaturated dialdehydes on cell membrane permeability in human neuroblastoma SH-SY5Y cells. Chemico-Biological Interactions 1992;84:85-95.

29. Grynkiewicz G., Poenie M. and Tsien R.Y. A new generation of Ca^{2+} indicators with greatly improved fluorescence properties. Journal of Biological Chemistry 1985;260:3440-3450.
30. Forsby A., Witt R. and Walum E. Sesquiterpenoid unsaturated dialdehydes increase the concentration of intracellular free Ca^{2+} in human neuroblastoma SH-SY5Y cells. Natural Toxins (accepted for publication).
31. Berridge M.J. Calcium oscillations (minireview). Journal of Biological Chemistry 1990;265:9583-9583.
32. Berridge M.J., Downes C.P. and Hanely M.R. Lithium amplifies agonist-dependent phosphatidylinositol responses in brain and salivary gland. Biochemical Journal 1982;206:587-595.
33. Forsby A. and Walum E. The effect of sesquiterpenoid unsaturated dialdehydes on inositol phosphate turnover and receptor signal transduction in human neuroblastoma SH-SY5Y cells. Journal of Neurochemistry (submitted).
34. Harootunian A.T., Kao J.P.Y., Paranjape S. and Tsien R.Y. Generation of calcium oscillations in fibroblasts by positive feedback between calcium and IP_3. Science 1991;251:75-78.
35. Bocchio F., Kalf-Hansen S., Dekermendjian K., Sterner O. and Witt R. The inhibitory effect of sesquiterpenoid unsaturated dialdehydes on dopamine D1 receptor, a quantitative structure-activity relationships study. Tetrahedron Letters 1992;33:6867-6870.

10

Human immune cells and *in vitro* immunotoxicity testing

I. Kimber and M. Cumberbatch

Zeneca Central Toxicology Laboratory, Alderley Park, Macclesfield, Cheshire, SK10 4TJ (UK)

Introduction

Immunotoxicology can be defined as the study of adverse health effects which may result from the interaction of chemicals or drugs with the immune system. Such adverse effects may be categorized broadly into two main types of insult. Immunosuppression resulting from the functional impairment of one or more components of the immune system is referred to usually as immunotoxicity. Here the concern is that depressed immune function may translate into enhanced susceptibility to infectious and/or malignant disease. The second major area is allergy; the adverse effects caused by the stimulation of specific immune responses.

There are available a number of test strategies that can be used to identify chemicals and drugs which have the potential to induce allergy or to cause immunosuppression. The majority of these tests, and almost without exception those which have gained general acceptance in toxicology, require the use of animals and measurement of effects either *in vivo* or *ex vivo*. The difficulty in deriving purely *in vitro* methods for the prospective identification of immunotoxicants or allergens is largely a function of the complexity of the immune system itself. The induction, regulation and expression of immune function demands the effective interaction between a variety of cells and molecules in the correct microenvironment. It has proven difficult to model accurately the immune system in culture. Such does not imply, however, that *in vitro* methods are not of considerable value in immunotoxicology. Despite limited progress with respect to the development of *in vitro* methods for predictive testing, culture systems using immune cells are used extensively for mechanistic investigation of immunotoxic processes. This article will focus upon allergy rather than immunotoxicity and the opportunities which exist to use immune cells for the identification and classification of sensitizing chemicals.

Chemical allergy

Chemicals are able to cause various forms of allergic disease in susceptible individuals; those of greatest importance in the context of occupational health being allergic contact dermatitis (skin sensitization) and respiratory allergy. There is now available a wide variety of guinea pig predictive tests for the identification of chemicals possessing skin sensitizing potential [1]. More recently murine test methods, such as the local lymph node assay [2] and the mouse ear swelling test [3] have been described also. The situation with respect to predictive tests for chemical respiratory allergens is rather different. There are, as yet, no well validated or widely applied methods. Some progress has been made, however, and the work of Karol and her colleagues has been instrumental in the development of methods for the investigation of chemical respiratory hypersensitivity in the guinea pig [4]. Based upon this work several approaches to predictive testing have been proposed [5-8]. In addition, a mouse assay system has recently been suggested [9].

The question posed here is whether there exist opportunities to measure the sensitizing potential of chemicals *in vitro*. The role of the skin during the induction phase of chemical allergy has attracted much attention. By definition, the skin is the route of exposure to contact sensitizing chemicals. It is possible also that the induction of immune responses necessary for efficient sensitization of the respiratory tract may also result from dermal exposure to the chemical allergen.

The skin and induction of allergic responses

Within the epidermis there exists a contiguous network of bone marrow derived Langerhans cells (LC) which are now considered to play a central role in the initiation of cutaneous immune responses to chemicals [10]. LC belong to a family known collectively as dendritic cells (DC) which are found in small numbers throughout lymphoid tissue and in those tissues, such as the skin and the respiratory and gastrointestinal tracts, which come into closest contact with the external environment [11-13]. In these tissues DC act as sentinels of the immune system, sampling the external environment and processing information for transmission to other immunologically active cells. It has been known for some time that epidermal LC form a trap for contact allergens in the skin [14]. Following skin sensitization, a proportion of local LC, many of which bear high levels of allergen, are induced to leave the epidermis and to migrate, via afferent lymphatics, to lymph nodes draining the site of exposure [15-19]. This migration is accompanied by a functional and phenotypic maturation such that by the time LC arrive in the lymph nodes they have acquired the characteristics of immunostimulatory dendritic cells and are able effectively to present antigen to responsive T lymphocytes [20-23].

It is now apparent that keratinocytes can produce constitutively, or can be stimulated to produce, a wide variety of cytokines [24]. Epidermal cytokines influence directly the activity and maturational status of LC and thereby the induction phase of skin sensitization. By analogy with *in vitro* studies it is hypothesized that granulocyte/macrophage colony-stimulating factor (GM-CSF), possibly acting in concert with interleukin 1 (IL-1), effects the changes to which LC are subject while in transit to the draining lymph nodes [25]. It is likely also that cytokines produced locally provide the initial signal for LC to leave the epidermis and move into the afferent lymphatics. We have shown recently that tumour necrosis factor α (TNF-α) may provide one such stimulus. Intradermal injection of mice with recombinant TNF-α causes an accumulation of DC in draining lymph nodes [26]. Moreover, systemic administration of a neutralizing anti-TNF-α antibody inhibits markedly the accumulation of DC in lymph nodes which results normally from topical sensitization with a skin allergen (unpublished observations).

Taken together these data suggest the following series of events is initiated after first contact with a sensitizing chemical. The inducing allergen associates with epidermal LC and either directly or indirectly provokes the production by keratinocytes of cytokines. Some of these cytokines are required for the movement and maturation of LC. The functional development of LC into active immunostimulatory DC is dependent upon the availability of GM-CSF (and possibly IL-1 and other cytokines) and TNF-α provides an important stimulus for LC migration.

On this basis it might be argued that skin sensitizing chemicals may be identified as a function of the cytokines that keratinocytes are induced to synthesize and secrete and which directly affect LC function. It must be borne in mind, however, that dermal trauma, other than that associated with skin sensitization, will also cause the local production of some cytokines. It has been found, for instance, that both irradiation with ultraviolet B light and topical exposure to the non-sensitizing skin irritant sodium lauryl sulphate (SLS) result in enhanced production by keratinocytes of TNF-α [27,28]. There may be some justification therefore to propose that it may be possible to screen chemicals for sensitizing activity on the basis of negative criteria. Chemicals which fail to induce the production of relevant cytokines such as TNF-α and GM-CSF are unlikely to stimulate the sequence of events necessary for effective sensitization.

Another approach is to consider whether exposure to skin sensitizing chemicals results in selective changes in epidermal cell (either keratinocyte or Langerhans cell) behaviour. It has been reported that exposure of mice to chemical allergens results in the activation of LC and enhanced absorptive endocytosis [29]. In the same study similar treatment with skin irritants caused only degenerative changes in LC [29]. There is evidence also that contact allergens modulate directly the expression by LC of MHC class II (Ia) antigens. Aiba and Katz found that treatment of mice with skin sensitizing chemicals, but not with SLS, resulted, 24 hours later, in a marked increase in Ia expression by a proportion (22-50%) of epidermal LC [30]. Consistent with this is the fact that contact allergens have been shown to provoke increased LC mRNA for Ia antigen within 6 hours of topical exposure [28]. Sensitizing chemicals may cause changes in the localization as well as production of Ia antigens. Contact allergens such as 2,4-dinitrofluorobenzene (DNFB) have been found to induce the internalization of Ia molecules; an endocytic process which may be important for the handling and presentation of the chemical hapten by activated LC [31,32]. Studies *in vitro* appear somewhat contradictory. Picut et al [33] reported that treatment of epidermal cell suspensions with contact allergens caused a rapid activation of LC characterized by a marked increase in the expression of Ia and the presence of rough endoplasmic reticulum and numerous ribosomes and lysosomes. In contrast, Becker et al. [32] found that culture of epidermal cells with DNFB resulted in decreased membrane expression of Ia associated with elevated intracellular levels of the molecule.

The cytokines described previously which are known or suspected to play an important role in the migration and maturation of LC (TNF-α and GM-CSF, respectively) are produced by keratinocytes in response to a number of stimuli. Thus, Enk and Katz [28] have reported that production of these cytokines is upregulated following the application of both allergens and primary irritants. There is preliminary evidence, however, that other epidermal cell-derived cytokines may be induced exclusively by chemical sensitizers. It has been found that epidermal mRNA for interferon (IFN)- induced protein 10 (IP-10), macrophage inflammatory protein 2 (MIP-2) and interleukin 1β (IL-1β) is increased only following topical exposure of mice to sensitizing chemicals [28]. Subsequently, interleukin 10 (IL-10), a product of keratinocytes, was shown also to be upregulated only by chemical allergens [34]. Importantly, recent evidence indicates that the production in the skin of one of these 'allergen-selective' epidermal cytokines (IL-1β) is essential for the induction of contact sensitization [35]. These studies suggest that the production of certain epidermal cytokines is induced or enhanced only following exposure to those chemicals which have the potential to cause skin sensitization. If these observations can be confirmed and extended using a wider range of chemicals possessing differing sensitizing activity and with non-sensitizing materials then it may be possible to identify chemical allergens on this basis employing epidermal cell cultures or isolated tissue slices.

At one time it was considered that dendritic cell populations failed to produce cytokines. Investigations during the last 2 years argue that this is not the case. Within epidermal cell populations it has been found that LC are the major, or exclusive, source of IL-1β [28,36-38] and macrophage inflammatory protein 1α (MIP-1α) [36,37] and that cultured LC (which are considered to be functionally equivalent to LC which have migrated to draining lymph nodes following skin sensitization) produce interleukin 6 (IL-6) [37,38]. Of particular interest is the production by LC of IL-1β. Not only is this cytokine produced solely by LC in unstimulated epidermal cell populations [36], but also production is increased markedly during culture [37]. As this is one of the cytokines considered to be upregulated only following exposure to chemical allergens [28], and in view of the fact that it appears to be essential for effective sensitization [35], IL-1β may provide a relevant and potentially very useful marker of sensitizing activity. If the induction of IL-1β results from the direct interaction of chemicals with LC then analysis *in vitro* is theoretically possible. The primary limitation of such an approach is the difficulty in obtaining sufficient quantities of LC for analysis. A solution may be provided by the recent demonstration that GM-CSF and TNF-α act together to drive the development of dendritic cells from CD34⁺ haemopoietic progenitors [39-42]. The ability to generate *in vitro* large numbers of dendritic cells paves the way to a more exacting analysis of their immunological characteristics and their use in toxicological investigations.

In summary, it can be argued that currently the most realistic approach to the identification of potential contact allergens by purely *in vitro* techniques is via analysis of local cytokine production in the skin following primary exposure to chemical. It remains to be confirmed formally that under all conditions of epicutaneous application only those chemicals with sensitizing activity provoke the production, or increased production, of certain cytokines such as IL-1β. Moreover, optimal conditions for *in vitro* studies will have to be identified and the relative merits of full-thickness skin, epidermal sheets, epidermal cell suspensions, purified LC and expanded populations of dendritic cells investigated. Such methods if validated and shown to be robust can accommodate the analysis of human cells and here the use of regenerative skin cultures (for keratinocyte-derived cytokines) and of dendritic cell cultures (for measurement of LC- and DC-derived cytokines) are particularly attractive.

Stimulation of T lymphocyte responses

It has been known for some time that, in the presence of the relevant chemical hapten and an appropriate source of antigen presenting cells, it is possible to provoke *in vitro* secondary proliferative responses by primed lymphocytes isolated from previously sensitized mice [43,44] More recently it has been found that such responses are more vigorous if either epidermal cell suspensions (including LC) or antigen-bearing DC isolated from the draining nodes of contact sensitized mice are used as the source of antigen presenting cells [45-47].

Similarly in man, peripheral blood lymphocytes prepared from contact sensitized individuals can be induced to proliferate *in vitro* in response to the relevant chemical hapten presented in an appropriate form [48]. This phenomenon forms the basis of the lymphocyte transformation test which has been used to investigate human allergic contact dermatitis to a variety of skin sensitizers including nickel [49-51], neomycin sulphate [51], 2,4-dinitrochlorobenzene [51,52] and thiurams [53].

Evidence exists that for the effective induction of primary rather than secondary T lymphocyte activation there is an absolute requirement that DC act as antigen presenting cells [54]. The activity of DC is such that they will provoke *in vitro* proliferative responses to contact allergens by lymphocytes isolated from naive (unsensitized) mice [16,55,56]. This raises the possibility of identifying prospectively potential chemical allergens as a function of their ability, when presented by activated LC or DC, to stimulate primary proliferative responses by mouse or human T lymphocytes *in vitro*.

Concluding comments

An increased understanding of the induction phase of contact sensitization and of the cellular and molecular events which are initiated in the skin following exposure to chemicals is providing new and realistic opportunities to consider *in vitro* approaches to the identification of potential allergens. Much work still needs to be done and many practical problems will have to be overcome. Nevertheless, continued effort may allow these opportunities to be realised with the development of methods which make use of dendritic cells, their stimulation following contact with sensitizing chemicals and their ability to provoke responses by lymphocytes.

References

1. Andersen K.E. and Maibach H.I. Guinea pig sensitization assays. An overview. In: Contact Allergy Predictive Tests in Guinea Pigs. Current Problems in Dermatology, Vol. 14 (Andersen K.E. and Maibach H.I., eds.) Karger, Basel, 1985:263-290.
2. Kimber I. and Weisenberger C. A murine local lymph node assay for the identification of contact allergens. Assay development and results of an initial validation study. Archives of Toxicology 1989;63:274-282.
3. Gad S.C., Dunn B.J., Dobbs D.W., Reilly C. and Walsh R.D. Development and validation of an alternative dermal sensitization test: The mouse ear swelling test (MEST). Toxicology and Applied Pharmacology 1986;84:93-114.
4. Karol M.H. Occupational asthma and allergic reactions to inhaled compounds. In: Principles and Practice of Immunotoxicology (Miller K., Turk J. and Nicklin S., eds.) Blackwell Scientific Publications, Oxford, 1992:228-241.

5. Karol M.H., Stadler J. and Magreni C. Immunotoxicologic evaluation of the respiratory system: animal models for immediate- and delayed-onset pulmonary hypersensitivity. Fundamental and Applied Toxicology 1985;5:459-472.
6. Botham P.A., Rattray N.J., Woodcock D.R., Walsh S.T. and Hext P.M. The induction of respiratory allergy in guinea-pigs following intradermal injection of trimellitic anhydride. A comparison with the response to 2,4-dinitrochlorobenzene. Toxicology Letters 1989;47:25-39.
7. Pauluhn J. and Eben A. Validation of a non-invasive technique to assess immediate or delayed onset of airway hypersensitivity in guinea pigs. Journal of Applied Toxicology 1991;11:423-431.
8. Sarlo K. and Clark E.D. A tier approach for evaluating the respiratory allergenicity of low molecular weight chemicals. Fundamental and Applied Toxicology 1992;18:107-114.
9. Dearman R.J., Basketter D.A. and Kimber I. Variable effects of chemical allergens on serum IgE concentration in mice. Preliminary evaluation of a novel approach to the identification of respiratory sensitizers. Journal of Applied Toxicology 1992;12:317-323.
10. Kimber I. and Cumberbatch M. Dendritic cells and cutaneous immune responses to chemical allergens. Toxicology and Applied Pharmacology 1992;117:137-146.
11. Sertl K., Takemura T., Tschachler E., Ferrans V.J., Kaliner M.A. and Shevach E.M. Dendritic cells with antigen-presenting capability reside in the airway epithelium, lung parenchyma and visceral pleura. Journal of Experimental Medicine 1986;163:436-451.
12. Pavli P., Woodhams C.E., Doe W.F. and Hume D.A. Isolation and characterization of antigen-presenting dendritic cells from the mouse intestinal lamina propria. Immunology 1990;70:40-47.
13. Pollard A.M. and Lipscomb M.F. Characterization of murine lung dendritic cells: Similarities to Langerhans cells and thymic dendritic cells. Journal of Experimental Medicine 1990;172:159-167.
14. Shelley W.B. and Juhlin L. Langerhans cells form a reticuloepithelial trap for external contact allergens. Nature 1976;261:46-47.
15. Silberberg-Sinakin I., Thorbecke G.J., Baer R.L., Rosenthal S.A. and Berezowsky V. Antigen-bearing Langerhans cells in skin, dermal lymphatics and in lymph nodes. Cellular Immunology 1976;25:137-151.
16. Macatonia S.E., Edwards A.J. and Knight S.C. Dendritic cells and the initiation of contact sensitivity to fluorescein isothiocyanate. Immunology 1986;59:509-514.
17. Kinnaird A., Peters S.W., Foster J.R. and Kimber I. Dendritic cell accumulation in the draining lymph nodes during the induction phase of contact allergy in mice. International Archives of Allergy and Applied Immunology 1989;89:202-210.
18. Kripke M.L., Munn C.G., Jeevan A., Tang J.-M. and Bucana C. Evidence that cutaneous antigen-presenting cells migrate to regional lymph nodes during contact sensitization. Journal of Immunology 1990;145:2833-2838.

19. Cumberbatch M. and Kimber I. Phenotypic characteristics of antigen-bearing cells in the draining lymph nodes of contact sensitized mice. Immunology 1990;71:404-410.
20. Cumberbatch M. and Kimber I. Antigen-bearing dendritic cells in the draining nodes of contact sensitized mice: cluster formation with lymphocytes. Immunology 1991;74:139-145.
21. Cumberbatch M., Gould S.J., Peters S.W. and Kimber I. MHC class II expression by Langerhans cells and lymph node dendritic cells: possible evidence for maturation of Langerhans cells following contact sensitization. Immunology 1991;74:414-419.
22. Cumberbatch M., Peters S.W., Gould S.J. and Kimber I. Intercellular adhesion molecule-1 (ICAM-1) expression by lymph node dendritic cells: comparison with epidermal Langerhans cells. Immunology Letters 1992;32:105-110.
23. Aiba S., Nakagawa S., Ozawa H., Kensuke M., Yagita H. and Tagami H. Up-regulation of α4 integrin on activated Langerhans cells: analysis of adhesion molecules on Langerhans cells relating to their migration from skin to draining lymph nodes. Journal of Investigative Dermatology 1993;100:143-147.
24. Kupper T.S. Role of epidermal cytokines. In: Immunophysiology (Oppenheim J.J. and Shevach E.M., eds.) Oxford University Press, New York, 1990:285-305.
25. Heufler C., Koch F. and Schuler G. Granulocyte/macrophage colony-stimulating factor and interleukin 1 mediate the maturation of murine epidermal Langerhans cells into potent immunostimulatory dendritic cells. Journal of Experimental Medicine 1988;167:700-705.
26. Cumberbatch M. and Kimber I. Dermal tumour necrosis factor-α induces dendritic cell migration to draining lymph nodes and possibly provides one stimulus for Langerhans cell migration. Immunology 1992;75:257-263.
27. Kock A., Schwarz T., Kirnbauer R., Urbanski A., Perry P., Ansel J.C. and Luger T.A. Human keratinocytes are a source for tumor necrosis factor α: Evidence for synthesis and release upon stimulation with endotoxin or ultraviolet light. Journal of Experimental Medicine 1990;172:1609-1614.
28. Enk A.H. and Katz S.I. Early molecular events in the induction phase of contact sensitivity. Proceedings of the National Academy of Sciences of the USA 1992;89:1398-1402.
29. Kolde G. and Knop J. Different cellular reaction patterns of epidermal Langerhans cells after application of contact sensitizing, toxic and tolerogenic compounds. A comparative ultrastructural and morphometric time-course analysis. Journal of Investigative Dermatology 1987;89:19-23.
30. Aiba S. and Katz S.I. Phenotypic and functional characteristics of *in vivo*-activated Langerhans cells. Journal of Immunology 1990;145:2791-2796.
31. Becker D., Neiss U., Neis S., Reske K. and Knop J. Contact allergens modulate the expression of MHC class II molecules on murine epidermal Langerhans cells by endocytic mechanisms. Journal of Investigative Dermatology 1992;98:700-705.

32. Becker D., Mohamadzadeh M., Reske K. and Knop J. Increased level of intracellular MHC class II molecules in murine Langerhans cells following in vivo and in vitro administration of contact allergens. Journal of Investigative Dermatology 1992;99:545-549.
33. Picut C.A., Lee C.S. and Lewis R.M. Ultrastructural and phenotypic change in Langerhans cells induced in vitro by contact allergens. British Journal of Dermatology 1987;116:773-784.
34. Enk A.H. and Katz S.I. Identification and induction of keratinocyte-derived IL-10. Journal of Immunology 1992;149:92-95.
35. Enk A.H., Angeloni V.L., Udey M.C. and Katz S.I. An essential role for Langerhans cell-derived IL-1β in the initiation of primary immune responses in the skin. Journal of Immunology 1993;150:3698-3704.
36. Matsue H., Cruz P.D. Jr., Bergstresser P.R. and Takashima A. Langerhans cells are the major source of mRNA for IL-1β and MIP-1α among unstimulated mouse epidermal cells. Journal of Investigative Dermatology 1992;99:537-541.
37. Heufler C., Topar G., Koch F., Trockenbacher B., Kampgen E., Romani N. and Schuler G. Cytokine gene expression in murine epidermal cell suspensions:Interleukin 1β and macrophage inflammatory protein 1α are selectively expressed in Langerhans cells but are differentially regulated in culture. Journal of Experimental Medicine 1992;176:1221-1226.
38. Schreiber S., Kilgus O., Payer E., Kutil R., Elbe A., Mueller C. and Stingl G. Cytokine pattern of Langerhans cells isolated from murine epidermal cell cultures. Journal of Immunology 1992;149:3525-3534.
39. Reld C.D.L., Stackpoole A., Meager A. and Tikerpae J. Interactions of tumor necrosis factor with granulocyte-macrophage colony-stimulating factor and other cytokines in the regulation of dendritic cell growth in vitro from early bipotent CD34$^+$ progenitors in human bone marrow. Journal of Immunology 1992;149:2681-2688.
40. Inaba K., Inaba M., Romani N., Aya H., Deguchi M., Ikehara S., Muramatsu S. and Steinman R.M. Generation of large numbers of dendritic cells from mouse bone marrow cultures supplemented with granulocyte/macrophage colony-stimulating factor. Journal of Experimental Medicine 1992;176:1693-1702.
41. Santiago-Schwarz F., Belilos E., Diamond B. and Carsons S.E. TNF in combination with GM-CSF enhances the differentiation of neonatal cord blood stem cells into dendritic cells and macrophages. Journal of Leukocyte Biology 1992;52:274-281.
42. Caux C., Dezutter-Dambuyant C., Schmitt D. and Banchereau J. GM-CSF and TNF-α cooperate in the generation of dendritic Langerhans cells. Nature 1992;360:258-261.
43. Phanuphak P., Moorhead J.W. and Claman H.N. Tolerance and contact sensitivity to DNFB in mice. I. In vivo detection by ear swelling and correlation with in vitro cell stimulation. Journal of Immunology 1974;122:115-123.
44. Kimber I., Botham P.A., Rattray N.J. and Walsh S.T. Contact sensitizing and tolerogenic properties of 2,4-dinitrothiocyanobenzene. International Archives of Allergy and Applied Immunology 1986;81:258-264.

45. Jones D.A., Morris A.G. and Kimber I. Assessment of the functional activity of antigen-bearing dendritic cells isolated from the lymph nodes of contact-sensitized mice. International Archives of Allergy and Applied Immunology 1989;90:230-236.
46. Robinson M.K. Optimization of an *in vitro* lymphocyte blastogenesis assay for predictive assessment of immunological responsiveness to contact sensitizers. Journal of Investigative Dermatology 1989;92:860-867.
47. Gerberick G.F., Ryan C.A., Fletcher E.R., Sneller D.L. and Robinson M.K. An optimized lymphocyte blastogenesis assay for detecting the response of contact sensitized or photosensitized lymphocytes to hapten or photohapten modified antigen presenting cells. Toxicology in Vitro 1990;4:289-292.
48. von Blomberg-van der Flier B.M.E., Bruynzeel D.P. and Scheper R.J. Impact of 25 years of *in vitro* testing in allergic contact dermatitis. In: Current Topics in Contact Dermatitis (Frosch P.J., Dooms-Goossens A., Lachapelle J-M., Rycroft R.J.G. and Scheper R.J., eds.) Springer-Verlag, Heidelberg, 1989:569-577.
49. Macleod T.M., Hutchinson F. and Raffle E.J. The uptake of labelled thymidine by leukocytes of nickel sensitive patients. British Journal of Dermatology 1970;82:487-492.
50. von Blomberg-van der Flier M., van der Burg C.K.H., Pos O., van de Plassche-Boers E.M., Bruynzeel D.P., Garotta G. and Scheper R.J. *In vitro* studies in nickel allergy: diagnostic value of dual parameter analysis. Journal of Investigative Dermatology 1987;88:362-368.
51. Kimber I., Quirke S. and Beck M.H. Attempts to identify the causative allergen in cases of allergic contact dermatitis using an *in vitro* lymphocyte transformation test. Toxicology in Vitro 1990;4:302-306.
52. Soeberg B. and Anderson V. Hapten-specific lymphocyte transformation in humans sensitized with NDMA or DNCB. Clinical and Experimental Immunology 1976;25:490-492.
53. Kimber I., Quirke S., Cumberbatch M., Ashby J., Paton D., Aldridge R.D., Hunter J.A.A. and Beck M.H. Lymphocyte transformation and thiuram sensitization. Contact Dermatitis 1991;24:164-171.
54. Inaba K. and Steinman R.M. Resting and sensitized T lymphocytes exhibit distinct (antigen presenting cell) requirements for growth and lymphokine release. Journal of Experimental Medicine 1984;160:1717-1735.
55. Knight S.C., Krejci J., Malkovsky M., Colizzi V., Gautam A. and Asherson G.L. The role of dendritic cells in the initiation of immune responses to contact sensitizers. I. *In vivo* exposure to antigen. Cellular Immunology 1985;94:427-434.
56. Hauser C. and Katz S.I. Activation and expansion of hapten- and protein-specific T helper cells from non-sensitized mice. Proceedings of the National Academy of Sciences of the USA 1988;85:5625-5628.

11

Human kidney cells in *in vitro* pharmaco-toxicology

S. Kastner*, M. Soose** and H. Stolte*

* Abteilung Nephrologie, Arbeitsbereich Exp. Nephrologie, Medizinische Hochschule Hannover, Konstanty-Gutschow-Str. 8, 30625 Hannover (Germany).
** Institut für Tierphysiologie, Justus-Liebig-Universität, Wartweg 91, 35392 Gießen (Germany).

Introduction

The principal function of the mammalian kidneys is the composition of the body fluids within narrow boundaries. In order to accomplish this, the kidneys receive 20% of the cardiac output, although they comprise only 0.4% of the body weight in most mammals [1]. This high blood flow dictates that large quantities of sytematically circulating xenobiotics will be delivered to the kidneys and predisposes the organ to damage by potential nephrotoxins [2]. The category of nephrotoxins includes large numbers of substances of different classes ranging from antibiotics, organic solvents, and poisons to metal ions (Table I).

Renal heterogeneity and target cell toxicity

To study and understand renal target cells toxicity it has to be taken into account that the kidney comprises a marked morphological, functional and biochemical heterogeneity, reflecting a high degree of organisation in this organ. Within the kidney the basic structural and functional unit is the nephron [6]. The term heterogeneity describes on the one hand the different nephron populations (superficial, cortical and juxtamedullary) which can be distinguished by their distribution within the kidney as

METALS

-Arsenic	-Cadmium	-Chromium
-Copper	-Germanium	-Gold
-Indium	-Lead	-Mercury
-Nickel	-Platinum	-Uranium
-Uranyl nitrate	-Zinc	

DRUGS

Cytostatics :
- **Adriamycin**
- **cis-Platin**

Analgetics :
- Acetaminophen
- Aspirin
- Phenacetine

Antibiotics :
- **Aminoglycosides**
- Amphotericin B
- Cephalosporins
- Polymyxin B
- Sulfonamides
- Tetracyclines

Immunosuppressives :
- **Cyclosporine**

ORGANIC CHEMICALS AND SOLVENTS

-Aniline	-Butyl ether	-Carbon tetrachloride
-Chloroform	-Cresol	-Diesel oil
-Dioxane	-Ethylene dichloride	-Ethylene glycol
-Lysol	-Naphtalene	-Perclorethylene
-Phenol	-Polyethylene glycol	-Toluene
-Trichlorethylene		

POISONS

Herbicides :
- Paraquat
- Lindan

Insecticides :
- DTT

Mycotoxins :
- Ochratoxin

OTHERS

-Aminonucleosides	-Biotech peptides	-Contrast media
-Fluorinated anesthetics		

Table I :
Summary of potentially nephrotoxic substances[3,4,5]
(**bold printed** compounds are described in further detail below)

well as by their anatomical and functional differences. However, the term heterogeneity not only applies to the different nephron populations, it is on the other hand also used to describe the different nephron segments and subsegments. The nephron consists of glomerulus, proximal tubule, loop of Henle, distal tubule and collecting duct; each of these segments has distinct structural, biochemical and functional characteristics. On the cellular level there are over 20 morphologically different cell types in the kidney, as well as a cellular heterogeneity both along and between the nephrons [7]. The term heterogeneity even applies to the tubular and peritubular cell membrane of epithelial cells [8] (Table II).

Functional heterogeneity means that each element of the kidney has specific functions, all of which may be differently influenced by nephrotoxicants. The characteristic functions of each single cell type

Morphological level	Heterogeneity
Total Kidney *Intrarenal distribution of different nephron populations*	-Superficial -Cortical -Juxtamedullary
Single nephron *Segments*	-Glomerulus -Tubular apparatus
Tubular apparatus *Subsegments*	-Proximal tubule (S_1, S_2, S_3 - segments) -Loop of Henle (thin descending limb, thick ascending limb) -Distal tubule -Collecting duct
Epithelium *Cellular sideness*	-Luminal side -Peritubular side

Table II :
Morphological heterogeneity of the kidney

might also be influenced individually by target cell selective nephrotoxic substances. The profile of biochemical and physiological characteristics define the function of the cell, but different cells also interact to maintain normal renal integrity.

The basis for the biochemical heterogeneity is the fact that enzymes capable of forming endogenous and exogenous chemicals are not uniformly distributed, but have discrete distribution among certain cell types. The unique biochemical characteristics predispose the target cell to injury, whereas adjacent, non-target cells, are unaffected.

This morphological, functional and biochemical heterogeneity is the basis for the selective targeting of nephrotoxic chemicals. The concept of target cell toxicity means that a compound preferentially affects a discrete group of target cells, or sometimes only a single cell type, along the nephron or in the interstitium, while adjacent cells are unaffected (Fig. 1). The reasons for this selectivity are the key for the understanding of the underlying mechanisms of nephrotoxicity and subsequently of prevention and therapy of renal damage.

The described heterogeneity within the nephron itself and the fact that most of the pathological and biochemical alterations in disease states are unique only for a particular nephron segment or even for a specific glomerular or tubular cell type has made the *in vivo* assessment of target cell nephrotoxicity and the study of underlying mechanisms difficult. Discrete renal target cell injury can, however, be exploited *in vitro* to study the interactions between the toxic compound and the specific target cell [9].

In vitro models in nephrotoxicity

Several *in vitro* models have been used to study the potential interactions between target cells and chemicals and to elucidate the pathomechanisms of nephrotoxicity [10,11,12] (Table III). Nevertheless, *in vivo* studies are of paramount importance because they determine whether certain conclusions based on *in vitro* experiments are relevant. However, a major problem with *in vivo* experiments is the fact that conditions can not easily be controlled as *in vitro*. Further implications are inter-individual variations, possible extra-renal influences and the lack of unambiguous parameters for estimating the extent of toxicity. With the different *in vitro* model systems these problems can be solved. The problem of inter-individual variations can be solved by obtaining many virtually identical samples of the same kidney. In this case individual animals serve as their own control. However, the deliberate exclusion of extra-renal influences is at the same time a major drawback of *in vitro* studies: the extra-renal effects may be responsible for/or modulate the ultimate nephrotoxicty [13]. For instance, the renal accumulation of cadmium which leads to severe nephrotoxicity is due to extra-renal incorporation of cadmium into metallothionein. The complex is selectively reabsorbed from the primary urine by the proximal tubular cells, whereas free Cd^{2+}, on the other hand, is primarily a heptatoxin [14].

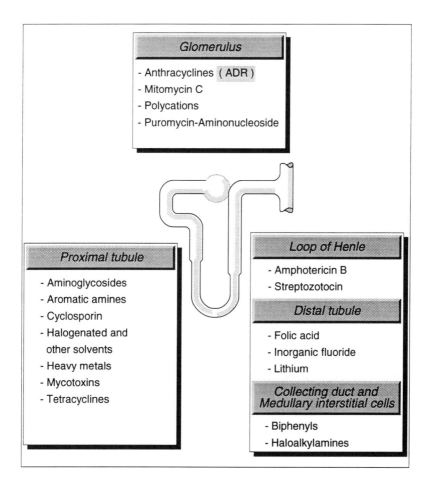

Figure 1:
Specific target regions or target cell types along the nephron affected by target selective nephrotoxins.

In vitro model	*References*
- Isolated perfused kidney	15, 16
- Kidney slices	17, 18
- Isolated nephron segments	
(glomeruli, tubules)	19, 20, 21, 22
- **Primary renal cell cultures**	23, 24, 25, 26, 27, 28
- **Kidney cell lines**	29, 30, 31, 32, 33, 34, 35
- Isolated organelles	36, 37, 38

Table III :

In vitro models in renal toxicology

Each *in vitro* model system possesses its own advantages and disadvantages and all have demonstrated their usefullness and application in renal toxicology. The model that resembles the *in vivo* situation the closest is the isolated perfused kidney (IPK). The IPK can provide data on clearance and transport of xenobiotics, but is still in many respects a black box. Renal slices have been in use for over 40 years [39] and can be obtained readily from a variety of species including man [40]. A substancial part of the present knowledge on renal toxicology has come from the use of renal slices [41,42]. However, this model suffers from two major disadvantages. Firstly, slices contain a heterogeneous cell population, which makes it cumbersome to assess functional changes in a distinct cell type. Secondly, many of the tubules on the exposed surface are damaged during the preparation and lack cellular integrity to various degrees [13]. Preparations of isolated glomeruli and tubules in suspension are widely employed and have been prepared from kidneys of various mammals [43,44,45] as well as from human kidneys [46,47,48]. *In vitro* studies with specific isolated nephron segments suffer from a lack of sufficient final cell quantity for detailed study and a limited viability of the preparation.

Kidney cell culture

An approach to overcome these limitations would be to prepare homogenous differentiated kidney cell cultures of defined nephronal origin able to be serially propagated *in vitro*. The introduction of kidney cell culture in the late seventies and early eighties has allowed a more specific approach to the role of individual kidney cell types in nephrotoxicity.

One of the major advantages of renal cell cultures is the yield of a sufficient cell mass. Both acute and chronic studies can be performed directly on the cellular level under normal and pathological conditions. To model the effects that may occur on chronic exposure *in vivo*, cultured kidney cells are exposed to low concentrations of nephrotoxins for long periods. Another advantage is the possibility to probate a controlled environment over a defined period of time to study the morphological and functional properties of a living single cell type. Thus, the interactions of several nephrotoxic chemicals can be studied, and probes can be used that are to toxic *in vivo*. Further, the response to and recovery from challenges can be studied with selected nephrotoxic compounds under controlled culture conditions.

The major disadvantage of renal cell culture studies is that the cells are taken out of their natural environment and are exposed to conditions not normally encountered *in vivo*. Thus, the loss of normal cell-cell and cell-matrix interactions may lead to morphological and functional dedifferentiation with subsequent changes in the biosynthetic profile and response to foreign chemicals. As with all *in vitro* systems, there is the questions of appropriateness of the test sytem and the parameters chosen for comparative purposes, i.e. kind of cells, media, exposure time and concentration, route of administration, choice of test parameters etc. Some of the potential advantages and disadvantages of renal cell culture compared to more traditional *in vitro* systems are summarized in Table IV. One way to overcome some of these disadvantages is to use multicellular *in vitro* systems instead of single cell systems.

Essentially two approaches to cell culture methodology are used to

Advantages	Disadvantages
- Sufficient yield of cellular material	- Reduced functional and metabolic capabilities compared to *in vivo* tissue
- Acute and chronic studies possible	
- Controlled environment	
- Direct exposure to toxic compounds	- Changes in morphologic identity
- Cell specific events/responses	- Artificial conditions *ex vivo*
- Extended viability	- Question of appropriateness
- No extra-renal influences	- Loss of cell-cell and cell-matrix interactions
- Bidirectional exposure/transport	

Table IV :
Advantages and disadvantages of renal cell cultures.

provide kidney cells. The first approach is using existing cell lines of kidney origin. Among those the MDCK[30,31], the LLC-PK[29,32,33] and the OK[34,35] cells are the most extensively studied cells lines. The major deficiencies of this approach is that the exact site of origin within the nephron is unknown, and that being a cell line, it may not be totally representative of the normal state and may in fact possess tumorigenic properties. However, there are no kidney cell lines of human origin available until present.

The second approach is to establish primary cultures of renal cells. The sources of human kidney tissue are usually samples of unaffected tissue obtained at a surgery for renal carcinoma, or material of biopsies and transplantion. Specific nephron segments (glomeruli, tubules) are mechanically isolated from kidney tissue by macro- or microdissection or sieving. Primary growth is established by explant techniques or protease digestion which is followed by cloning or plating the cells according to their differential growth capacities in a defined medium to assure uniform cell types. Cloning greatly facilitates defining the site of origin within the nephron [24,26,27,49] but has as a limitation the number of cells which can be grown for study since, when cloned, many generations of potential cell division are expended [50]. The explantation of kidney tissue in a hormonally and serum defined culture medium encourages the growth of certain cells whereas the growth of other cells is limited or even eliminated [51,52,53]. The advantage of this type of approach is the possibility that depending on media composition only a defined type of cells may be able to proliferate. This would further the possibility that defined segments of the nephron could be cultured simply by adjusting media composition. Primary cultures of epithelial cells, for example, usually do best in medium with little or no serum, whereas the growth of non-epithelial cells is encouraged in serum-containing medium [54]. Another approach to select kidney cells for culture is the use of monoclonal antibodies directed against cell-surface proteins that are specific for a certain cell type [55].

In general, to establish a kidney cell strain of defined origin in culture several criteria must be considered and fulfilled. Firstly, as described above, there are over 20 different renal cell types; thus, one must be certain that homogenous cultures have been obtained before beginning experiments. Secondly, the cell strain developed must proliferate well in culture and has to be able of extended subculture, such that laboratories with limited culture facilities can routinely grow and maintain their own cultures. Thirdly, the isolated cell strain must retain many of the *in vivo* properties it exhibits within the intact nephron if it is to serve as an *in vitro* model for kidney metabolism. But once established, kidney cells of defined origin, able to be propagated *in vitro*, might be a valuable tool for defining the pathological and biochemical alterations of renal function in diseases and disorders of the kidney.

Properties of cultured kidney cells

In this chapter the function, culture conditions and markers for characterization of kidney cells *in vitro* are summarized. Since there is still a lack of information, based on studies in human kidney cell cultures, many of the described properties of renal cells in normal and disease states are derived from studies performed in rat or rabbit renal cell cultures. If informations or data from studies in human renal cell cultures are available this will be particulary mentioned.

Glomerulus

Structure and function. The renal glomerulus is composed *in vivo* of at least four cell types: (1) glomerular epithelial cells, (2) endothelial cells, (3) parietal epithelial cells, and (4) two types of cells residing in the mesangium, the contractile mesangial cells and the phagocytic, bone marrow derived monocytes [24]. The glomerulus acts as a filter allowing water and small molecules to pass and retaining large molecules. It also modulates the blood flow to the rest of the nephron via the afferent and efferent arteries.

Isolation and purification. Glomeruli are isolated from human kidneys by forcing the minced kidney tissue through sieves with graded mesh sizes [28,56]. Glomerular cells can be grown from either intact glomeruli by directly plating the whole isolated glomeruli into culture for outgrowth of cells, or by enzymatic collagenase dissociation of the glomeruli and plating the dissociated cells in culture [26,28]. In either case, one has at least three glomerular cell types present in culture, and further purification procedures are necessary to ensure homogeneity.
Several methods have been used to obtain purified cultures of these different glomerular cell types [24,28]. One of such techniques is cloning. Cells are diluted with a sufficient volume of tissue culture medium to allow the addition of single cells to the culture. Colonies of cells, derived

from a single cell are individually subcultured and transferred to other dishes. Three cell types from explanted human glomeruli have been obtained by cloning [57]. Two of these cells types have been identified as glomerular epithelial and mesangial cells, respectively [57]. Another method for isolating cultures of glomerular epithelial and mesangial cells from explants of whole glomeruli is based on the differential growth capacities of these cells [24,26]. This procedure has been referred to as the 'mosaic theory'; it states that any explant tissue contains cells with low and high growth potential [58]. According to its proponents, glomerular epithelial cells represent a vast majority of emigrating cells from explanted glomeruli for the first 6 days of growth and mesangial cells represent 100% of the culture at day 30 [24,26]. The outgrowth can then further be enriched by dilute plating and/or cloning.

Epithelial cells (Table V)
Functions. Glomerular epithelial cells are attributed with several functions: (1) They participate in the synthesis of the glomerular basement membran (GBM) [59]; (2) they participate in the filtration process through pinocytosis of filtered proteins that may have leaked through the glomerular basement membrane [60]; (3) they participate in the filtration process by restricting the passage of negatively charged macromolecules because of its cell coat rich in sialoglycoproteins [61,62].
Culture conditions. One way to obtain purified, homogenous cultures of glomerular epithelial cells is by cloning. Epithelial cells can be isolated for cloning from human glomeruli by collagenase digestion. Glomeruli are incubated for 30 minutes with 750 U/ml collagenase [27,28]. The cells in the supernatant are a 90% pure fraction of epithelial cells [63,64], which grow well when further plated in Waymouth's medium supplemented with 20% fetal calf serum (FCS) or pooled human serum [27,28]. Another way is to explant whole glomeruli for initial outgrowth in RPMI 1640 supplemented with 20% FCS dilute in half with conditioned medium obtained from Swiss 3T3 fibroblasts. After 6 - 10 days of growth polyglonal cells are seen growing from glomeruli which can be plated as single cells for further cloning without serum [65].
Characterization. Epithelial cells in culture can be identified by the following criteria: (1) the polyglonal shape as viewed by phase contrast microscopy and a "cobblestone" - like appearance of the culture when confluency is reached [65,66,67]; (2) the presence of cilia on the surface and junctional complexes [65]; (3) the ability to form domelike structures, which are a morphological indicator for a vectorial transport of salt and

Serum requirements	Low or none
Cell surface antigens	CALLA, C3b, PHM5, renal tubular epithelial antigen
Morphology	Monolayer, polygonal, desmosome-like cell junctions
Cytoskeleton	Cytokeratin, actin
Susceptibility to trypsin	Very susceptible
Response to agents	Puromycin aminonucleoside
Biosynthetic profile	
-Extracellular matrix	Collagen I & IV Heparan sulfate Fibronectin
-Cyclooxygenase products	$PGI_2 > PGE_2$ (rat) TxA_2 (rat) human: none
-Lipoxygenase products	12-hydroxyeicosatetrenoic acid (rat)

Table V :
Properties of epitelial cells *in vitro* [24,26,28,66,71,72]

water [68]; and (4) the presence of intermediate filaments containing cytokeratin [27,28]. Since many epithelial cells display these features *in vitro*, specific markers to identify glomerular epithelial cells must be used. One is the cytotoxic response to the aminonucleoside of puromycin (PAN) [65], which is in accordance with preferential injury of glomerular epithelial cells and not other glomerular cells *in vivo* [62,69]. In addition, this cell type does not contain factor VIII antigen, a marker for the epithelium [65,67]. It has been described that only human glomerular epithelial cells bear receptors for C3b *in situ* and bind circulating antigen-antibody complexes. These receptors should serve as a suitable marker for cultured human glomerular epithelial cells [65,70].

Metabolism and disease processes. Epithelial cells are known to produce several components of the GBM and the extracellular matrix (ECM) *in vivo* and *in vitro*. The major collagenous protein is collagen IV [71]; the principal sulfated glycosaminoglycan is heparan sulfate [72]. Fibronectin

(FN) is found in both the cell layer and medium of epithelial cell cultures [71].

Epithelial cells have been implicated in several diseases both in humans and experimental animals. Of special note is the glomerular charge barrier, which is thought to be lost in the so-called minimal-change nephrotic syndrome in humans. Experimental diseases resulting in albuminuria such as aminonucleoside nephrosis are assumed to be mainly governed by epithelial cell integrity and particulary by their synthesis of GBM components [27,28]. One of the components of the GBM which have been postulated to play a role in the glomerular charge barrier are the proteoglycans. Since heparan sulfate-containing proteoglycans are found to be synthesized by epithelial cells *in vitro* [72], this might be one parameter to monitor the influences of toxic compounds on GBM synthesis *in vitro*.

Endothelial cells (Table VI)

Functions. The endothelial cells which line the glomerular capillary wall form a layer with fenestrae of approximately 1000 A in diameter. They may participate in the restriction of macromolecules from passing across the capillary wall [73].

Culture conditions. Until recently the isolation and propagation of glomerular endothelial cells in continuous culture was not possible. This is probably due to the particular conditions these highly differentiated cells require for growth, which are unavailable in the media presently in use. Human glomerular endothelial cells could, however, recently be cloned and propagated in culture in Waymouth's medium supplemented with 20% FCS containing 2 ng/ml platelet-derived growth factor (PDGF) [74].

Characterization. The cells are positively identified as endothelial cells by the presence of von Willebrand factor (factor VIII) antigen and angiotensin converting enzyme (ACE) activity. Weibel-Palade bodies, a marker for endothelial cells *in vivo*, are only rarely found *in vitro*. Neither cytokeratin nor keratin can be detected, however actin and tubulin are present. In contrast to mesangial cells, microfilaments are observed only in the vicinity of the cell surface [74].

Disease processes. It has been found that glomerular endothelial cells exhibit a dose-dependent detachment in response to endotoxins, whereas umbilical vein endothelial cells and mesangial cells are unaffected [75]. These data support a direct, specific effect of endotoxin on human glomerular endothelial cells and may help to explain the glomerular thrombotic lesion found in some septic patients.

Serum requirements	20 %
Cell surface antigens	Factor VIII
Morphology	Monolayer, polygonal, tight junctions
Cytoskeleton	Actin, tubulin
Susceptibility to trypsin	Very susceptible
Response to agents	Platelet products Endotoxins
Biosynthetic profile	Angiotensin converting enzyme

Table VI :
Properties of endothelial cells *in vitro*[24,26-28,74]

Mesangial cells (Table VII)
Functions. The mesangium has been shown to contain at least two functionally distinct subgroups of cell types both *in vivo* and *in vitro*; one resembles a bone-marrow derived macrophage and the second a smooth muscle cell. Here, we will only focus on the smooth muscle cell-like mesangial cells. Glomerular contractile mesangial cells are attributed with several functions: (1) the clearing of debris from mesangial regions by phagocytosis[76], (2) the control of glomerular size and blood flow by contraction[77], (3) mediator production, and (4) matrix synthesis.

Culture conditions. Contractile mesangial cells are relatively easy to isolate and have successfully be grown from human and animal glomeruli in homogenous culture[24,26,27,28]. Mesangial cells are most often grown from explants and can be further separated from glomerular epithelial cells by their differential growth capacities. As described above, after 30 days of growth the cultures are nearly pure glomerular mesangial cells. Therefore, if one passages and subcultures glomerular cells until day 30, one should obtain primarily mesangial cells. Absolute purity can be achieved by further cloning. The growth medium most commonly used is RPMI 1640 tissue culture medium supplemented with 20% FCS and with 0.66 IU of insulin per ml medium[24,26].

Characterization. The characterization of mesangial cells *in vitro* depends on their phase-microscopic appearance and the absence of markers characteristic of the other glomerular cell types. Multilayered cells lack factor VIII-related and cytokeratin antigens. In primary culture and after early passages mesangial cells are of spindle shape in culture [78]. The positive identification of glomerular mesangial cells is based on (1) its contractile behaviour, (2) surface receptors for angiotensin II (A II), and (3) on the presence of microfilaments containing the contractile proteins actin and myosin [24,26,27,28].

Metabolism and disease processes. Smooth muscle mesangial cells in culture have been shown to secrete both interstitial and basement membrane collagens, mainly types I and III, but also small amounts of collagen IV [71]. The biosynthetic profile of glycosaminoglycans includes dermatan sulfate, chondroitin-4-sulfate and 6-sulfate, and small amounts of heparan sulfate [72,79]. With regard to glycoproteins, both laminin and fibronectin are synthesized *in vitro* [71,80]. In addition to secreting matrix

Serum requirements	10 - 20 %
Cell surface antigens	Ia, Thy 1-1, A II receptor
Morphology	Multilayer, stellate
Cytoskeleton	Actin, myosin
Susceptibility to trypsin	Relatively resistant
Response to agents	Angiotensin II Mitomycin Interferon 1 Macrophage supernatants Platelet lysates
Biosynthetic profile	
-Extracellular matrix	Collagen I, III & IV Dermatan sulfate, Heparan sulfate, Chondroitin-4-sulfate, Chondroitin-6-sulfate Fibronectin, Laminin
-Cyclooxygenase products	PGE2 (rat) human: PGE2 > PGF2α
-Lipoxygenase products	12-hydroxyeicosatetrenoic acid (rat)
-Others	Neutral proteinase Erythropoietin

Table VII :
Properties of contractile mesangial cells *in vitro* [24,26-28,71,72,79-81]

proteins, mesangial cells *in vitro* release a latent metalloendoprotease into the medium [81].

Many glomerular diseases in humans and in animals are characterized by mesangial disturbances. Many of these can be monitored *in vitro*. Outlined below are the various biological functions of mesangial cells *in vitro* that may play a role in the development of glomerular pathology *in vivo* (Table VIII). This table may help to extrapolate *in vitro* findings in mesangial cell cultures on possible *in vivo* effects.

Mesangial cell function *in vitro*	Possible effects *in vivo*
Mediator production	
-Cytokines, Prostaglandins	-Chemoattractant, cellular proliferation, altered matrix metabolism
-Platelet activating factor	-Vascular alterations
-Reactive oxygen species	-Oxidative tissue damage
Proliferation	Mesangium expansion
Phagocytosis	Antigen trapping Antigen presentation
Matrix synthesis	*Matrix accumulation* *Glomerulosclerosis* *Alteration of cellular function*
Contractility	Alteration of glomerular blood flow

Table VIII :
Function of mesangial cells *in vitro* and the effects that these functions may have in the development of pathological changes of the glomerulus *in vivo* [82]

Immune glomerular injury, both in man and in animal models, is often characterized by infiltration of polymorphs and mononuclear inflammatory cells. And while the role of local glomerular cells in the induction of these overtly inflammatory forms of glomerulonephritis remains unclear, several important pro-inflammatory functions of mesangial cells have been established. These include (1) the capacity to produce cytokines, which have numerous chemo-attractant and inflammatory actions, such as the platelet derived growth factor (PDGF), interleukin 1 (IL-1), tumor necrosis factor (TNF); (2) the capacity to localize antigens in the mesangium, and possibly initiate an immune response by presentation of deposited antigen to T-lymphocytes; and (3) the ability to alter glomerular haemodynamics by contraction in response to vasoactive stimuli [82].

Our interest is mainly focused on alterations in matrix synthesis of mesangial cells *in vitro* and related disturbances of glomerular function *in vivo*. The mesangial matrix is composed of a variety of extracellular matrix (ECM) proteins, including type IV and I collagen, fibronectin, laminin, heparan sulfate and chondroitin sulfate[83,84], shown to be synthesized by both mesangial and epithelial cells *in vivo* and *in vitro*. Many diseases of the glomerulus are characterized by an increase in mesangial matrix, as well as by an increase in mesangial cell number. Accumulation of matrix proteins leads to the progressive scarring of the glomerulus known as glomerulosclerosis. Glomerular mesangial cells and epithelial cells directly regulate the nature and amount of extracellular matrix present in the glomerulus, and it is also becoming clear that the matrix in turn influences the mesangial cell behaviour [85]. Therefore, mesangial cells *in vitro* are a valuable tool to study the effects of nephrotoxins on the metabolism of extracellular matrix proteins for modelling possible events during the development of glomerulosclerosis *in vivo*.

Tubular apparatus

Structure and function. The tubular apparatus is consisting of the proximal tubule, loop of Henle, distal tubule and collecting duct systems. It is involved in the selective reabsorption of the bulk of the filtrate with approximately 98-99% of the salts and water being reabsorbed. There is virtually complete reabsorption of filtered sugars and amino acids and selective elimination of waste materials. Furthermore, the tubular element actively secretes organic compounds, potassium and hydrogen ions into the urine.

Isolation and purification. In principle, all procedures for the isolation of tubular cells are based on mechanical or enzymatic dispersion of the kidneys followed by one or more purification steps. For mechanic disruption the tissue is simply minced with scissors or with a homogenizer. For enzymatic disruption the kidneys are preperfused via the renal artery with collagenase (0.05-0.2%) or trypsin. To obtain single cell supensions it is necessary to loosen the tight junctions between the cells in the tubules by perfusion of the kidney with Ca^{2+}-chelating agents (EDTA or EGTA) before protease treatment. Due to the cellular heterogeneity along the nephron tubular cell preparations are usually highly intermingled. This makes it impossible to isolate a specific cell type without purification procedures, irrespective of the previous isolation method. Several purification techniques have been developed, such as simple filtration or density sedimentation on gradients of non-toxic materials (Ficoll or Percoll)[22,86]. More complex methods are free-flow electrophoresis[87,88] and immunological selection[55,89,90]. However, it should be noted that the purification procedures described result in an enrichment rather than in complete elemination of unwanted cell types. Therefore, further subcloning is necessary to produce homogenous cell populations.

The simplest way to set up a primary culture of tubular cells is to explant the enzymatically or mechanically dispersed fragments for initial outgrowth. This technique has a limited application for defined renal tubular cultures because of the extreme heterogenous nature of the kidney, which would result in the outgrowth of numerous cell types. It has, however, been reported that minced explants of human renal cortex result in the outgrowth of epithelial monolayers with proximal tubular properties[25].

To overcome these limitations a more sophisticated technique uses explanted micro-dissected defined tubular fragments without proteolytic digestion[91,92]. This method has the advantage of absolute specificity of choice and isolation of cell types with standard criteria of tubular morphology and anatomical distribution. Outgrowing cells are subcultured in a hormonally defined and/or serum-supplemented medium[93] without any need for further purification. Primary cultures from these individually isolated tubules seem to retain more of the characteristic functions related to transport, enzymes, and sensitivity to hormones, even after several passages, than digested or fractionated cells. Using the micro-dissection technique primary cultures of some types of the human nephron have been set up, including cells of the proximal tubule, cortical thick ascending limb of Henle, and collecting tubule[94].

A recent and novel approach, described as immunodissection, has adapted the monoclonal antibody technology to the problem of picking out individual tubular cell types from the heterogenous organ[55,95]. This type of technique offers the advantage of the production of large cell numbers in culture and is potentially quite specific since it is based on antigen-antibody interactions. The full potential of immunodissection will be realized if purified antibodies can be produced which are specific for a single tubular cell typ with specific antigenic sites [26].

Culture conditions. The growth of fibroblasts, often overgrowing the primary cell cultures, poses a major problem in renal tubular cell culture [96]. An important development, enabling the establishment of defined epithelial cell cultures, without fibroblast overgrowth, was the definition of hormonal and growth factor supplements required to support growth in serum-free media [97]. Renal tubular epithelial cells have receptors for a wide variety of growth factors, many of which are circulating hormones. The segmental epithelial preference for certain combinations of these factors suggests that a particular balance of these factors may be the key to stimulating growth *in vitro* for defined tubular cells. There is a universal requirement for transferrin and hydrocortisone and a substantial selectivity of requirement for additional supplements (prostaglandin E_1, insulin, triiodothyronine, insulin, dexamethasone) depending on epithelial cell type and origin [52,98,99,100,101].

In addition to the importance of hormones and growth factors for the initiation of growth and maintainance of differentiated function of renal tubular cells, the extracellular matrix has also been shown to exert important effects on epithelial growth and function [102]. The provision of certain substrates such as collagens, laminin, and the matrix laid down by the mouse-derived endodermal line PF-HR-9 favours epithelial cell proliferation [26]. *In vivo*, all renal tubular epithelia lie on a basement-membrane of specific composition and it appears from recent studies that the provision of basement membrane adhesion factors is necessary and desirable for the continued proliferation of fully differentiated renal tubular cells with normal function and morphology. These adhesion factors may be provided in the form of interstitial collagen, which stimulates epithelia to produce their own basement membrane, or in the form of basement membrane, collagen gels or sheep amnion [94,98,100,101].

Polarity. Cells of transporting epithelia exhibit both structural and functional polarity, reflected by an asymmetric distribution of proteins, lipids, enzymes, transport activities, and hormone receptors between distinct apical and basolateral domains of the plasma membranes which are separated by tight junctions [103,104]. The establishment and maintainance of this polarity is essential for renal tubules, both *in vivo* and *in vitro* to fulfill their normal functions of selective permeability and vectorial transport. Microdissected renal tubules in primary culture have been shown to express several of these characteristics of well-polarized epithelia [94]. Ultrastructurally, microvilli are seen only on the apical surface, facing the medium in the dish, while basement membrane material is associated only with the basal cell surfaces, adjacent to the dish. Marker enzyme analysis has also shown polarized distribution *in vitro*, identical to that seen *in vivo* alkaline phosphatase and γ-glutamyl transpeptidase in cultured proximal tubules are located as ectoenzymes on apical cell membranes, while Na-K-ATPase, an integral membrane protein, is only located on basolateral membranes. Basolateral receptor-mediated responses of adenylat cyclase to parathyroid hormone (PTH) in proximal tubules and to arginine-vasopressin (AVP) in collecting tubules are also normal in primary cultures [101].

Proximal Tubule (Table IX)
Functions. The proximal tubular cells are mainly involved in the iso-osmotic reabsorption and secretion of organic anions, organic cations, inorganic electrolytes, sugars and water. The structure of the cell is therefore modified to this end. In particular, the surface area of both the apical and basal surface is increased by the presence of a brush border and basal infoldings respectively, while the enzymatic make-up of the two surfaces is quite different.
Culture conditions. Proximal tubular cells from various species, including man, can be maintained in primary culture. It has been described that macrodissected fragments of human renal cortex can be explanted on a collagen/fibronectin matrix. The explants were incubated in a serum free medium (Dulbecco's modified Eagles' medium and Ham's F12, 1:1) supplemented with transferrin, selenium, insulin, hydrocortisone, triiodothyronine and epidermal growth factor for the inital outgrowth of epithelial monolayers [25]. Microdissected fragments from human kidney tubules explanted on collagen-coated dishes in hormone-supplemented (transferrin, insulin, dexamethasone), serum-free RPMI 1640 medium have also been described to produce monolayers in culture [94].
Characterization. Proximal tubular cells are characterized structurally by the presence of apical microvilli and numerous mitochondria. Further characterization can be done by the demonstration of the presence of differentiated proximal tubular functions like transport processes (glucose, phosphate, amino acids, and organic

ions) [95,105,106,107,108,109], specific metabolism (cytochrom P-450 dependent oxidation) [109,110], and responsiveness to hormones (parathyroid hormone-stimulated cAMP production) [107,111], as well as by specifc enzymes (alkaline phosphatase, acid phosphatase, glucose-6-phosphatase) [109,111]. Preferentially the absence of markers for several possible contaminating other cell types like glomerular, distal tubular and collecting duct cells should be demonstrated. This may be done by confirming the absence of e.g. endothelial factor VIII, hexokinase or Tamm-Horsfall-glycoproteins [25,94,107,111,112].

Metabolism and disease processes. Glucose uptake is an important and specific function of the proximal tubular cells. Since glucosuria is one of the early symptoms of proximal tubular dysfunction [113], one might expect that nephrotoxins which specifically affect the proximal tubule will reduce glucose uptake by proximal tubular cells *in vitro*. However, this is not the fact since glucose is actively taken up at the apical membrane, but is secreted at the basolateral membrane by facilated transport. Thus glucose enters and leaves the cells but is not accumulated. However, α-methylglucose can be used instead since it is a non-metabolizable glucose analogue with high affinity for the glucose transporter at the apical membrane, but no affinity for the basolateral carrier [114].

Human polycystic kidney disease is an autosomal dominant trait and individual cysts have been microdissected and successfully cultured from end-stage kidneys [115]. Comparison of these cultured cyst epithelia with cells from proximal tubules and cortical collecting ducts from normal human kidneys revealed accelerated growth. Several morphological and functional abnormalities were seen in cystic cultured epithelium including enhanced Na-K-ATPase activity, modified polarity,

Transport processes	Hormone response	Enzyme pattern
Amino acids Na-Glucose Na-Phosphate	Angiotensin II Calcitonin Parathyroid hormone	Acid phosphatase Alkaline phosphatase Glucose-6-phosphatase Leucin aminopeptidase Na-K-ATPase γ-Glutamyl-transferase

Table IX :
Properties of proximal tubular cells in primary culture[25-27,94]

a decreased responsiveness to AVP and PTH, and a grossly modified basement membrane. Alterations were also seen in the morphological response to and requirements for specific extracellular matrix proteins. This culture system promises to provide a model for the study of human polycystic disease and the role of matrix proteins in the regulation of growth and differentiated function.

Loop of Henle

Function. The loop of Henle consists of two limbs, a thin descending limb and a thick ascending limb. The thick ascending limb (TAL) is mainly involved in the active reabsorption of water, Na^+ and Cl^-. It functionally plays a significant role in the counter-current mechanism related to the concentration of urine. The cells in this region have a very high mitochondrial densitiy and a great sensitivity to drugs which inhibit Na^+-transport.

Culture conditions and characterization. Cultures from cells of the medullary thick ascending limbs can be grown on human amnion in a Coon's modification of Ham's F-12 medium plus Lebowitz's L-15 medium supplemented with 0.5% rabbit serum and 0.5% FCS [98]. Cortical thick ascending limb cells have successfully been cultured from microdissected explants of human kidneys in serum-free RPMI 1640 medium supplemented with transferrin, dexamethasone, insulin, and triiodothyronine [94].

TAL cells are characterized (Table X) by the presence of large mitochondria, large amounts of Na-K-ATPase, and lack of stimulation of adenylate cyclase by arginine vasopressin. Tamm-Horsfall protein (THP) is a membrane glycoprotein characteristicly synthesized by cells of the thick ascending limb [116] *in vivo*. The expression of THP can be demonstrated in TAL cell cultures by immunofluorescence [98]. Anti-THP antibodies might also be usefull to select TAL cells for culture by immunodissection.

Hormone response	Enzyme pattern	Other characteristics
Calcitonin Parathyroid hormone	Na-K-ATPase	Furosemide-sensitive Tamm-Horsfall antigen

Table X :
Properties of thick ascending limb cells in primary culture [25-27,94,98]

Distal and collecting tubule (Table XI)
Function. The distal tubule has a histologic profile similar to the proximal tubule albeit with less mitochondria and a less distinct brush border. It is involved in the reabsorption of ions not already taken up at the proximal tubular sites. After the short distal tubule several nephrons drain into collecting ducts, consisting of a cortical and a medullary part. This structure is the site of active K^+-secretion, Na^+, Cl^- and HCO_3^--reabsorption and it is the prime site of action of the anti-diuretic hormone (ADH).

Hormone response	Enzyme pattern	Other characteristics
Aldosterone Arginine vasopressin Bradikinin Calcitonin	Cytochrome-oxidase	PGE_2 production

Table XI :
Properties of collecting tubular cells in primary culture[26,27,94]

Culture conditions and characterization. Several methods have been employed to isolate cortical and medullary collecting tubular cells. (1) The unique characteristic of medullary collecting duct cells to resist hypotonic lysis has been utilized to isolate these cells for subsequent culture [117,118]. (2) In another approach, monoclonal antibodies raised against MDCK cells were found to cross react with cortical collecting duct cells. Dishes coated with the monoclonal antibody were then used to bind and thereby select cortical collecting duct cells from a suspension of cells prepared from collagenase-treated kidney cortex [55,90]. (3) Microdissected cortical collecting tubules grown in defined medium (RPMI 1640 medium, supplemented with transferrin and dexamethasone) produce cell monolayers in culture [94].

Cortical collecting tubular cells have characteristicly only few organelles and poor staining for cytochrom-oxidase. The stimulation of adenylat cyclase by arginine vasopressin but not to parathyroid hormone also demonstrates that these cells remain characteristics similar to the *in vivo* situation [94].

Human kidney cells in *in vitro* pharmaco-toxicology

The main purposes of toxicity tests are to provide a data base that can be used to assess the risk potential to humans associated with a situation in which the drug, the subject and the exposed conditions are defined. The most frequently chosen species for nephrotoxicity is the rat. The rat kidney has many basic similarities to human renal structure and function, but also a number of differences. Differences such as in metabolic rates and susceptibility to toxins may cause uncertainties when extrapolating the results from animals to man. Therefore, to minimize or even to avoid these uncertainties it is essential to foster the use of human kidney cells in *in vitro* pharmaco-toxicological studies. Since human kidney cells in culture are a comparatively new tool in the field of *in vitro* pharmaco-toxicology [119] and their use in studying mechanisms of drug-induced nephrotoxicty and in screening new drug candidates for nephrotoxic potential is just beginning to be described, there is not much information available in this field until present. In this chapter, some examples of the use of human renal cell cultures in *in vitro* pharmaco-toxicology will be given.

Glomerulus

The glomerulus is the first nephron structure that comes into contact with circulating chemicals. Therefore, the glomerulus is the primary site of action of several chemicals and is also susceptible to immunologic injury [10].

Anticancer drugs

Adriamycin. The anticancer drug Adriamycin (ADR) is a potent nephrotoxin targeting primarily the glomerulus. The ADR-induced nephrotic syndrome is documented in detail in rodents, and it is mainly characterized by an increased proteinuria and a decreased glomerular filtration rate (GFR) [120]. Morphological studies revealed a mesangium proliferation, an accumulation of mesangial matrix [121,122] and ultra-structural changes such as fusion and detachment of foot processes and a thickening of the glomerular basement membrane [120,121,123]. The molecular and cellular mechanisms responsible for the ADR-nephrotoxicty, however, are not clearly defined yet.
A causal relationship between ADR-caused permeability changes of the

glomerular filtration barrier and the turnover of one of its constituent molecules, fibronectin (FN), was recently demonstrated in an *in vivo* study. Focusing on renal fibronectin excretion, the enhanced glomerular permeability for plasma FN in ADR-treated rats was found to be accompanied by a loss of urinary degradation products of FN [124]. These data are compatible with a proliferation of the glomerular mesangium in chronic ADR-nephrosis [121,122], suggesting a disturbed metabolism of glomerular extracellular matrix proteins by ADR. As indicated above, the extracellular matrix (ECM) protein fibronectin, which plays a major role in the development of structural alterations of the glomerular filtration barrier is produced by mesangial cells both *in vivo* and *in vitro* [71]. A follow up *in vitro* study was therefore designed to establish the role of extracellular matrix proteins as a specific cellular target of pharmaceutical substances[125]. In this study confluent cultures of human mesangial cells (HMC) were incubated for 24 hours in the presence of ADR (0.5 - 2 µg/ml).

HMC synthesize cellular fibronectin which amounts to approximately 2% of total protein synthesis. Newly synthesized fibronectin is both secreted into the culture medium and incorporated into a fibrillar extracellular matrix. After incubation with ADR an accumulation of FN in the ECM was revealed by immunostaining (Fig. 2). Correspondingly, radioactively labeled, immunoprecipitable FN was significantly increased in the extracellular compartments (ECM and culture medium) by 23% compared to controls. Concomitantly with the ADR-induced accumulation of newly synthesized FN in extracellular compartments, immunoprecipitable intracellular FN was reduced by 22%. (Fig. 3). In contrast to the quantitative changes of newly synthesized FN in the three culture compartments, the total amount of newly synthesized FN was not elevated in ADR-treated cultures compared to controls; there was only a shift from the intracellular to the extracellular compartment. Qualitative characterization of the FN pattern revealed a diminished number of degradation products in the culture medium of ADR-treated HMC, which is assumed to be due to an inhibition of FN-degradating proteases.

These data suggest that ADR exerts different effects on FN metabolism of HMC *in vitro*. By interfering with the degradation of FN secreted by the cells, ADR induces an extracellular FN accumulation. This is answered by the cells via a negative feedback (cell-matrix interactions) with a reduced intracellular FN synthesis. However, this regulatory mechanisms is regarded to be insufficient during long term ADR-treatment, resulting

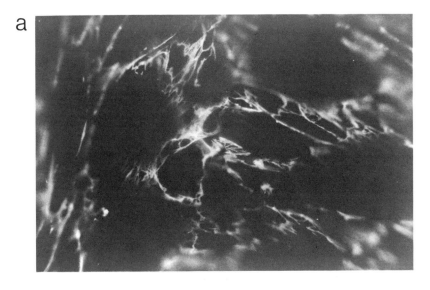

2 A

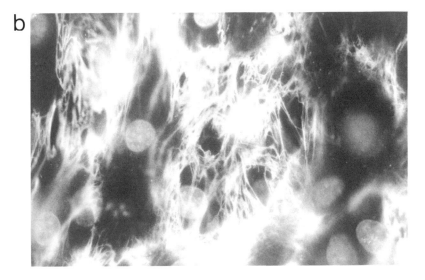

2 B

Figure 2 :
Fibronectin in the extracellular matrix of control and ARD-treated human mesangial cells (HMC) detected by indirect immunofluorescence (x420)
a) control; b) HMC treated with 2 µg ADR/ml.

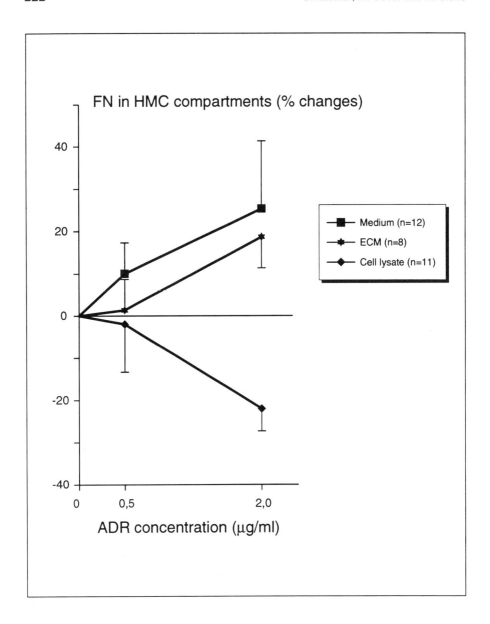

Figure 3 :
Effect of ADR on the fibronectin fractions in extracellular and intracellular compartments of human mesangial cells. Immunoprecipitable radioactivity recovered from the respective compartment after 24 hrs labeling with ^{35}S-methionine. Results are expressed as % of control ± SD

in an accumulation of extracellular matrix proteins. These *in vitro* findings are in accordance with a diminished excretion of renal FN fragments in ADR-treated rats [124] and with the proliferation of mesangial matrix in chronic ADR-nephrosis [121,122] as indicated above.

In conclusion, human mesangial cell provide a usefull *in vitro* model to elucidate the primary targets, the pathomechanisms, and the cascade of toxic events of nephrotoxins affecting the metabolism of extracellular matrix proteins during development of nephrotoxic-induced glomerulopathies. Further, fibronectin is regarded as a valuable marker protein to study the effects of nephrotoxins on mesangial cells *in vitro*. Since HMC were shown to preserve essential features of FN synthesis and processing *in vitro*, they provide a suitabel model to study FN-turnover and its pharmaco-toxicologically-induced alterations.

Cyclosporine. As described below in further detail, Cyclosporine A (CsA) possesses a powerful immunomodulating activity effecting an amelioration in graft rejection of transplanted organs in humans. It is nevertheless able to induce such dramatic side effects as hypertension and nephrotoxicity [126]. Whether the etiology of the nephrotoxicity lies in a defect in renal tubular function or in a decreased renal blood flow and/ or glomerular filtration rate is unknown.

Therefore, a study in human mesangial cells was aimed to confirm the direct vasoactive effect of CsA [127]. When HMC are incubated with various concentrations of CsA (10^{-6} to 10^{-10} M) a reduction of the planar surface area and a disappearance of myosin stress fibers could be observed.

Contraction of mesangial cells *in vitro* could at least partly explain the dramatic vasoconstriction observed *in vivo* in animals or in humans. HMC therefore provide an usefull experimental *in vitro* model to study the vasoactive effects of nephrotoxins and to explain haemodynamic changes *in vivo*.

Tubular apparatus

The prerequisite for studies of normal renal tubular cell function in culture is the establishment of a homogenous epithelial cell population of known tubular segmental origin, which is capable of normal, differentiated function. Therefore, most studies of human tubular cell cultures have focused on the development of appropriate cell models and on the investigation of normal cell biology. There is now, however, a growing body of investigations applying the established cell cultures for pathophysiology and toxicology studies [128].

Many nephrotoxins appear to have their primary site of action in/on the proximal tubule. This is reasonable since most of the blood flow to the kidney is delivered to the cortex, which is predominantly proximal tubule. In addition, active secretion of compounds occurs in the proximal tubule and by reabsorption of water and salts, the materials remaining in the tubular lumen (including the potential toxicant) are concentrated. Thus, a non-toxic concentration of a compound in the plasma can become toxic in the kidney subsequent to concentration within the urine [10]. These processes predispose especially late proximal tubular cells (PTC) to very high concentrations of the agent and cause toxicity.

Aminoglycosides. The nephrotoxic potential of aminoglycoside antibiotics is well documented in man. For example, at least 10% of all cases of acute renal failure in humans have been attributed to the use of aminoglycosides [129,130]. It is well known that the nephrotoxic lesions that occur *in vivo* during aminoglycoside-induced nephrotoxicity are both dose- and time-dependent. The proximal tubule is the primary site affected in aminoglycoside-nephrotoxicity and the lysosomes are one major intracellular target. Sequestration of aminoglycosides in lysosomes leads to 'myeloid body'-formation due to an impairment of phospholipid degradation [129,131,132]. These myeloid bodies have also been reported to be excreted into the urine by aminoglycoside-treated animals [133], and many researchers believe that these bodies are the earliest morphological evidence of aminoglycoside nephrotoxicity. Subsequently lysosomal membrane integrity is reduced, and release of lysosomal enzymes into the cytosol and digestion of cytoplasmic components and organelles may occur [129]. Additionally, aminoglycosides produce numerous biochemical and functional abberations in proximal tubular cells. They alter membrane phospholipid composition, permeability, Na-K-ATPase activity, adenylate cyclase activity and cation transport [134] and the release of tubular proteins into the urine [135].

To elucidate the cellular targets and possible mechanisms of aminoglycoside nephrotoxicity human proximal tubular cells have been used in several *in vitro* studies [136,137,138,139,140,141]. For studying dose- and time dependent relationships, actively dividing and resting human PTC were exposed to increasing concentrations of streptomycin, kanamycin, gentamycin, and neomycin for monitoring cell growth and toxicity over an 18 day period of exposure [139]. The order of toxicity of the aminoglycosides was neomycin > kanamycin > gentamycin > streptomycin. Both actively dividing and resting cultures of human PTC displayed dose- and time-dependency with regard to toxicity and the ability to regenerate in the continued presence of aminoglycoside exposure [139]. Prolonged exposure to gentamycin severely decreased sphingomyelinase activity in human PTC, causing an accumulation of phopholipids in the lysosomes, morphologically visible as myeloid bodies [141]. Another paper reports the effects of gentamycin (0.01 - 1.0 mg/ml) on certain aspects of lysosomal function and integrity, i.e. endocytotic activity, pH, and membrane fragility, in cultured human PTC using *in vitro* conditions associated with the morphologic observation of myeloid bodies [138]. Gentamycin treatment caused a slight decrease in endocytotic activity, measured by the rate with which PTC accumulated Fluorescein-isothiocyanat-labeled dextran. Intralysosomal pH was slightly increased, whereas fragility of the lysosomes, estimated by the release of N-acetyl-β-glucosaminidase, was only effected after longterm treatment (≤ 10 days) with gentamycin [138].

The reproducible findings *in vivo* and *in vitro* provide strong evidence of the validity of this model system. It is further proposed from these studies that cultured proximal tubular cells could be a useful model system to extend current research avenues assessing the mechanisms of aminoglycoside nephrotoxicity.

Cyclosporine. Cyclosporine A is a potent immunosuppressive agent that has been shown in animals and humans to prolong graft survival presumably via preferential suppresion of T-lymphocytes [142]. However, CsA is associated with a reversible dose-related nephrotoxicity in humans that has been estimated to occur in 60% to 80% of all patients. The nephrotoxicity manifests itself in the form of an insidious rise in serum creatinine [143]. Kidneys examined 21 days after CsA application showed focal proximal tubular cell vacuolation and necrosis. Ultrastructural studies exhibited dilatation of the endoplasmic reticulum, increased number of lysosomes including the presence of myeloid bodies, and large lipid droplets that affect the whole length of the proximal tubule [144]. Several studies are conducted in human proximal tubular cells to elucidate the pathogenic mechanisms of CsA-induced cell injury [145,146]. These include biochemical and ultrastructural studies of subcellular loci of injury, i.e., target organelles (plasma membrane, mitochondria, lysosomes endoplasmic reticulum), as well as possible mediators (lipid peroxidation and altered calcium homeostasis). By phase microscopy cultures of human renal tubular cells appeared to contain increased numbers of cytoplasmic vacuoles as the concentration (0.4 - 10 µg/ml) and exposure time (3 - 21 days) of CsA was increased. This is in accordance with the *in vivo* findings in biopsy materials, indicating that tubular vacuolation may be an early manifestation of Cyclosporine A toxicity. Lipid hydroperoxide production and intracellular calcium were measured after CsA incubation of monolayer human PTC cultures with fluorescent probes, revealing an increase in hydroperoxide production and a decrease in cytosolic calcium. These results, however, were not statistically significant, but indicate a causal relationship between CsA toxicity and these parameters.

It is concluded that human proximal tubular cells in culture provide a means of defining the temporal sequence of CsA-induced alterations and their progression in response to dose and duration. Simultaniously, they provide a valuable means of verification and comparison of nephrotoxicity data derived from animal studies. These studies in a human *in vitro* system are particulary important in the case of CsA nephrotoxicity in which the suitability of animal models is still in question.

Heavy metals. cis-Platin. Nephrotoxicity is frequently a complication of therapy with cis-Platin, a platinum coordination complex with antineoplatic properties [147]. Proximal tubular damage has been observed in humans and animals, associated with acute proximal tubular necrosis, leading to enzymuria, proteinuria and altered organic ion transport[147]. Electron microscopical studies reveal several ultrastructural changes such as thinning of the brush border and rounded mitochondria [148].

The cytotoxicity of cis-Platin (0.1 - 100 µg/ml) was assessed in primary cultured tubular cells. Membrane damage was established by the release of two specific proximal tubular brush border membrane enzymes (γ-glutamyl-transferase, GGT, and alkaline phosphatase, ALP) and lysosomal damage by the release of a specific lysosomal enzyme (N-acetyl-β-D-glucosaminidase, NAG) into the culture medium. Nuclear dysfunction was assessed by inhibition of DNA-synthesis with the ^{3}H-thymidine incorporation test [149,150]. The results revealed that cis-Platin targets for the DNA, shown by a decreased thymidine incorporation, and also causes membrane damage, characterized by an increased release of GGT and ALP.

This study confirms again the use of cultured human tubular cells to evaluate the nephrotoxicity of xenobiotics by comparing cytotoxicity affecting membrane and nuclear integrity to help define subcellular targets of toxic compounds.

Despite unique and universal challenges involved in extrapolating any *in vitro* data to the *in vivo* situation, these summarized studies all strongly indicate that human renal cells in culture provide usefull *in vitro* models to elucidate the mechanisms of renal injury induced by pharmaco-toxicological substances.

Future perspectives

Although significant challenges remain in the development of cultured renal cell systems, their immediate utility is evident. Perhaps the greatest challenges facing renal cell culture development involve (1) the maintenace of *in vivo* metabolic capabilities and (2) the establishment of polarized, bidirectional exposure systems [119].

The later area is under active investigation and development as the technology has become available to grow cells on porous filter membranes. Such systems will permit investigators to study the bidirectional aspects of drug or chemical accumulation and toxicity which are thought to be of paramount importance in a polarized cell such as the kidney tubular epithelium [119]. LLC-Pk$_1$ monolayers grown on such membranes have been applied to investigate transport characteristics of organic ions and glucose [151,152]. This technique will help to understand the mechanisms involved in the biogenesis of a distinct apical and basolateral membrane structure.

Coming back to the first point, one of the major problems of toxicity screening *in vitro* is the rapid de-differentiation of primary cell cultures. This is especially the case for renal cortical cells, where the enzyme profile changes markedly over a few days [153]. There is a need to control the biochemical properties of stable cell lines in such a way as predispose them to certain types of specific injury. For example, the coexistence of peroxidase activity and lipid droplets in 3T3 fibroblasts makes them a potentially usefull system in which to screen papillotoxic chemicals [154]. The possibility that no single cell type will contain all of the factors that may predispose them to 'target selective' injury can be adressed by several molecular biological approaches including the fusion of two different cells to combine desirable functions (such as transport process and metabolic activation system). Cell hydrids formed by electrofusion have already been used to produce monoclonal antibodies [155]. It may be possible to hybridize renal cells with stable lines to provide cells that reflect the characteristics of different renal cell types for nephrotoxicity testing. The establishment of an array of cells with such properties would provide the potential to learn more about the mechanisms of injury in these model chimeral systems and hence in renal and other cell types [9].

Established renal cell lines, although possessing an indefinitive life span, have some limitations. They have lost a number of properties of their *in vivo* ancestor cells, like gluconeogenesis or specific transporters. Furthermore, no untransformed continuous cell lines of human origin are available so far. For this reason the pig proximal tubular cell line LLC-PK$_1$ was fused with primary cultures of human proximal tubular cells using the fusogen polyethylen glycol (PEG) [156]. The produced hybridoma cells retain most of the structural and functional features of the primary cells and may be considered as permanent if they survive more than 35 passsages. Furthermore, for the first time, a permanent cell line with characteristics of the human proximal tubular cell is available. Such cell lines may provide more reliable models for *in vitro* testing of nephrotoxic compounds in the future.

References

1. Brod J. The kidney. Butterworth, London, 1973:53.
2. Maher J.F. Toxic nephropathy. In: The Kidney (Brenner B.B. and Rector F.C., eds.) W.B. Saunders, Philadelphia, 1976:1355.
3. Thurau K., Mason J. and Gstraunthaler G. Experimental acute renal failure. In: The Kidney: Physiology and Pathophysiology (Seldin D.W. and Giebisch G., eds.) Raven Press, New York, 1985:1885-1899.
4. Stolte H. and Fels L.M. Selten, aber relevant. Münchener Medizinische Wochenschrift 1993;135:15-16.
5. Heintz R. Erkrankungen durch Arzneimittel. Thieme, Stuttgart, 1978.
6. Brod J. The Kidney. Butterworth, London, 1973:26.
7. Bach P.H. and Lock E.A. Renal heterogeneity and target cell toxicity. Wiley, Chichester, 1985.
8. Stolte H. and Alt J.M. Regulatory mechanisms and heterogeneity in the kidney. In: Nuklearmedizin. Nuklearmedizin und Biokybernetik (Oeff K. and Schmidt H.A.E., eds.) Medico Informationsdienste, Berlin, 1978:597-608.
9. Bach P.H. and Kwizera E.N. Nephrotoxicity: A rational approach to target cell injury *in vitro* in the kidney. Xenobiotica 1988;18:685-698.
10. Hook J.B. and Hewitt W.R. Toxic responses of the kidney. In: Casarett & Doull's Toxicology. The basic science of poisons (Klaassen C.D., Amdur M.O. and Doull J., eds.) MacMillan, New York, 1986:310-319.

11. Bach P.H., Ketley C.P., Benns S.E., Ahmed I. and Dixit M. The use of isolated and cultured cells in nephrotoxicity-Practice, potential and problems. In: Renal heterogeneity and target cell toxicity (Bach P.H. and Lock E.A., eds.) Wiley, Chichester, 1985:505-518.
12. Smith M.A., Hewitt W.R. and Hook J.R. *In vitro* methods in renal toxicology. In: In vitro methods in toxicology (Atterwill C.K. and Steele C.E., eds.) Press Syndicate of the University of Cambridge, New York, 1987:13-36.
13. Boogaard P.J., Nagelkerke J.F. and Mulder G.J. Renal proximal tubular cells in suspension or in primary culture as *in vitro* models to study nephrotoxicity. Chemico-Biological Interactions 1990;76:251-292.
14. Cain K. Metallothionein and its involvement in heavy metal induced nephropathy. In: Nephrotoxicity in the experimental and clinical situation (Bach P.H. and Lock E.A., eds.) Nijhoff, Dordrecht, 1987:473-531.
15. Bekersky I. The isolated perfused kidney: A model to study biochemical aspects of nephrotoxicity. Review in Biochemical Toxicology 1985;7:139-157.
16. Maak T. Renal clearance and isolated kidney perfusion techniques. Kidney International 1986;30:142-151.
17. Carpenter H.M. and Mudge G.H. Acetaminophen nephrotoxicity: Studies on renal acetylation and deacetylation. Journal of Pharmacology and Experimental Therapeutics 1981;218:161-167.
18. Smith J.H. The use of cortical slices from the Fisher 344 rat as an *in vitro* model to evaluate nephrotoxicity. Fundamental and Applied Toxicology 1988;132-142.
19. Kastner S., Wilks M.F., Soose M., Bach P.H. and Stolte H. Metabolic studies on isolated rat glomeruli. A valuable tool to study glomerular damage. In: Nephrotoxicity: Mechanisms, early diagnosis, and therapeutic management (Bach P.H., Gregg N.J., Wilks M.F. and Delacruz L., eds.) Marcel Dekker, New York, 1991:467-473.
20. Kastner S., Wilks M.F., Gwinner W., Soose M. and Bach P.H. Metabolic heterogeneity of isolated cortical and juxtamedullary glomeruli in Adriamycin nephrotoxicity. Renal Physiology and Biochemistry 1991;14:48-54.
21. Hjelle J.T., Morin J.P. and Trouet A. Analytical cell fractionation of isolated rabbit renal proximal tubules. Kidney International 1981;20:71-77.
22. Gesek F.A., Wolff D.W. and Strandhoy J.W. Improved separation method for rat proximal and distal renal tubules. American Journal of Physiology 1987;253:F358-F365.
23. Tay L.K., Bregman C.L., Masters B.A. and Williams P.D. Effects of cis-diammine dichloroplatinum on rabbit kidney *in vitro* and on rabbit proximal tubule cells in culture. Cancer Research 1988;48:2538-2543.
24. Kreisberg J.I. and Karnovsky M.J. Glomerular cells in culture. Kidney International 1983;23:439-447.
25. Detrisac C.J., Sens M.A., Garvin A.J., Spicer S.S. and Sens D.A. Tissue culture of human kidney epithelial cells of proximal tubule origin. Kidney International 1984;25:383-390.
26. Kreisberg J.I. and Wilson P.D. Renal cell culture. Journal of Electron Microscopy Technique 1988;9:235-263.

27. Striker L.J., Tannen R.L., Lange M.A. and Striker G.E. The contribution of cell cultures to the study of renal diseases. In: International Review of Experimental Pathology (Richter G.W. and Solez K., eds.) Academic Press, San Diego, 1988:55-105.
28. Striker G.E. and Striker L.J. Biology of disease. Glomerular cell culture. Laboratory Investigation. 1985;53:122-131.
29. Holohan P.D., Sokol P.P., Ross C.R.,Coulson R., Trimble M.E., Laska D.A. and Williams P.D. Gentamycin-induced increases in cytosolic calcium in pig-kidney cells (LLC-PK_1). Journal of Pharmacology and Experimental Therapeutics 1988;247:349-354.
30. Taub M., Chuman L., Saier M.H. and Sato G.H. The growth of a kidney epithelial cell line (MDCK) in hormone-supplemented serum-free media. Proceedings of the National Academy of Sciences USA 1979;76:3338-3342.
31. Gausch C.R., Hark W.L. and Smith T.F. Characterization of an established line of canine kidney cells (MDCK). Proceedings of the Society for Experimental Biology and Medicine 1966;122:931-935.
32. Hull R.N., Cherry W.R. and Weaver G.W. The origin and characteristics of a pig cell line LLC-PK. In Vitro 1976;12:670-677.
33. Perantoni A. and Berman J.J. Properties of Wilms' tumor line (TuWi) and pig kidney line (LLC-PK_1) typical of normal kidney tubular epithelium. In Vitro 1979;15:446-454.
34. Koyama H., Goodpasture C., Miller M.M., Teplitz R.L. and Riggs A.D. Establishment and characterization of a cell line from the American Opossum (Didelphys virginiana). In Vitro 1978;14:239-246.
35. Malstrom K., Stange G. and Murer H. Identification of proximal tubular functions in the established kidney cell line, OK. Biochimica et Biophysica Acta 1987;902:269-277.
36. Grassl S.M. and Aronson P.S. Na^+/HCO_3^- - Co-transport in basolateral membrane vesicles isolated from rabbit renal cortex. Journal of Biological Chemistry 1986;2:8778-8783.
37. Hilden S.A., Johns C.A., Guggino W.B. and Madias N.E. Techniques for isolation of brush border and basolateral membrane vesicles from dog kidney cortex. Biochimica et Biophysica Acta 1989;983:77-81.
38. Wallin A., Jones T.W., Vercesi A.E., Cotgreave I., Ormstad K. and Orrenius S. Toxicity of S-V pentachlorobutadienyl-1-cysteine studied with isolated rat renal mitochondria. Archives of Biochemistry and Biophysics 1987;258:365-372.
39. Forster R.P. Use of thin kidney slices and isolated renal tubules for direct study of cellular transport kinetics. Science 1984;108:65-67.
40. Roth K.S., Holtzapple P., Genel M. and Segal S. Uptake of glycine by human kidney cortex. Metabolism 1979;18:677-681.
41. Berndt W.O. Use of renal slice technique for evaluation of renal tubular transport process. Environmental Health Perspectives 1976;15:73-88.
42. Kacew S. and Hirsch G.H. Evaluation of nephrotoxicity of various compounds by means of *in vitro* techniques and comparison to *in vitro* methods. In: Toxicology of the kidney (Hook J.B., ed.) Raven Press, New York, 1981:77-98.

43. Brendel K. and Meezan E. Properties of a pure metabolically active glomerular preparation from rat kidney. II. Metabolism. Journal of Pharmacology and Experimental Therapeutics 1973;187:342-351.
44. Ashkar S., Kennedy J. and Mendicino J. Regulation of gluconeogenesis in swine kidney proximal tubule cells. Molecular and Cellular Biochemistry 1989;87:105-118.
45. Lyerla T.A., Gross S.K., Shea T.B., Daniel P.F. and McCluer R.H. Biochemical and morphological characterization of primary kidney cell cultures from beige mutant mice. Cell and Tissue Research 1987;250:627-632.
46. Rudo K.M., Dauterman W.C. and Langenbach R. Human and rat kidney cell metabolism of 2-acetylaminofluorene and benzo(a)pyrene. Cancer Research 1989;49:1187-1192.
47. Atkins R.C., Glasgow E.F., Holdswoth S.R., Thomson N.M. and Hancock W.W. Tissue culture of isolated glomeruli from patients with glomerulonephritis. Kidney International 1980;17:515-527.
48. Fish A.F., Michael A.F., Vernier R.L. and Brown D.M. Human glomerular cells in tissue culture. Laboratory Investigation 1975;33:330-341.
49. Ishikawa Y., Wada T. and Sakaguchi H. The possibility of three types of cells in cultured glomeruli *in vitro*. American Journal of Pathology 1980;100:779-790.
50. Hayflick L. The limited *in vitro* lifetime of human diploid cell strains. Experimental Cell Research 1965;37:614-619.
51. Taub M. and Sato G. Growth of functional primary cultures of kidney epithelial cells in defined medium. Journal of Cellular Physiology 1980;105:369-378.
52. Chung D.C., Alavi N., Livingston D., Hiller S. and Taub M. Characterization of primary rabbit kidney cultures that express proximal tubule functions in a hormonally defined medium. Journal of Cell Biology 1982;95:118-126.
53. Chuman L., Fine L.G., Cohen A.H. and Saier M.H. Continuous growth of proximal tubular kidney epithelial cells in hormone-supplemented free medium. Journal of Cell Biology 1982;94:506-510.
54. Handler J.S. Studies of kidney cells in culture. Kidney International 1986;30:208-215.
55. Smith W.L. and Garcia-Perez A. Immunodissection: Use of monoclonal antibodies to isolated collecting tubule cells. American Journal of Physiology 1985;248:F1-F7.
56. Foidart J.B., Dechenne C., Dubois C., Deheneffe J. and Mahieu P. Tissue culture of isolated renal glomeruli: Present and future. In: Advances in Nephrology (Hamburger J., Crosnier J., Grunfeld J.-P. and Maxwell M.H., eds.) Year Book Publishers Inc., Chicago, 1981:267-292.
57. Scheinmann J.I. and Fish A.J. Human glomerular cells in culture: three subcultured types bearing glomerular antigens. American Journal of Pathology 1978;92:125-146.
58. Soukupova M. and Holeckova E. The latent period of explanted organs of newborn, adult and senile rats. Experimental Cell Research 1964;33:361-367.

59. Kurtz S.M. and Feldman I.D. Experimental studies on the formation of the glomerular basement membrane. Journal of Ultrastructural Research 1962;6:19-27.
60. Farquhar M.G. The primary glomerular filtration barrier-basement membrane or epithelial cells? Kidney International 1975;8:197-211.
61. Blau E.B. and Haas M.E. Glomerular sialic acid and proteinuria in human renal disease. Laboratory Investigation 1977;28:477-481.
62. Ryan G.B. and Karnovsky M.J. An ultrastructural study of the mechanisms of proteinuria in aminonucleoside nephrosis. Kidney International 1975;8:219-232.
63. Quadracci L.J. and Striker G.E. Growth and maintenance of glomerular cells in vitro. Proceedings of the Society for Experimental Biology and Medicine 1970;135:947-950.
64. Striker G.E., Killen P. and Farin F.M. Human glomerular cells in vitro: Isolation and characterization. Transplantion Proceedings 1980;12:88-99.
65. Kreisberg J.I., Hoover R.L. and Karnovsky M.J. Isolation and characterization of rat glomerular epithelal cells in vitro. Kidney International 1978;14:21-30.
66. Killen P. and Striker G.E. Human glomerular visceral epithelial cells synthesize a basal lamina collagen in vitro. Proceedings of the National Academy of Sciences of the USA 1979;76:3518-3522.
67. Scheinman J.I., Fish A.J., Kim Y. and Michael A.F. C3b receptors on human glomeruli in vitro. American Journal of Pathology 1978;92:147-154.
68. Kreisberg J.I., Patel P.Y., Venkatachalam M.A. and Taylor G. Elevation of cAMP results in a change in cell shape that resembles dome formation in cultured rat glomerular epithelial cells. In Vitro 1986;22:393-396.
69. Grisham E. and Churg J. Focal glomerulosclerosis in nephrotic patients. An electron microscopic study of glomerular podocyts. Kidney International 1975;7:111-122.
70. Kasinath B.S., Maaba M.R., Schwartu M.M. and Lewis E.J. Demonstration and characterization of C3 receptors on rat glomerular epithelial cells. Kidney International 1986;30:852-861.
71. Foidart J.M., Foidart J.B. and Mahieu P.R. Synthesis of collagen and fibronectin by glomerular cells in culture. Renal Physiology 1980;3:183-190.
72. Foidart J.B., Pirad Y.S., Winard R.J. and Mahieu P.R. Tissue culture of normal rat glomeruli: glycosaminoglycan biosynthesis by homogeneous epithelial and mesangial cell populations. Renal Physiology 1980;3:169-182.
73. Ryan G.B. and Karnovsky M.J. Distribution of endogenous albumin in the rat glomerulus: Role of hemodynamic factors in glomerular barrier function. Kidney International 1976;9:36-45.
74. Striker G.E., Soderland C., Bowen-Pope D.F., Grown A.M., Schmer G., Johnson A., Luchtel D., Ross R. and Striker L.J. Isolation, characterization, and propagation in vitro of human glomerular endothelial cells. Journal of Experimental Medicine 1984;160:323-328.
75. Raghu G., Striker L. and Striker G. Lipopolysaccharide-mediated injury to cultured glomerular endothelial cells. Clinical Immunology and Immunopathology 1986;38:275-281.

76. Farquhar M.G. and Palade G.E. Functional evidence for the existence of a third cell type in the renal glomerulus: Phagocytosis of filtration residue by a 'distinct' third cell type. Journal of Cell Biology 1962;13:55-87.
77. Barger A.C. and Herd J.A. The renal circulation. New England Journal of Medicine 1971;284:482-490.
78. Kreisberg J.I., Venkatchalam M.A. and Troyer D.A. Contractile properties of cultured glomerular mesangial cells. American Journal of Physiology 1985;249:F457-F463.
79. Templeton D.M. and Sheepers J. Effects of Ni and Cd on proteoglycan synthesis by the isolated glomerulus and glomerular cells in culture. In: Nephrotoxicity: Mechanisms, early diagnosis, and therapeutic management (Bach P.H., Gregg N.J., Wilks M.F. and Delacruz L., eds.) Marcel Dekker, New York, 1991:377-382.
80. Sterzel R.B., Lovett D.H., Foellmer H.G., Perfetto M., Biemesclerfer D. and Kashgarian M.C. Mesangial cell hillocks: Nodular foci of exaggerated growth of cells and matrix. American Journal of Pathology 1986;125:130-140.
81. Lovett D.H., Sterzel R.B., Kashgarian M. and Ryan J.C. Neutral proteinase activity produced *in vitro* by cells of the glomerular mesangium. Kidney International 1983;23:342-349.
82. Hawkins N.J., Wakefield D. and Charlesworth J.A. The role of mesangial cells in glomerular pathology. Pathology 1990;22:24-32.
83. Courtoy P.J., Timpl R. and Farquhar M.G. Comparative distribution of laminin, type IV collagen and fibronectin in the rat glomerulus. Journal of Histochemistry and Cytochemistry 1982;30:874-886.
84. Kanvar Y.S. and Farquhar M.G. Presence of heparan sulfate in glomerular basement membrane. Procceedings of the National Academy of Sciences of the USA 1979;76:1303-1307.
85. Foellmer H.G., Perfetto M., Kashgarian M. and Sterzel R.B. Matrix constituents promote adhesion and proliferation of glomerular mesangial cells in culture. Kidney International 1987;31:318A.
86. Boogard P.J., Mulder G.J. and Nagelkerke J.F. Isolated proximal tubular cells from rat kidney as an *in vitro* model for studies on nephrotoxicity. I. An improved method for preparation of proximal tubular cells and their functional characterization by α-methylglucose uptake. Toxicology and Applied Pharmacology 1989;101:135-143.
87. Heidrich H.G. and Dew M.E. Homogenous cell populations from rabbit kidney cortex. Proximal, distal tubule and renin-active cell isolated by free-flow electrophoresis. Journal of Cell Biology 1977;74:780-788.
88. Toutain H., Fillastre J.P. and Morin J.P. Preparative free flow electrophoresis for the isolation of two populations of proximal cells from the rabbit kidney. European Journal of Cell Biology 1989;49:247-280.
89. Vandevalle A., Taub M., Clueaud F., Ronco P., Chatelet F., Verroust P. and Poujeol P. Indirect immunodissection of late distal cell populations from rabbit kidney cortex. American Journal of Physiology 1986;250:F387-F395.
90. Garcia-Perez A. and Smith W.L. Use of monoclonal antibodies to isolate cortical collecting tubule cells: AVP induces PGE release. American Journal of Physiology 1983;244:C211-C220.

91. Burg M., Grantham J., Abramow M. and Orloff J. Preparation and study of segments of single rabbit nephrons. American Journal of Physiology 1966;210:1293-1298.
92. Horster M. Hormonal stimulation and differential growth response of renal epithelial cells cultivated *in vitro* from individual nephron segments. International Journal of Biochemistry 1980;12:29-35.
93. Blackburn J.G., Hazen-Martin D.J., Detrisac C.J. and Sens D.A. Electrophysiology and ultrastructure of cultured human proximal tubular cells. Kidney International 1988;33:508-516.
94. Wilson P.D., Dillingham M.A., Breckon R.D. and Anderson R.J. Defined human renal tubular epithelia in culture: Growth, characterization and hormonal response. American Journal of Physiology 1985;248:F436-F443.
95. Stanton R.C., Mendrick D.L., Rennke H.G. and Seifter J.L. Use of monoclonal antibodies to culture rat proximal tubular cells. American Journal of Physiology 1986;251:C780-C786.
96. Jefferson D.M., Cobb M.H., Gennaro J.F. and Scott W.N. Transporting epithelium: Culture in hormonally defined serum-free medium. Science 1980;210:912-914.
97. Hayashi I. and Sato G.H. Replacement of serum by hormones permits growth of cells in defined medium. Nature 1976;256:132-134.
98. Green N., Algren A., Hoyer J., Triche T. and Burg M. Differentiated lines of cells from rabbit renal medullary thick ascending limbs grown on amnion. American Journal of Physiology 1985;249:C97-C104.
99. Wilson P.D. and Horster M.F. Differential response to hormones of defined distal nephron epithelial in culture. American Journal of Physiology 1983;244:C166-C174.
100. Valentich J.D. and Stokols M.F. An established cell line from mouse kidney medullary thick ascending limb. I. Cell culture techniques, morphology, and antigenic expression. II. Transepithelial electrophysiology. American Journal of Physiology 1986;251:C299-C322.
101. Wilson P.D., Anderson R.J., Breckon R.D., Nathrath W. and Schrier R.W. Retention of differentiated characteristics by cultures of defined rabbit kidney epithelia. Journal of Cellular Physiology 1987;130:245-254.
102. Kleinman H.K., Klebe R.J. and Martin G.R. Role of collagenous matrices in the adhesion and growth of cells. Journal of Cell Biology 1981;88:473-485.
103. Matlin K.S. The sorting of proteins to the plasma membrane in epithelial cells. Journal of Cell Biology 1986;103:2565-2568.
104. Simons K. and Fuller S.D. Cell surface polarity in epithelia. Annual Reviews of Cell Biology 1985;1:243-288.
105. Trifillis A.L., Regec A.L. and Trump B.F. Isolation, culture and characterization of human renal tubular cells. Journal of Urology 1985;133:324-329.
106. Kempson S.A., McAteer J.A., Al-Mahrouq H.A., Dousa T.P., Dougherty G.S. and Evan A.P. Proximal tubule characteristics of cultured human renal cortex epithelium. Journal of Laboratory and Clinical Medicine 1989;3:285-296.

107. Chen T.C., Curthoys N.P., Lagenaur C.F. and Puschett J.B. Characterization of primary cell cultures derived from rat renal proximal tubules. In Vitro Cellular and Developmental Biology 1989;25:714-722.
108. States B., Foreman J., Lee J. and Segal S. Characteristics of cultured human renal cortical epithelia. Biochemical Medicine and Metabolic Biology 1986;3:151-161.
109. Bruggeman I.M., Mertens J.J.W.M., Temmink J.H.M., Lans M.C., Vos R.M.E. and van Bladeren P.J. Use of monolayers of primary rat kidney cortex cells for nephrotoxicity studies. Toxicology in Vitro 1989;3:261-269.
110. Bell C.L., Tenenhouse H.S. and Scriver C.R. Inition and characterization of primary mouse kidney epithelial cell cultures. In Vitro Cellular and Developmental Biology 1988;24:83-95.
111. Hatzinger P.B. and Stevens J.L. Rat kidney proximal tubule cells in defined medium: The roles of cholera toxins, extracellular calcium and serum in cell growth and expression of γ-glutamyltransferase. In Vitro Cellular and Developmental Biology 1989;25:205-212.
112. Chen J.C., Stevens J.L., Trifillis A.L. and Jones T.W. Renal cysteine conjugate β-lyase mediated toxicity studied with primary cultures of human proximal tubular cells. Toxicology and Applied Pharmacology 1990;103:463-473.
113. Lauwerys R. and Bernard A. Preclinical detection of nephrotoxicity: Description of the tests and appraisal of their health significance. Toxicology Letters 1989;4:13-29.
114. Silverman M. Glucose transport in the kidney. Biochimica et Biophysica Acta 1976;457:303-351.
115. Wilson P.D., Schrier R.W., Breckon R.D. and Gabow P.A. A new method for studying human polycystic kidney disease epithelial in culture. Kidney International 1986;30:371-378.
116. Hoyer J.R. and Seiler M.W. Pathophysiology of Tamm-Horsfall protein. Kidney International 1979;16:279-289.
117. Grenier F.C., Rollins T.E. and Smith W.L. Kinin-induced prostaglandin synthesis by renal papillary collecting tubule cells in culture. American Journal of Physiology 1981;241:F94-F104.
118. Sato M. and Dunn M.J. Osmolality, vasopressin-stimulated cAMP, and PGE_2-synthesis in rat collecting tubule cells. American Journal of Physiology 1986;250:F802-F810.
119. Williams P.D. The application of renal cells in culture in studying drug-induced nephrotoxicity. In Vitro Cellular and Developmental Biology 1989;25:800-805.
120. Bertani T., Poggi A., Pozzoni R., Delani F., Sacchi G., Thoua Y., Mecca G., Remuzzi G. and Donati M.B. Adriamycin induced nephrotic syndrome in rats. Sequence of pathologic events. Laboratory Investigation 1982;46:16-23.
121. Fajardo L.F., Eltringham J.R., Steward J.R. and Klauber M.R. Adriamycin nephrotoxicity. Laboratory Investigation 1980;43:242-253.
122. Robison T.W., Giri S.N. and Wilson D.W. Effects of chronic administration of Doxorubicin on myocardial creatine phosphokinase and antioxidant defenses and levels of lipid peroxidation in tissues and plasma of rats. Journal of Biochemical Toxicology 1989;4:87-94.

123. Van Vleet J.F. and Ferrans V.F. Clinical and pathologic features of chronic Adriamycin toxicosis in rabbits. American Journal of Veterinary Research 1980;41:1462-1469.
124. Soose M., Gwinner W., Grotkamp J., Hansemann W. and Stolte H. Altered renal fibronectin excretion in early Adriamycin nephrosis in rats. Journal of Pharmacology and Experimental Therapeutics 1991;257:493-499.
125. Soose M., Wenzel S., Oberst D. and Stolte H. Fibronectin turnover in human mesangial cell cultures as affected by Adriamycin. Cell Biology and Toxicology 1993;9:149-164.
126. Myers B.D., Sibley R., Newton L., Tomlanovich S.J., Boshkos C., Stinson E., Luetscher J.A., Whitney D.J., Krasny D., Coplon N.S. and Perlroth M.G. The long-term course of Cyclosporine-associated chronic nephropathy. Kidney International 1988;33:590-600.
127. Gonzales R., Redon P., Lakhdar B., Potaux L., Cambar J. and M. Aparicio. Cyclosporine nephrotoxicity assessed in isolated human glomeruli and cultured mesangial cells. Toxicology in Vitro 1990;4:391-395.
128. Wilson P.D. Use of cultured renal tubular cells in the study of cell injury. Mineral and Electrolyte Metabolism 1986;21:71-84.
129. Humes H.D., Weinberg J.M. and Knauss T.C. Clinical and pathophysiological aspects of aminoglycoside nephrotoxicity. American Journal of Kidney Diseases 1982;11:5-29.
130. Bennett W.M. Aminoglycoside nephrotoxicity. Nephron 1983;35:73-77.
131. Hostetter K.Y. and Hall C.B. Inhibition of kidney lysosomal phospholipase A and C by aminoglycoside antibiotics: Possible mechanism of aminoglycoside toxicity. Proceedings of the National Academy of Sciences of the USA 1982;79:1663-1667.
132. Kosek J.C., Mazze R.I. and Cousins M.J. Nephrotoxicity of gentamycin. Laboratory Investigation 1974;30:48-57.
133. Sufian S. and Katz S.M. Urinary myelin figures in gentamycin: Treated vs ischemic kidney. American Surgeon 1983;49:254-260.
134. Luft F.C., Patel V., Yum M.N., Patel B. and Kleit S.A. Experimental aminoglycoside nephrotoxicity. Journal of Clinical Medicine 1975;86:213-220.
135. Schentag J.J., Suftin T.A., Plant M.E. and Jusko W.J. Early detection of aminoglycoside nephrotoxicity with urinary beta-2-microglobulin. Journal of Medicine 1978;9:201-210.
136. Williams P.D., Laska D.A. and Hottendorf G.H. Comparative toxicity of aminoglycoside antibiotics in cell cultures derived from human and pig kidney. Toxicology in Vitro 1986;1:23-32.
137. Chatterjee S., Trifillis A.L. and Regec A.L. Morphological and biochemical effects of gentamycin on cultured human renal tubular cells. In: Renal Heterogeneity and target cell toxicity (Bach P.H. and Lock E.A., eds.) Wiley, Chichester, 1985:549-552.
138. Regec A.L., Trump B.F. and Trifillis A.L. Effect of gentamycin on the lysosomal system of cultured human proximal tubular cells. Endocytotic activity, lysosomal pH and membrane fragility. Biochemical Pharmacology 1989;38:2527-2534.

139. Sens M.A., Hazen-Martin D.J., Blackburn J.G., Hennigar G.R. and Sens D.A. Growth characteristics of cultured human proximal tubule cells exposed to aminoglycoside antibiotics. Annals of Clinical and Laboratory Science 1989;19:266-279.
140. Sens M.A., Hennigar G.R., Hazen-Martin D.J., Blackburn J.G. and Sens D.A. Cultured human proximal tubule cells as a model for aminonucleoside nephrotoxicity. Annals of Clinical and Laboratory Science 1988;18:204-214.
141. Gosh P. and Chatterjee S. Effects of gentamycin on sphingomyelinase activity in cultured human proximal tubular cells. Journal of Biological Chemistry 1987;262:12550-12556.
142. Britton S. and Palacios R. Cyclosporine A - Usefulness, risks and mechanisms of action. Immunological Reviews 1982;65:5-22.
143. Sibley R.K., Rynasiewicz J., Ferguson R.M., Fryd D., Sutherland D.E., Simmons R.L. and Najarian J.S. Morphology of Cyclosporine nephrotoxicity and acute rejection in patients immunosuppressed with Cyclosporine and Prednisone. Surgery 1983;94:225-302.
144. Thomson A.W. Immunbiology of Cyclosporine - A review. Australian Journal of Experimental Biology and Medical Science 1983;61:147-172.
145. Trifillis A.L. and Kahng M.W. Effect of Cyclosporine A on cultured human kidney cells: Lipid peroxidation and cytosolic calcium. Transplantation Proceedings 1988;20:717-721.
146. Trifillis A.L., Regec A.L., Hall-Graggs M. and Trump B.F. Effects of Cyclosporine on cultured human renal tubular cells. In: Renal heterogeneity and target cell toxicity (Bach P.H. and Lock E.A., eds.) Wiley, Chichester, 1985:545-548.
147. Goldstein R.S. and Mayor G.H. The nephrotoxicity of cis-Platin. Life Science 1983:32:685-690.
148. Laurent G., Yernaux V., Nonclercg D., Toubeau G., Maldague P., Tulkens P.M. and Heuson-Stiennon J.A. Tissue injury and proliferation response induced in rat kidneys by cis-diamminedichloroplatinum (II). Virchows Archiv 1988;55:129-145.
149. Castaing N., Merlet D. and Cambar J. Cis-platin cytotoxicity in human and rat tubular cell cultures. Toxicology in Vitro 1990;4:396-398.
150. Merlet D., Merlet J.P. and Cambar J. Differential heavy metal cytotoxicity in human normal and tumoral cultured tubular cells. In: Nephrotoxicity: Mechanisms, early diagnosis, and therapeutic management (Bach P.H., Gregg N.J., Wilks M.F. and Delacruz L., eds.) Marcel Dekker, New York, 1991:355-360.
151. Fauth C., Rossier B. and Roch-Ramel F. Transport of tetraethylammonium by a kidney epithelial cell line (LLC-PK_1). American Journal of Physiology 1988;254:F351-F357.
152. Mullin J.M., Mc Ginn M.T., Snock K.V. and Kofeldt L.M. Na^+-independent sugar transport by cultured renal (LLC-PK_1) epithelial cells. American Journal of Physiology 1989;257:F11-F17.

153. Belleman P. Primary monolayer cultures of liver parenchymal cells and kidney tubules as a useful new model for biochemical pharmacology and experimental toxicology. Studies *in vitro* on hepatic membrane transport, induction of liver enzymes and adaptive changes in renal cortical enzymes. Archives of Toxicology 1980;44:63-84.
154. Bach P.H., Ketley C.P., Dixit M. and Ahmed I. The mechanisms of target cell injury in nephrotoxicity. Food and Chemical Toxicology 1986;24:775-779.
155. Zimmermann U., Scheurich P., Pilwat G. and Benz R. Cells with manipulated functions: New perspective for cell biology, medicine and technology. Angewandte Chemie 1981;20:325-344.
156. Netzer A., Weirich-Schwaiger H., Pfaller W. and Gstraunthaler G. Establishment of new proximal tubular cell lines obtained by cell fusion. Pflügers Archiv 1993;422:R91.

12

Isolated human heart cells

M. Borgers and L. Ver Donck

Life Sciences, Janssen Research Foundation, Turnhoutseweg 30, 2340 Beerse (Belgium).

Introduction

The isolated cell has become a very popular and well accepted tool in basic and applied research, and also in the cardiovascular discipline. Single cells indeed provide a number of advantages over the use of intact tissue [2]: the experimental conditions can be easily controlled in various aspects; the homogeneity of the isolated cell population makes it a suitable tool for biochemical assays and subcellular fractionation studies; it is possible to evaluate cellular properties in the absence of external influences such as neuronal modulation, cell-cell interactions or mechanical stress, and single cells are very suitable for patch and voltage clamp studies. Furthermore, the multitude of cells that are usually obtained from a donor organ allows the investigator to perform an almost unlimited series of experiments, thereby using only a very low number of experimental animals.

Limitations for the broad use of human cardiomyocytes

Although a widespread use of cardiomyocytes isolated from experimental animals (rat, guinea pig, rabbit, chicken, hamster, frog, etc.) has emerged since the late seventies [6], to date there is only a limited number of laboratories involved in isolation of cardiomyocytes from adult human myocardium. This may sound rather unexpected, since the majority of basic and applied research resides within in the framework of human physiology and pathology. The reason for the discrepancy is related to a number of practical and scientific limitations inherent to such an approach.

Origin of samples and isolation techniques

The restricted opportunities to obtain cardiac samples from human heart in conditions such that they can be optimally used for pharmacological and toxicological studies is a serious drawback. Frequency, uniformity and sample size on the one hand, and inherent difficulties in isolating viable cells from the very small amount of myocardial tissue on the other, represent the main obstacles today.
Other, more practical limitations are that, in view of the dependency on surgery, tissue availability is often unscheduled and that the lab facility needs to be near the operating theatre, as tissues need to be processed as soon as possible upon excision.
The major problem encountered by most groups active in the field is the procedure to dissociate cells. It is safe to say that isolation of adult cells is an empirical art and laboratories routinely isolating cells from animal hearts frequently encounter unexpected and inexplicable problems. Such is even more the case when cells are isolated from human myocardium, because of specific inherent problems. Most isolation techniques used for human myocytes are inspired by those applied to disperse cells from animal hearts : these are based upon an enzymic digestion of the tissue by means of coronary artery perfusion [7]. Human tissue is almost exclusively available as a biopsy obtained during surgery. As a consequence, cells need to be set apart according to the 'chunk' method : incubation of small tissue pieces in an enzyme solution, eventually combined with mechanical agitation. Such methods are known to generally provide a very small if not zero yield of viable cells [18]. In this regard, it is understandable that in most of the studies reported hitherto the yield of viable cells is not mentionned and the type of experiments which are performed always require a limited number of cells only. In theory, only when larger pieces of myocardium are available from explanted hearts or from donor hearts rejected for transplantation, the classical perfusion technique to isolate cells can be applied.

Variability in quality of human cells

Apart from the technicalities of the isolation procedure, there are other factors that set limits to an unconstrained use of human cardiomyocytes in cardiovascular research. First of all, the nature of the myocardial tissue is not under the control of the investigator: unlike the wide and well defined diversity in genetic strains of laboratory animals, one cannot control characteristics such as the age and genetic constraints of tissue donors.

Secondly, since tissue is exclusively available through surgery, a variety of underlying pathologies has to be taken into account. These include various elements from the wide spectrum of myocardial diseases such as hypertrophic cardiomyopathy, acute ischaemic heart disease, hibernating or stunned myocardium, etc.... Indeed, the underlying substructure of the myocardium represents a plethora of cellular and extracellular characteristics that vary in quality and quantity from patient to patient. Tissue samples may be obtained during coronary bypass surgery, heart transplantation, mitral valve replacement, correction of tetralogy of Fallot or from endocardial biopsies taken for diagnostic purposes. Figures 1-3 illustrate this variety of cellular morphology in normal (Fig. 1), hibernating (Fig. 2) and cardiomyopathic myocardium (Fig. 3). The success of an experiment with isolated cells thus highly depends on whether the underlying structure is 1) normal; 2) remodelled as a consequence of a previous acute ischaemic event (stunning or infarction); 3) changed during chronic exposure to a low oxygen environment (hibernation); 4) adapted as a consequence of underlying pathology (cardiomyopathies with different etiology). So, it is practically impossible to yield a population of isolated cells, that one would expect to react uniformly to any aggression given during the 'in vitro' experiment. Other aspects to be taken into consideration are whether the tissue is from ventricular or atrial origin. In addition, the effects of the patient's medical treatment on the properties of isolated cells remain largely unknown.

Thirdly, a question that also remains unanswered is to what extent the limited number of isolated cardiomyocytes are representative of the whole heart. One has to consider the possibility that these cells represent a selection of the most viable ones, which survived the stress involved with the isolation procedure.

These reflections clearly illustrate that it is rather complicated to compare the cellular properties observed with matched controls, since

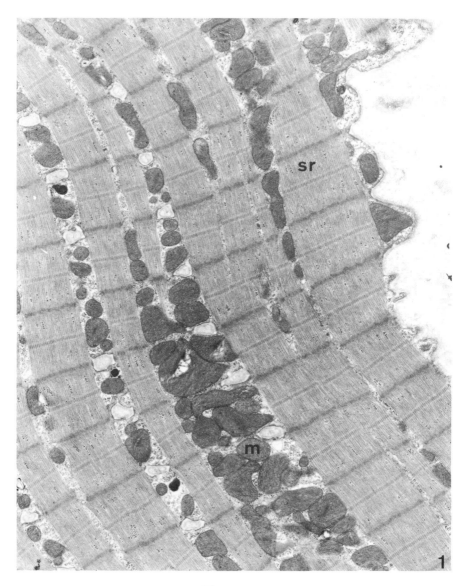

Figure 1 :
Ultrastructural characteristics of human cardiac cells in situ.
Biopsies were taken from a normal donor heart.
Normal ultrastructure of a cardiomyocyte showing regularly arranged rows of sarcomeres (sr) and mitochondria (m) (x 12600).

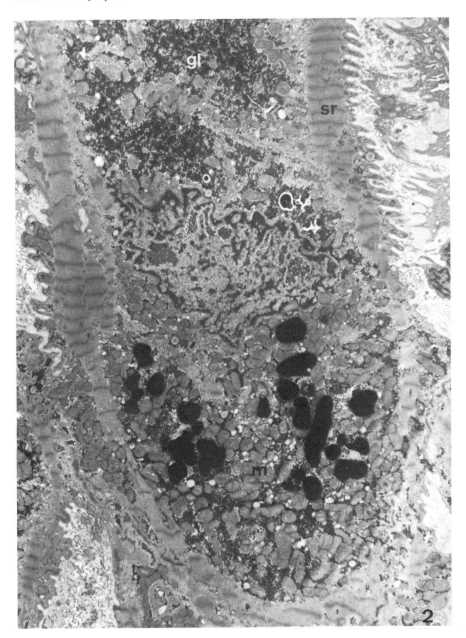

Figure 2:
Ultrastructural characteristics of human cardiac cells in situ. Biopsies were taken from a hypokinetic area in the ventricular wall of hibernating myocardium. Sarcomeres (sr) are only present at the cell periphery. The bulk of the cytoplasm is occupied by glycogen (gl) and mitochondria (m). Nucleus (n). (x 5250)

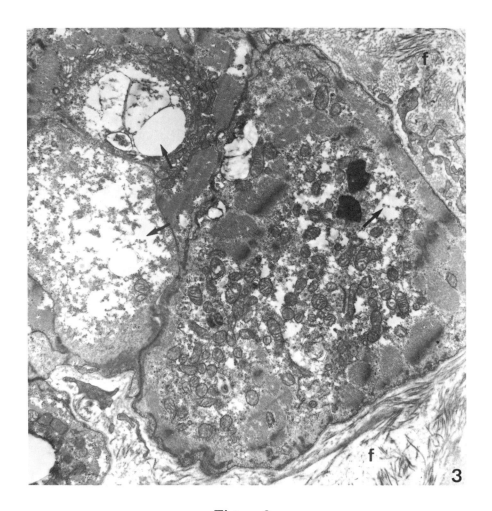

Figure 3 :
Ultrastructural characteristics of human cardiac cells in situ. Biopsies were taken from a cardiomyopathic patient (3). The diversity of structural remodeling in the diseased hearts is evident, and supports the scepsis as to whether cells successfully isolated from such tissue samples actually represent the diseased status of the respective myocardium. Note the severe degeneration of the cytosol (arrows) in cells in a fibrotic (f) environment. (x 9730)

the latter are only infrequently available from hearts initially intended as transplant donors where transplantation was cancelled for reasons of incompatibility. Occasionally, post-mortem material from patients who had died from non-myocardial causes is used as a control in comparative studies [3,28]. Obviously, there is only little room for useful applications in the latter case.
Long term culturing of the cells is usually not possible because of the generally low yield of viable cells, since adult cardiomyocytes are in a differentiated state. Culturing of such cells inevitably leads to dedifferentiation and phenotypic changes [5,23].
This summary of problems and limitations, however, should not cause scepticism towards research projects on isolated human cardiomyocytes. In the following paragraphs we will present an overview on studies with isolated human cardiomyocytes, which contributed to current knowledge in this field. This demonstrates that it is a feasable area, providing indispensable knowledge with regard to human cardiovascular disease and therapy.

Overview of studies performed with human cardiomyocytes

As mentioned earlier, only a few centres in the world have published data from experiments on isolated human cardiomyocytes. The majority of these reports comes from laboratories on the European continent (Table I). Most of the studies report on various aspects of the diseased heart (usually heart failure), sometimes in comparison with the normal human heart. In the following paragraphs, we will review these papers which cover the fields of toxicology, pharmacology, physiology, electrophysiology, morphology and biochemistry (see Table II).

Pharmaco-toxicology and pharmaco-physiology

The inotropic state of the myocardium is of utmost importance for the functional performance of heart muscle: an adequate contractile response of the heart indeed governs the overall mechanical properties of the cardiac system. Because the heart's contractile function is mainly the result of a concerted action of the individual myocytes within the muscle layers, the isolated ventricular cardiomyocyte is a very attractive object for the investigation of the heart's ability to contract under various pathophysiological conditions, in the absence of any extracellular

Country	number of centers	number of publications
EUROPE	13	35
- France	3	7
- U.K.	2	13
- Germany	1	3
- Italy	1	1
- Belgium	1	2
- C.I.S.	5	9
USA*	10	10
CANADA	5	7
JAPAN	1	1
Total	28	53

Table I :
Centers involved in research on human myocardial cells [1]

[1] according to publications retrieved by a computer assisted literature search in the Medline database in May 1993.
* mainly refers to cultures from human foetus.

constraints.
Poole-Wilson's laboratory in London, in particular, contributed greatly to the understanding of cellular contractility in the normal and diseased human heart. In several studies from this group, the contractile performance of isolated myocytes from both healthy and hypertrophic or failing human hearts has been reported. The characteristics of unloaded twitch shortening upon electrical field stimulation is measured via a video-edge detection system. Their first paper reported on contractile properties of single cells from various animal species and man [12]: although there was only little species variation in cell and sarcomere length, myocytes from larger animals tended to contract and relax more slowly than those from smaller ones, and the velocity of shortening correlated with basal heart rate. Even within species, they also observed differences in kinetics from left and right ventricular tissue. An interesting extension of this work was a comparison of contractile properties in papillary muscles and isolated cardiomyocytes from the same failing and non-failing human hearts [13]. Although basic contractile function

number of publications	France	U.K.	Germany	Italy	Belgium	C.I.S.	Total
Morphology and morphometry		1				8	9
Biochemistry		1					1
Physiology and pharmacology		9					9
Electrophysiology	7	2	3	1	2	1	16
Toxicology							0
Total	7	13	3	1	2	9	35

Table II :

Topics of research with human isolated cardiac myocytes in Europe [1]

[1] according to publications retrieved by a computer assisted literature search in the Medline database in May 1993.

does not differ, human papillary muscles were less sensitive to isoprenaline stimulation, showed a 4-5 times larger variability in absolute responses, had a longer relaxation time, and had much less isoprenaline-induced aftercontractions than did isolated cells. However, such differences were not observed between rabbit muscles and myocytes. In a subsequent study, Harding et al.[14] compared contractile and electrophysiological parameters of cells from normal and failing human hearts. A striking observation was that, as in papillary muscle, differences for most of these parameters correlated well with the degree of heart failure. Furthermore, a decreased response to β-stimulation was observed in cells from failing hearts. This was further confirmed by two studies on β-adrenoreceptor desensitization in failing hearts, which showed a better correlation with the degree of the disease and with patient's age, than with the etiology of heart failure [15]. Brown and Harding [4] pinpointed this difference to an increased level or activity of inhibitory G-protein levels in the failing human heart.

Isolated human heart cells have not been used sofar for pure toxicological assessments of chemical and pharmacological compounds.

Electrophysiology

The very first paper ever published on isolated human cardiomyocytes dealt with electrophysiological measurements [24]. The isolation of single cells from adult myocardial tissue made it possible for the first time to record trans-sarcolemmal ion currents, and electrophysiologists have taken great advantage of this possibility to identify the nature of various sarcolemmal ion currents in various animal species, including man. Together with the fact that this kind of studies suffer the least from the limited yield of viable cells, because only a few cells are required for successful measurements, electrophysiological studies account for the majority of papers dealing with isolated human cardiomyocytes (Table II). A number of laboratories have reported on the pharmacological modulation of ion currents in atrial or ventricular cells isolated from normal and/or diseased myocardium. These include recordings of calcium current [1,21,22]; potassium current [17]; slow inward current [9]; transient outward current [10]; and effects of acetylcholine or noradrenaline [16,20].

Morphology and biochemistry

The reports on morphological aspects of human isolated cardiomyocytes thus far deal with cells from diseased origin. The first report stems from an Armenian team demonstrating a correlation between myocardial hypertrophy and polyploidy [26]. These findings were investigated in more detail in biopsies from patients with rheumatic heart disease by Erokhina *et al.* [8]. These authors also observed a high degree of ploidy in NYHA-class IV patients, but no direct correlation existed between ploidy level and degree of cell degeneration, or between degeneration and ejection fraction. The ploidy level in cells obtained from normal hearts was reported to vary from 3.2c to 7.3c in different layers from the ventricular anterior left wall [3].

Shperling *et al.* [27] also reported a morphometrical analysis of myocytes isolated from concentric and excentric hypertrophic hearts. The changes in dimensions of these cells appear to be proportional to the degree of hypertrophy. An interesting finding on morphometrical characteristics of cells isolated from ventricular aneurysms was observed by Harding *et al.* [11] : cells from these dyskinetic areas had significantly increased sarcomere lengths, but were unable to contract upon stimulation. This correlated with a surprisingly high yield (80-100%) of rod shaped cells obtained from these tissues, in contrast to other tissue types where only a few, but contractile, cells could be isolated.

As far as metabolic studies dealing with isolated cells are concerned, an investigation of the nucleotide catabolism in human cardiomyocytes by Smolenski *et al.* [29] is the only biochemical report available to date. These investigators observed that adenosine accounted for 70 % of all intra- and extracellular degradation products, suggesting that adenosine production represents the principal route in nucleotide catabolism in human heart cells.

Alternatives to human cardiomyocytes

The limitations described above have fostered the search for valid alternatives to isolated human cardiac cells. The most useful alternative reported so far is the use of small trabeculae from the right atrium. Such trabeculae can be obtained during routine cannulation of the heart for cardiopulmonary bypass prior to CABG or valvular replacement. They are very suitable for the pharmacological evaluation of drugs that influence the contractile state of the heart and for the generation of physiological parameters. Moreover, they offer a more than valid alternative to isolated human cells and animal cardiac tissue because of the relative ease with which they can be obtained and because they can be manipulated in a very reproducible way to perform '*in vitro*' experiments. The toxic influence of high concentrations of calcium, which lead to degenerative Ca^{2+}-overload, has been compared between human atrial trabeculae and guinea-pig atrial muscle strips [19]. In a subsequent study, the same material was used to evaluate the potential of cytoprotective interventions to prevent cardiomyocyte dysfunction caused by Ca^{2+}-overload [25]. So far as we are aware, human heart trabeculae have not been used in attempts to solve toxicological problems.

Conclusion

In view of the considerations above, the broad use of human cardiomyocytes for toxico-pharmacological purposes is not envisaged in the near future, but the scanty material will certainly be used for specific problem solving for which cells from other species are not suitable.

Among these problems are: 1) Validation of the use of animal cells for human disease. This necessitates an initial comparative study between human and animal cardiomyocytes. For example, the sensitivity to hypoxic / ischaemic insults, the distribution of receptors, and the tolerance to drugs should be verified for interspecies differences; 2) Research aiming at the identification of the fundamental cause(s) of the dysfunction, e.g. cardiomyopathic subtypes; 3) Molecular biological approach in search for phenotypic changes in diseased states.

References

1. Beuckelmann D.J., Näbaeur M. and Erdman E. Characteristics of Ca-channel in isolated human ventricular myocytes from patients with terminal heart failure. Journal of Molecular and Cellular Cardiology 1991;23:929-937.
2. Borgers M., Ver Donck L. and Vandeplassche G. Pathophysiology of cardiomyocytes. Annales of the New York Academy of Science 1988;522:433-453.
3. Brodsky V.Y., Chernyaev A.L. and Vasilyeva I.A. Variability of the cardiomyocyte ploidy in normal human hearts. Virchows Archives. B. Cell Pathology 1991;61:289-294.
4. Brown L.A. and Harding S.E. The effect of pertussis toxin on beta-adrenoceptor responses in isolated cardiac myocytes from noradrenaline-treated guinea-pigs and patients with cardiac failure. British Journal of Pharmacology 1992;106:115-122.
5. Bugaisky L.B. and Zak R. Differentiation of adult rat cardiac myocytes in cell culture. Circulation Research 1989; 64:493-500.
6. Clark W.A., Decker R.S. and Borg T.K. Biology of isolated adult cardiac myocytes. Elsevier, New York, 1988: 441.
7. Dow J.W., Harding N.G.L. and Powell T. Isolated cardiac myocytes: I Preparation of adult myocytes and their homology with the intact tissue. Cardiovascular Research 1981;15:483-514.
8. Erokhina I.L., Selivanova G.V., Vlasova T.D., Komarova N.I., Emel-ianova O.I., Aleshkin N.G. and Soroka V.V. Changes in the ultrastructure and DNA and protein content in human atrial myocytes in cardiac hyperfunction due to mitral valve defects. Tsitologiia 1991;33:38-50.

9. Escande D., Coulombe A., Faivre J.F. and Coraboeuf E. Characteristics of the time-dependent slow inward current in adult human atrial single myocytes. Journal of Molecular and Cellular Cardiology 1986;18:547-551.
10. Escande D., Coulombe A., Faivre J.F., Deroubaix E. and Coraboeuf E. Two types of transient outward currents in adult human atrial cells. American Journal of Physiology 1987;252:H142-H148.
11. Harding S.E., Vescovo G., Jones S.M., Bennett G., Yacoub M. and Poole-Wilson P.A. Morphological and functional characteristics of myocytes isolated from human left ventricular aneurysms. Journal of Pathology 1989;159:191-196.
12. Harding S.E., O-Gara P., Jones S.M., Brown L.A., Vescovo G. and Poole-Wilson P.A. Species dependence of contraction velocity in single isolated cardiac myocytes. Cardioscience 1990;1:49-53.
13. Harding S.E., MacLeod K.T., Jones S.M., Vescovo G. and Poole-Wilson P.A. Contractile responses of myocytes isolated from patients with cardiomyopathy. European Heart Journal 1991;12(Suppl D):44-48.
14. Harding S.E., Gurden J.M. and Poole-Wilson P.A. A comparison of contractile function between papillary muscles and isolated myocytes from the same human hearts. Cardioscience 1991;2:141-146.
15. Harding S.E., Jones S.M., O-Gara P., del Monte F., Vescovo G. and Poole-Wilson P.A. Isolated ventricular myocytes from failing and non-failing human heart; the relation of age and clinical status of patients to isoproterenol response. Journal of Molecular and Cellular Cardiology 1992; 24:549-564.
16. Heidbüchel H., Vereecke J. and Carmeliet E. The electrophysiological effects of acetylcholine in single human atrial cells. Journal of Molecular and Cellular Cardiology 1987;19:1207-1219.
17. Heidbüchel H., Vereecke J. and Carmeliet E. Three different potassium channels in human atrium : contribution to the basal potassium conductance. Circulation Research 1990;66:1266-1286.
18. Jacobson S.L., Altschuld R.A. and Hohl C.M. Muscle cell cultures from human heart. In: Cell culture techniques in heart and vessel research (Piper H.M., ed.), Springer Verlag, Berlin,1990:75-98.
19. Liu G.S., Ravens U., Sadony V., Vandeplassche G. and Borgers M. Functional and structural impairment in human, rat and guinea-pig atrial muscle in response to *in vitro* calcium overload: a cytochemical study on cellular calcium distribution. Journal of Molecular and Cellular Cardiology 1991;23:795-805.
20. Mitchell M.R., Powell T., Sturridge M.F., Terrar D.A. and Twist V.W. Electrical properties and response to noradrenaline of individual heart cells isolated from human ventricular tissue. Cardiovascular Research 1986;20:869-876.
21. Ouadid H., Seguin J., Chaptal P.A., Ricard S. and Nargeot J. Properties of Ca-channels in adult human atrial cells. Journal of Molecular and Cellular Cardiology 1991;23:41-54.
22. Ouadid H., Seguin J., Dumuis A., Bockaert J. and Nargeot J. Serotonin increases calcium current in human atrial myocytes via the newly described 5-hydroxytryptamine 4 receptors. Molecular Pharmacology 1992;41:346-351.

23. Piper H.M., Jacobson S.L. and Schwartz P. Determinants of cardiomyocyte development in long-term primary culture. Journal of Molecular and Cellular Cardiology 1988;20:825-835.
24. Powell T., Sturridge M.F., Suverna S.K., Terrar D.A. and Twist V.W. Intact individual heart cells isolated from human ventricular tissue. British Medical Journal 1981;283:1013-1015.
25. Ravens U., Liu G.S., Vandeplassche G. and Borgers M. Protection of human, rat and guinea-pig by mioflazine, lidoflazine and verapamil against the destructive effects of high concentrations of Ca^{2+}. Cardiovascular Drugs and Therapy 1992;6:47-58.
26. Shperling I.D., Mirakian V.O. and Petrosian D.G. Characteristics of isolated cardiomyocytes of the left regions of the human heart in hypertrophy. Arkhiv Patologii 1983;45:52-55.
27. Shperling I.D. and Arakelian L.A. Characteristics of isolated cardiomyocytes in concentric and eccentric hypertrophy of the human heart ventricle. Arkhiv Patologii 1988;50:37-40.
28. Shperling I.D. and Arakelian L.A. The number and some other characteristics of isolated human ventricular cardiomyocytes under pathological conditions. Cor et Vasa 1990;32:327-334.
29. Smolenski R.T., Suitters A. and Yacoub M.H. Adenine nucleotide catabolism and adenosine formation in isolated human cardiomyocytes. Journal of Molecular and Cellular Cardiology 1992;24:91-96.

13

Human chondrocyte culture in pharmaco-toxicological research

M. Adolphe*, B. Benoit*, G. Verbruggen** and E.M. Veys**

* Laboratoire de Pharmacologie Cellulaire, 15, Rue de l'Ecole de Médecine, 75006 Paris (France).
** Afdeling Reumatologie, Universitair Ziekenhuis, De Pintelaan 185, 9000 Gent (Belgium).

Introduction

Chondrocytes are the unique cell type of cartilage. This tissue, which derives from embryonic mesoderm, plays an important role in skeletal protection by withstanding pressure and absorbing shocks. Two types of cartilage can be distinguished : growth cartilage in embryogenesis, and extraskeletal and articular cartilage in post-natal life.

As with all connective tissues, cartilage may be divided into cellular and intercellular components. The latter category, which is produced by the chondrocyte, is responsible for the mechanical properties of the cartilage. The culture of chondrocytes has been undertaken from a large variety of tissue sources since the beginning of tissue culture. Many reports have been published on chondrocytes derived from animals. However, human chondrocytes maintained *in vitro* have also been described, particularly for physiopathological research and also for drug toxicity assessment.

Main *in vivo* functions of chondrocytes

Although proliferative capacity is important in cartilage growth, cell growth is infrequent in normal adult cartilage except during the first steps of tissue repair after damage.

The main function of chondrocytes is to produce matrix. Matrix structure is heterogeneous and made up of several components linked one to another. The two major constituents are collagen fibers and aggregates of proteoglycans.

Although type II collagen (3 α_1(II) chains) is the dominant type, other types have been described from different cartilaginous tissues, such as type IX in articular cartilage [1], type X in growth plate cartilage [2] and type XI which appears to be localized on the chondrocyte surface.

Cartilaginous proteoglycans consist of a central core protein along which chondroitin sulfate and keratan sulfate are located. These subunits interact with hyaluronic acid to form aggregates stabilized by link proteins. Several other glycoproteins, such as chondronectin and thrombospondin have also been found in cartilage matrix.

In addition, it should be mentioned that chondrocytes synthesize enzymes which are implicated in the degradation of their matrix, including metalloproteinases (collagenase, stromelysin, gelatinase) and proteoglycanases.

Various types of human chondrocyte culture

The culture of human chondrocytes was performed either from normal articular tissue (foetal or adult) or from pathological tissues such as arthritic, osteoarthritic or chondrosarcoma cells. Whatever the tissue origin, different types of culture can be used, such as cartilage fragments, monolayer, high density and three dimensional culture. Recently, attempts have been made to obtain an immortalized human cell line of articular chondrocytes.

Cartilage fragments

It is possible to obtain, by careful dissection of cartilage of various origins, cartilage slices, that are free of extraneous cell types. This type of culture permits the study of chondrocytes in the presence of normal cell/matrix interactions since the tissue remains intact. According to Verbruggen *et al.* [3,4], the cells, which are in their original environment, are able to synthesize and accumulate abundant matrix macromolecules in the extracellular space. Synthetic activity and accumulation of macromolecules reach an optimum after 4-6 weeks. After this period increasing catabolic activity and decreasing synthesis rates make the tissue culture system less reliable. It is possible that the lack of mechanical influences causes impaired cellular function. Furthermore this type of tissue culture system allows the maintainance of the chondrocyte phenotype, as is demonstrated by the fact that the cells continue to synthesize cartilage-specific proteoglycans.

The major drawback of this tissue culture system are the large standard deviations of the mean for most of the variables tested (proteoglycan synthesis rates, relative amounts of proteoglycan subtypes and so forth). Coefficients of variation of 20-40% are the rule rather than the exception. This variability can be the consequence of the sampling of the cartilage explants from different sites in the joint and the difficulty in obtaining full-depth cartilage samples.

Monolayer culture

Monolayer culture is the type of chondrocyte culture referred to most frequently in the literature. Release of cartilaginous cells from joint tissue is usually achieved using the technique of Green, which is based on serial enzymatic digestions [5] with hyaluronidase, trypsin and finally collagenase in order to degrade the collagenous matrix. Benya et al. described a modification of this technique using a short collagenase step followed by an overnight treatment with collagenase at a lower concentration in the presence of foetal calf serum (FCS) [6]. This procedure permits the release of approximatively 90% of the chondrocytes present in rabbit cartilage slices.

After their release, cells are seeded in a rich synthetic medium such as DMEM or Ham F12 supplemented with 10% FCS. In these media, chondrocytes divide with a doubling time related to the age of the donor.

The main disadvantage of monolayer culture is that the matrix produced in culture is quite different from the one produced *in vivo*. The chondrocyte phenotype is labile with respect to collagen synthesis. It has been shown in rabbit chondrocyte culture that a switch from type II to type I collagen occur [7,8]. This phenomenon, which appears as soon as the end of the primary culture, is particularly evident in the first and subsequent subcultures [9]. With regards to proteoglycan synthesis, it has been shown that decreasing proportions of proteoglycans and increasing proportions of hyaluronan are synthesized when the number of passages in culture increases. The proteoglycans have a lower avidity for hyaluronan. Consequently, relatively less proteoglycan aggregates are formed. Furthermore, chondroitinsulfate in the proteoglycans is replaced by dermatansulfate and the glycosaminoglycans in the proteoglycan macromolecule are less sulfated [10]. However, this dedifferentiation is reversible. Benya and Schaffer showed that dedifferentiated chondrocytes can reexpress the differentiated phenotype in three-dimensional culture [11].

Three-dimensional culture

Three dimensional cell culture is achieved either by embedding the chondrocytes in a gel (collagen, agarose or alginate) or through the use of particular culture conditions (suspension or high density culture) in which chondrocytes themselves produce their three-dimensional environment.

This first type of culture system (chondrocytes embedded in a gel) has been studied at the fundamental level by various authors [11, 12-15] who have shown that it gives rise to cells which retain the chondrocyte phenotype. Furthermore, it is claimed that redifferentiation of dedifferentiated chondrocytes was possible. Cartilage cells suspended in agarose continue to produce cartilage-specific proteoglycans [16]. These proteoglycans form aggregates which can be removed from the artificial matrix with associative solvents. This permits the study of the native proteoglycan aggregate [17,18].

The major drawback of this culture system is the low rate of cell proliferation which limits the availability of this system. Moreover, the cells are not in their original environment.

Chondrocyte aggregates, obtained by culturing cell suspensions in spinner bottles or gyratory shakers, were also shown to retain the differentiated phenotype of chondrocytes. This last model appears more suitable for the obtention of larger quantities of cells than chondrocytes suspended in gel.

High-density cultures are obtained by seeding chondrocytes at a concentration of 10^5 cells/cm^2. At this density, cells reestablish a territorial matrix rich in collagen and proteoglycans. The importance of seeding density has been studied by Watt on pig articular chondrocytes, showing the evident relationship between the number of cells and the stability of the differentiated phenotype [19].

Immortalized chondrocytes

Studies on cultured chondrocytes are limited by their relative short life span and the frequent instability of their differentiated properties. The dream of obtaining a chondrocyte cell line possessing both the capacity for infinite proliferation and maintenance of specific functions has stimulated research in this field. An immortalized chondrocyte cell line would be particularly interesting because there are very few continuous cell lines of this type. The most famous one is a tumorigenic cell line, the swarm rat chondrosarcoma. Takigawa et al. have also established a cell line from human chondrosarcoma [20]. However, these cell lines are cancerous and present a low growth capacity.

Several attempts have been made to immortalize chondrocytes from animals (bird-rabbit) using virus infection or oncogenic transfection [21-26]. Although immortalization of mammalian chondrocytes has been easily obtained by these different means, maintenance of all differentiated functions and their regulation are quite imperfect.

Because of a variety of control mechanisms, such as an efficient repair system, the human genome is quite stable compared to most animal species. It has been reported that two stages are involved in the immortalization of human cells with SV40 Large T antigen. After the initial step of transformation, their proliferative capacity is very limited during a latency phase named 'crisis'. A further step is required for those rare cells which escape crisis and become immortal. To the best of our knowledge, human articular chondrocyte immortalization has never been achieved. Immortalization of this cell type is the aim of a European research programme (BRIDGE). The immortalization procedure used involves the transfection of human articular chondrocytes by the calcium phosphate method as described by Graham & van der Eb [27]. The transfections are performed with several immortalizing oncogenes, including SV40 Large T, temperature sensitive SV40 (*tsA48* mutation), polyoma Large T and *c-myc*. To date, we have obtained immortalized articular chondrocytes from 3 adult donors after transfection of human chondrocytes with temperature sensitive SV40 Large T antigen. However, their differentiated functions appear to be altered.

Applications of human condrocyte culture in pharmacology and toxicology

Human chondrocyte culture has been used quite frequently for pharmacotoxicological studies. The main end points studied are the following: proliferation and DNA synthesis; production of proteoglycan and collagen typing by biochemistry or Northern blotting; and production of various enzymes such as collagenase, stromelysin, gelatinase and proteoglycanase. All of these end points evaluate the *in vivo* functions of chondrocytes. On the other hand, several papers studied the interaction of drugs on some cell mediators such as prostaglandins and cytokines. The substances most frequently tested on human chondrocyte culture belong to the family of antiinflammatory drugs as a result of the involvement of inflammatory processes in the pathology of articulations. The effects of non-steroïdal antiinflammatory drugs (NSAID), *e.g.* tiaprofenic and acetylsalicylic acid [28], etodolac [29,30], piroxicam [31] and naproxen [32], on DNA synthesis, proteoglycan metabolism and type II collagen synthesis have been mostly evaluated in three dimensional culture. At therapeutic concentrations, acetylsalicylic acid depressed DNA synthesis and proteoglycan release in culture medium, whereas type II collagen was not modified. Tiaprofenic acid did not affect chondrocyte function. The same results were found with etodolac and naproxen. By contrast, piroxicam inhibited the proliferation and synthesis of proteoglycans by healthy and osteoarthritic chondrocytes cultured to high density. These types of studies should be checked and validated for other drugs before they can be said to have a predictive value for the testing of negative side effects of some antiinflammatory drugs.

Organ culture demonstrated the heterogeneity of human cartilaginous tissue according to the donors with regard to the effects of NSAID [33]. More interesting was the difference of response between tissues from normal and pathological joints. Using cartilage samples, no clear effects of niflumic acid were observed on normal cartilage; on the contrary, synthesized proteoglycans were retained in the intercellular matrix from fibrillated cartilage in the presence of this drug [34].

Steroidal drugs have been studied on cultured chondrocytes originating from various animals (rabbit, pig and rat). On human chondrocytes, it has only been demonstrated that proteoglycan synthesis was reduced by hydrocortisone [35]; although this phenomenon has been previously described on animal chondrocyte culture, cortisol suppression of proteoglycan synthesis remains controversal.

Bassleer et al. [36], using cultures of aggregated cells, demonstrated that a peptidic-glycosaminoglycan (PGAG) complex, isolated from calf cartilage and bone marrow, stimulated proliferation and production of matrix components (type II collagen and proteoglycans). In the same culture conditions, calcitonin at pharmacological concentrations had no proliferative effect on human articular chondrocytes, but displayed a stimulatory action on proteoglycans and type II collagen production [37]. High density culture of human chondrocytes originating from osteoarthritic articulations [38] showed that S-adenosylmethionine seemed to induce a higher synthesis rate for proteins and also for proteoglycans. These drugs may thus have chondroprotective properties.

With regards to toxicology, research has been focused most particularly on two types of drugs: retinoids and quinolones.

The dedifferentiative effect of retinoids on animal chondrocyte culture has been extensively described. For example, Benya and Padilla [39] have shown that retinoic acid treatment of rabbit articular chondrocytes led to the complete loss of the type II collagen synthesis and the induction of type I-trimer collagen in parallel with a eight-fold decrease in collagen and proteoglycan synthesis. With respect to human tissue, retinol was shown to suppress proteoglycan synthesis by young cartilage but to stimulate proteoglycan synthesis by old cartilage. It appeared that the effects of retinol are related to the high or low metabolic state of the chondrocyte [40].

In addition to their valuable antibacterial properties, all quinolones appeared to damage the articular cartilage of immature animals. This *in vivo* phenomenon has also been observed on chondrogenesis in murine cartilage organoid culture; type II collagen decreased in a dose-dependent manner after ofloxacin treatment. Some experiments on fluoroquinolone toxicity have been performed on human chondrocyte cultures in the Laboratory of Cellular Pharmacology. However, these studies have not yet permitted the elucidation of the mechanism of the toxic effects exerted by this type of agents.

Some tests were also performed to evaluate the effects of various cytokines on human cultured chondrocytes. The most frequently studied cytokines are interleukin-1 (IL-1), tumor necrosis factor (TNF) and interferon-gamma. All the papers dealing with IL-1 demonstrated that human articular chondrocytes cultured in the presence of this cytokine displayed an increased production of latent metalloproteinases and a proteoglycan release from cartilage [41-45]. A stimulation of prostaglandin E and interleukin-6 production has also been described [46,47]. TNF seemed to produce similar effects [44-48]. The effects of interferon are less evident. It seemed to suppress collagen synthesis [49,50] and induced a dose dependent decrease of cell proliferation and proteoglycan synthesis due to an inhibition of the proteoglycans core protein production and to a down regulation of the glycosaminoglycan chain elongation [51].

Conclusion

Human chondrocyte culture is an efficient target system for the evaluation of the pharmacological and toxicological effects of drugs acting on cartilaginous tissue. Many types of culture exist and have their own advantages and drawbacks. For example, in monolayer culture, chondrocytes do not retain all of their specific functions. Cartilage fragments and three-dimensional culture maintain chondrocytes in a differentiated state but without noticeable cell division. In spite of this disadvantage, most recent pharmacotoxicological experiments have been performed on these latter two models using various end points with respect to matrix anabolism or catabolism.

Antiinflammatory and antiosteoarthritic drugs have been especially studied on human cultured chondrocytes. Furthermore, the interaction of vitamin A derivatives and various cytokines with cartilaginous tissue should permit an increase in our knowledge of the complex regulations of chondrocytes and open the way to new antirheumatic drugs. However, the scope of the experiments are limited due to the difficulty of maintaining the chondrocytes in a differentiated state. A human immortalized chondrocyte cell line retaining all differentiative properties through the use of expression vectors in which the oncogen sequence is driven by tissue specific regulatory sequences could be the perfect cellular model of the future.

References

1. Ricard-Blum S., Tiollier J., Garrone R. and Herbage D. Further biochemical and physiochemical characterization of minor disulfide bonded (type IX collagen, extract from foetal calf cartilage). Journal of Cellular Biochemistry 1985;27:347-358.
2. Mayne I.R. and Irwin M.H. Collagen types in cartilage. In: Articular Cartilage Biochemistry (Kuettner K.E., Schleyerbach R. and Hascall V.C., eds.), Raven Press, New York, 1985:23-38.
3. Verbruggen V., Luyten F.P. and Veys E.M. Renewal of intercellular matrix proteoglycans by longterm organ culture of human articular cartilage. In: Degenerative joints, vol. II. (Verbruggen G. and Veys E.M., eds.), Excerpta Medica, Amsterdam, 1985:227-248.
4. Verbruggen G., Luyten F.P. and Veys E.M. Repair function in organ cultured human cartilage. Replacement of enzymatically removed proteoglycans during longterm organ culture. Journal of Rheumatology 1985;12:665-673.
5. Green W.T. Behaviour of articular chondrocytes in cell culture. Clinic Orthopaedics and Related Research 1971;75:248-260.
6. Benya P.D. Chondrocyte culture, introduction and survey of techniques for chondrocyte culture. In: Methods in Cartilage Research (Kuettner K. and Maroudas A., eds.), Academic Press, London, 1990:85-89.
7. Von der Mark K., Gauss V., Von der Mark H. and Muller P. Relationship between cell shape and type of collagen synthesized as chondrocytes lose their cartilage phenotype in culture. Nature 1977; 267:531-532.
8. Benya P.D., Padilla S.R. and Nimmi M.E. The progeny of rabbit articular chondrocytes synthesize collagens type I and III and type I trimer, but not type II. Verification by cyanogen bromide peptide analysis. Biochemistry 1977;16:865-872.
9. Benya P.D., Padilla S.R. and Nimmi M.E. Independent regulation of collagen types by chondrocytes during the loss of differentiated function in culture. Cell 1978;15:1313-1321.
10. Verbruggen G. and Veys E.M. Proteoglycan metabolism of connective tissue cells. An *in vitro* technique and its relevance to *in vivo* conditions. In: Degenerative joints. (Verbruggen G. and Veys E.M., eds.) Excerpta Medica, Amsterdam, 1980:113-129.
11. Benya P.D. and Shaffer J.D. Dedifferentiated chondrocytes reexpress the differentiated collagen type when cultured in agarose gels. Cell 1982;30:215-224.
12. Yasui N., Osawa S., Ochi T., Nakashima H. and Ono K. Primary culture of chondrocytes embedded in collagen gels. Experimental Cell Biology 1982;50:92-100.
13. Gibson G.J., Schor S.L. and Grant M.E. Effects of matrix macromolecules on chondrocyte gene expression : synthesis of a low molecular weight collagen species by cells cultured within collagen gels. Journal of Cellular Biology 1982;93:767-774.

14. Thomas J.T. and Grant M.E. Cartilage proteoglycan aggregate and fibronectin can modulate the expression of type X collagen by embryonic chick chondrocytes cultured in collagen gels. Bioscience Reports 1988;8:163-171.
15. Dewilde B., Benel L., Hartmann D.J. and Adolphe M. Subculture of rabbit articular chondrocytes within a collagen gel: growth and analysis of differentiation. Cytotechnology 1988;1:123-132.
16. Verbruggen G., Veys., E.M., Wieme N., Gijselbrecht L., Nimmegeers J., Almquist K.L. and Broddelez C. The synthesis and immobilisation of cartilage-specific proteoglycan by human chondrocytes in different concentrations of agarose. Clinical and Experimental Rheumatology 1990;8:371-378.
17. Cornelissen M., Verbruggen G., Malfait A.M., Veys E.M., Dewulf M., Hellebuyck P. and De Ridder L. Size distribution of native aggrecan aggregates of human articular chondrocytes in agarose. In Vitro Cellular and Developmental Biology 1993 (in press).
18. Cornelissen M., Verbruggen G., Malfait A.M., Veys E.M., Broddelez C. and De Ridder L. The study of representative populations of native aggregan aggregates synthesized by human chondrocytes *in vitro*. Journal of Tissue Culture Methods 1993 (in press).
19. Watt F.M. Effect of seeding density on stability of the differentiated phenotype of pig articular chondrocytes in culture. Journal of Cell Sciences 1988;89: 373-378.
20. Takigawa M., Tajima K., Pan H.O., Enomoto M., Kinoshita A., Suzuki F., Takano Y. and Mori Y. Establishment of a clonal human chondrosarcoma cell line with cartilage phenotypes. Cancer Research 1989;49:3996-4002.
21. Gionti E., Pontarelli G. and Cancedda R. Avian myelocytomatosis virus immortalizes differentiated quail chondrocytes. Proceedings of the National Academy of Sciences of the USA 1985;82:2756-2760.
22. Gionti E., Jullien P., Pontarelli G. and Sanchez M. A continuous cell line of chicken embryo cells derived from a chondrocyte culture infected with RSV. Cell Differentiation and Development 1989;27:215-223.
23. Horton W.E., Cleveland J., Rapp U., Nemuth G., Bolander M., Doege K., Yamada Y. and Hassel J.R. An established rat cell line expressing chondrocyte properties. Experimental Cell Research 1988;178:457-468.
24. Adolphe M. and Thenet S. Le concept d'immortalité cellulaire, un mythe ou une réalité. Exemple de chondrocytes articulaires 'immortalisés'. Bulletin de l'Académie Nationale de Médecine 1990;174:139-146.
25. Thenet S., Demignot S. and Adolphe M. Modulation de l'expression des fonctions différenciées chez des chondrocytes immortalisés par SV40. Médecine/Sciences 1991;4:XXII-XXIII.
26. Thenet S., Benya P.D., Demignot S., Feunteun J. and Adolphe M. SV40-immortalization of rabbit articular chondrocytes. Alteration of differentiated functions. Journal of Cellular Physiology 1992;150:158-16.
27. Graham F.L. and van der Eb A.J. A new technique for the assay of infectivity of human adenovirus 5 DNA. Virology 1973; 52:456-467.
28. Bassleer C.T., Henrotin Y.E., Reginster J.L. and Franchimont P.P. Effects of tiaprofenic acid and acetylsalicylic acid on human articular chondrocytes in 3-dimensional culture. Journal of Rheumatology 1992;19:1433-1438.

29. Henrotin Y., Bassleer C., Reginster J.Y. and Franchimont P. Effects of etodolac on human chondrocytes cultivated in three dimensional culture. Clinical Rheumatology 1989;8:36-42.
30. Bacon P.A. Etodolac: efficacy in osteoarthritis and effects on chondrocyte function. Rheumatology International 1990;10:3-7.
31. Bulstra S.K., Kuijer R., Buurman W.A., Terwindt-Rouwenhorst E., Guelen P.J. and van der Linden A.J. The effects of piroxicam on the metabolism of isolated human chondrocytes. Clinic Orthopaedics 1992;277:289-296.
32. Bassleer C., Henrotin Y. and Franchimont P. Effects of sodium naproxen on differentiated human chondrocytes cultivated in clusters. Clinical Rheumatology 1992;11:60-65.
33. Verbruggen G., Veys E.M., Malfait A.M., Cochez P., Schatteman L., Wieme N., Heynen G. and Broddelez C. Proteoglycan metabolism in tissue cultured human articular cartilage. Influence of piroxicam. Journal of Rheumatology 1989;16:355-362.
34. Verbruggen G., Veys E.M., Malfait A.M., Schatteman L., Wieme N., Nimmegeers J., Gerin M.G. and Broddelez C. Proteoglycan metabolism in tissue-cultured human articular cartilage. Influence of niflumic acid. Scandinavian Journal of Rheumatology 1990;19:257-268.
35. Pelletier J.P., Cloutier J.M. and Martel-Pelletier J. In vitro effects of tiaprofenic acid, sodium salicylate and hydrocortisone on the proteoglycan metabolism of human osteoarthritic cartilage. Journal of Rheumatology 1989;16:645-655.
36. Bassleer C., Gysen P., Bassleer R. and Franchimont P. Effects of peptidic glycosaminoglycans complex on human chondrocytes cultivated in three dimensions. Biochemical Pharmacology 1988;37:1939-1945.
37. Franchimont P., Bassleer C., Henrotin Y., Gysen P. and Bassleer R. Effects of human and salmon calcitonin on human articular chondrocytes cultivated in clusters. Journal of Clinical Endocrinology and Metabolism 1989;69:259-266.
38. Harmand M.F., Vilamitjana J., Maloche E., Duphil R. and Ducassou D. Effects of S-adenosylmethionine on human articular chondrocyte differentiation. An in vitro study. American Journal of Medicine 1987;83:48-54.
39. Benya P.D. and Padilla S.R. Modulation of the rabbit chondrocyte phenotype by retinoic acid terminates type II collagen synthesis without inducing type I collagen : the modulated phenotype differs from that produced by subculture. Developmental Biology 1986;118:296.
40. Huber-Bruning O., Wilbrink B., Vernooij J.E., Bijlsma J.W., Den Otter W. and Huber J. Contrasting in vitro effects of retinol and mononuclear cell factor on young and old human cartilage. Journal of Pathology 1986;150:21-27.
41. Hubard J.R., Steinberg J.J., Bednar M.S. and Sledge C.B. Effect of purified human interleukin-1 on cartilage degradation. Journal of Orthopaedic Research 1988;6:180-187.
42. Shinmei M., Kikuchi T., Masuda K. and Shimomura Y. Effects of interleukin-1 and anti-inflammatory drugs on the degradation of human articular cartilage. Drugs 1988;35:33-41.

43. Shinmei M., Masuda K., Kikuchi T. and Shimomura Y. The role of cytokines in chondrocyte mediated cartilage degradation. Journal of Rheumatology 1989;18:32-34.
44. Verbruggen G., Veys E.M., Malfait A.M., De Clercq L., van den Bosch F. and de Vlam K. Influence of human recombinant interleukin-1 beta on human articular cartilage. Mitotic activity and proteoglycan metabolism. Clinical and Experimental Rheumatology 1991;9:481-488.
45. Malfait A.M., Verbruggen G., Veys E.M., Lambert J., De Ridder L. and Cornelissen M. Comparative and combined effects of interleukin-6, interleukin-1 beta and tumor necrosis factor alpha on proteoglycan metabolism of human articular chondrocytes cultured in agarose. Journal of Rheumatology 1993 (in press).
46. Goldring M.B. Control of collagen synthesis in human chondrocyte cultures by immune interferon and interleukin-1. Journal of Rheumatology 1987;14:64-66.
47. Campbell I.K., Piccoli D.S. and Hamilton J.A. Stimulation of human chondrocyte prostaglandin E2 production by recombinant human interleukin-1 and tumor necrosis factor. Biochimica et Biophysica Acta 1990;1051:310-318.
48. Bunning R.A. and Russell R.G. The effect of tumor necrosis factor alpha and gamma-interferon on the resorption of human articular cartilage and on the production of prostaglandin E and of caseinase activity by human articular chondrocytes. Arthritis and Rheumatism 1989;32:780-784.
49. Goldring M.B., Sandell L.J., Stephenson M.L. and Krane S.M. Immune interferon suppresses levels of procollagen mRNA and type II collagen synthesis in cultured human articular and costal chondrocytes. Journal of Biological Chemistry 1986;261:9049-9055.
50. Goldring M.B. Control of collagen synthesis in human chondrocyte cultures by immune interferon and interleukin-1. Journal of Rheumatology 1987;14:64-66.
51. Verbruggen G., Malfait A.M., Veys E.M. Gyselbrecht L., Lambert J. and Almquist K.F. Influence of interferon-gamma on isolated chondrocytes from human articular cartilage. Journal of Rheumatology 1993 (in press).

14

Use of human pulmonary cells in pharmaco-toxicology

B. Nemery and P.H.M. Hoet

Laboratory of Pneumology (Unit of Lung Toxicology), K.U. Leuven, Kapucijnenvoer 35, 3000 Leuven (Belgium).

Introduction

In recent years, there has been a tendency to extend the notion of 'lung' - and certainly its adjective 'pulmonary' - to the entire respiratory tract, starting from the nose and the upper airways (i.e. above the larynx), along the trachea and large bronchi, down to the bronchioles and the actual lung tissue with its gas exchange units [1]. This is a relatively logical extension since all these 'lung'structures share the property that they are all primarily affected by inhaled compounds. Such compounds may be inhaled either from the personal, 'self-inflicted' environment (tobacco and other smoked drugs), or from the occupational, domestic or general environment. The respiratory tract thus represents a major target for the toxicity, carcinogenicity and allergenicity of inhaled environmental chemicals. Indeed, smoking-related diseases mainly involve the respiratory tract, lung disorders rank among the main occupational diseases, bronchial asthma caused by various inhaled allergens is a condition affecting a growing number of people and urban air pollution essentially causes respiratory problems. It is, therefore, not surprising that inhalation toxicology has always featured prominently in toxicological research.

In pharmacology too, a great deal of research effort is presently devoted to the lung, particularly in the important field of understanding the mechanisms of asthma, in order to develop appropriate drug treatment. Moreover, the lungs are also an important target for the toxicity of pharmaceuticals. Indeed a considerable number of compounds, some of which are widely used, can induce serious pulmonary side-effects for reasons that, for the great majority, are still unclear [2,3].

Research in environmental pulmonary disease and in pulmonary pharmacology involves clinical and epidemiological studies, on the one hand, and laboratory studies, on the other. In the past, most of the latter research was carried out using experimental animals and there is no doubt that such studies have contributed a great deal to our present understanding of lung pharmacology and toxicology. However, various arguments, of which the difficulties of species extrapolation are the most pervasive, plead for experimental studies with a more direct relevance to human health and disease. For obvious ethical reasons, such studies can in most instances only be carried out *in vitro* on material obtained or derived from human sources. One of the most promising avenues in this field is the use of cell cultures [4].

A characteristic feature of the respiratory tract is the diversity of the cells composing both the airways and the lung parenchyma. Each cell population has specific physiological functions and may exhibit different responses and susceptibilities to toxic chemicals [5,6]. Figure 1 indicates, in schematic form, the main morphologic characteristics of the cells of the lung and airways. The cells that have received the greatest attention in human pharmaco-toxicology, partly because of their importance in various disease processes and partly because of their amenability to investigation, are the alveolar macrophage, the bronchial epithelial cells and the type II alveolar epithelial cell.

In this review we will summarize and illustrate some of the main recent achievements in the *in vitro* use of these categories of human lung cells. We will focus on and refer explicitly only to those investigations in which cells of human origin have been studied, although it has to be recognized that the methods used for obtaining human cells have been essentially derived and adapted from work on respiratory cells from laboratory or large domestic animals (ovine, porcine or bovine lung).

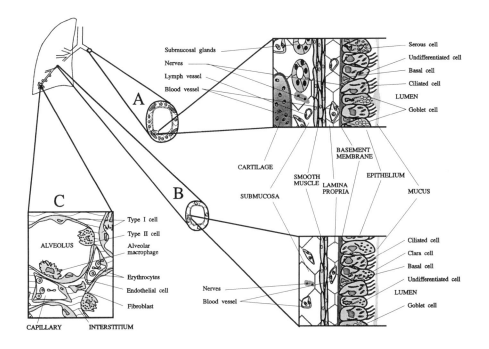

Figure 1 :
Schematic representation of:
A: tracheobronchial mucosa, B: bronchiolar mucosa, C: lung parenchyma
(relative dimensions of cells are not precise)

Airway epithelial cells

Cellular characteristics

Ciliated cells and mucus secreting (goblet) cells make up the bulk of the tracheobronchial epithelium [7]. The tracheobronchial secretions, including mucin glycoproteins, originate from both surface secretory cells and submucosal glands. Adequate ciliary function of the ciliated cells is essential to clear the respiratory tract from these secretions, as well as from foreign material deposited in the lung.

Airway epithelial cells have been mainly studied in relation to the pathogenesis of cystic fibrosis (a disease caused by a defective apical membrane chloride ion transport) and the mechanisms of bronchial asthma (characterized by epithelial eosinophilic inflammation) and in relation to their response to inhaled pollutants.

Methodological aspects

Human airway epithelial cells can be derived and cultured from nasal, tracheal or bronchial tissue. Large quantities of nasal mucosa are widely available by utilizing surgically removed nasal turbinates or polyps. It has been established that, at least for some physiologic functions, nasal epithelial cells are probably valid substitutes for tracheobronchial epithelial cell [8]. Tracheal and bronchial tissue may be obtained during surgery or at autopsy; the cells may be collected following immediate enzymatic dissociation of the tissues or later from outgrowths of explants of these tissues. More recently, bronchial epithelial cells have been obtained from living, healthy donors by suction or by brushing of the bronchial mucosa during fiberoptic bronchoscopy [9,10]. In the study of Kelsen et al. [10] 14 million cells were yielded per subject (24% ciliary, 11% secretory, 29% basal, 36% non identifiable cells); the mean cellular viability was only 36% (and was markedly reduced by the use of lidocaine for topical anaesthesia) and the plating efficiency was 50-60%.

The methodological and technical issues in relation to the *in vitro* study of animal and human airway epithelial cells have been recently reviewed and discussed by Jorissen et al. [11]. Techniques have mainly involved organ cultures, cells dissociated from the outgrowth of explants, and monolayer cultures of dissociated cells. The physiological function which is maintained most easily in culture is that of ion and water transport. Thus, culture conditions (medium and growth supports) have been described for an optimal retention, in culture and subculture, of the electrical properties of normal and cystic fibrosis epithelial cells [12,13]. Other important cellular functions, such as ciliary beating and mucous secretion, are usually rapidly lost in culture. Nevertheless, some groups have successfully developed methods to obtain cells maintaining functional cilia. Thus, ciliary beat frequency has been used as an endpoint of pharmacologic action [14,15] or toxicity [16] in cultured bronchial epithelial cells. Jorissen et al. [11] have shown that nasal epithelial cells grown in suspension, rather than as monolayers, exhibit ciliogenesis followed by active ciliary beating for several months. Wu et al. [17] have also improved their original procedure of culturing human tracheo-bronchial epithelial cells so as to obtain mucin secreting cells. Recently, Benali et al. [18] have described how nasal epithelial cells cultured on three-dimensional collagen lattices form tubular structures with cells exhibiting polarity and either secretory or ciliary activity. Other groups have studied secretory processes in human tracheobronchial submucosal gland cells [19-22].

Transformation of human airway epithelial cells into stable, proliferative cell lines has been achieved: a frequently used line is the BEAS line, obtained by transformation with a SV40/adenovirus hybrid [23].

A cell type which has received a great attention in toxicology is the non-ciliated bronchiolar (Clara) cell, because this cell contains a considerable amount of cytochrome-P450 activity in laboratory animals [24,25]. However, it is still unclear whether the Clara cell (or an equivalent cell) has this capacity in the human lung and, as yet, no reports exist on the successful isolation and culture of pure Clara cell populations from the human lung [26].

Applications

Cultured airway epithelial cells have been extensively studied with regard to their possible involvement in immune-inflammatory processes such as asthma. Thus human nasal or tracheobronchial cells have been shown to secrete metabolites of arachidonic acid [27-32] and various cytokines and other products [33-42]. These cells also possess, to some extent, the receptors for intercellular adhesion [43] and antigen presentation [9,44]. They have been shown to be relatively resistant to cellular damage by e.g. eosinophils or neutrophils [45,46] and the process of wound repair has been elegantly studied [47].

Human nasal or tracheobronchial cells have in fact not yet been used widely in pharmacology, toxicology or carcinogenicity studies, at least not as much as animal cells. Effects of drugs used in asthma, such as β-adrenergic drugs [48] or corticosteroids [38,49], have been studied. Samet et al. [50] and McKinnon et al. [51] have recently bescribed how *in vitro* exposure of cultured airway epithelial cells to ozone effects the release of platelet-activating factor (PAF) and arachidonic acid products. Similarly, Mattoli et al. [29,30,36,52] have investigated extensively the effects of exposure of cultured human bronchial epithelial cells to isocyanates, compounds which are responsible for a large proportion of chemically-induced occupational asthmas.

Grafström [53] has compared differences in cytotoxicity, induction of differentiation and genotoxicity between formaldehyde and acrolein, two aldehydes of considerable environmental relevance.

Pulmonary alveolar macrophages

Cellular characteristics

No pulmonary cell has been investigated so extensively as the alveolar macrophage. The reason is that this cell plays a very important role in various lung diseases and that this free cell can be harvested easily from the respiratory tract by the technique of bronchoalveolar lavage (BAL).

Pulmonary alveolar macrophages make out the great majority (85% or more) of the cells recovered by bronchoalveolar lavage in normal subjects. Their main physiological function is to defend the distal airways and alveoli against micro-organisms and particulates, mainly via phagocytosis [54]. This defensive role involves a vast array of surface receptors and secretory products, including oxygen metabolites, proteolytic enzymes and various mediators, such as polypeptides (cytokines) or bioactive lipids (arachidonic acid-derived and PAF). These functions may be impaired by toxic agents, thus potentially resulting in defective clearance and increased susceptibility to pulmonary infections.

Methodological aspects

BAL has now become a widely used clinical tool for the assessment of many respiratory diseases. Because of its safety and minimal invasiveness BAL may be carried out, even in normal volunteers, without great ethical reservations, according to guidelines issued by a report of the European Respiratory Society [55]. The technique consists of instilling, through a fiberoptic bronchoscope, aliquots (30-50 ml) of usually a saline solution into a segment of the lung and to retrieve that fluid for analysis of the recovered cellular population and soluble components. Alterations in the distribution of inflammatory cells in the BAL fluid are reasonably good reflections of the tissue inflammation and are used as adjuncts for the diagnosis of various lung disorders such as hypersensitivity pneumonitis, sarcoidosis, interstitial fibrosis, etc. The cells obtained by BAL may also be cultured and their function studied or their response to various stimuli investigated.

Thanks to BAL it has been possible to establish that the alveolar macrophage plays a pivotal role in a number of pulmonary inflammatory diseases of evidently exogenous origin, such as smoking-induced emphysema or dust pneumoconioses, and also in diseases of a still obscure origin such as sarcoidosis and idiopathic pulmonary fibrosis. The good availability of these cells has undoubtedly allowed this area to be the most successful one with regard to the use of pulmonary cells in toxicology.

Applications

In practice, few studies have shown macrophage functions to be suppressed by toxic agents in humans, e.g. in smokers [56-58]. More often the converse has been observed, i.e. activation of macrophage functions leading to inflammation and tissue destruction as a result of exposure to cigarette smoke or dust particles [54]. Thus, smokers not only have increased numbers of macrophages in their alveoli, they also have increased numbers of polymorphonuclear neutrophils, attracted by the release of chemoattractants by the macrophages. A recent study using human alveolar macrophages has shown that these cells and neutrophils synergize in causing the oxidative inactivation of $\alpha 1$-proteinase inhibitor, thus leading to protease-antiprotease imbalance in the lung, a mechanism thought to be responsible for the development of pulmonary emphysema [59].

The inhalation of inorganic mineral particles and fibres is also associated with chronic inflammation of the alveoli. Rom *et al.* [60] have shown in non-smoking subjects with asbestosis, coal worker's pneumoconiosis or silicosis that this inflammation is dominated by the presence of macrophages. These macrophages exhibited signs of activation, in that they spontaneously released increased amounts of superoxide anion and hydrogen peroxide, as well as fibrogenic mediators. Moreover, it was established subsequently that there is a relationship between the severity of the pneumoconiosis and the release of mediators by macrophages *in vitro* [61-63]. Exposure of normal human alveolar macrophages to coal dust *in vitro* was further shown to induce the release of mediators (TNF-α and IL-6) having a probable relevance in the causation of lung damage [64]. Similarly, *in vitro* exposure of normal human alveolar macrophages to chrysotile and crocidolite asbestos leads to the release of superoxide anion and this was enhanced by the presence of IgG [65].

Exposure to gaseous pollutants such as ozone also leads to alveolitis, but this alveolitis is mainly characterized by increased numbers of neutrophils and there is no measurable macrophage dysfunction [66,67].

Other pollutants, such as NO_2, have been studied *in vitro* by Wallaert and Voisin [68], using their system for exposure of cells to gaseous compounds.

Macrophages are not normally considered to have much xenobiotic metabolizing activity, although older studies have shown that human alveolar macrophages were able to metabolize benzo(a)pyrene [69] and their aryl hydrocarbon hydroxylase activity could be induced *in vitro* by benzanthracene [70]. It has also been shown that human macrophages could reduce Cr(VI) to Cr(III), a process thought to be critical for the carcinogenic effects of chromates [71].

Alveolar epithelial cells

Cellular characteristics

The alveolar epithelium is made up of two types of cells: alveolar type I and type II pneumocytes. The largest part of the epithelial surface is covered by type I pneumocytes which are terminally differentiated cells with a very thin cytoplasm and little known functional activity, other than that of offering the least possible resistance to the diffusion of oxygen and carbon dioxide to and from the capillaries; type I cells have not yet been successfully isolated from mammalian lungs, but similar cells may be obtained by culturing their progenitor cells, the type II pneumocytes. Type II cells are cuboidal cells located in the corners of the alveoli, which in addition of being progenitor cells for the type I cells, have important physiological roles such as the secretion of the pulmonary surfactant, the regulation of ion and water fluxes across the alveolo-capillary membrane and other metabolic functions, including xenobiotic biotransformation [72].

Methodological aspects

Cancer cells of either bronchial or alveolar origin, isolated from patients with various types of malignant lung disease, are made to grow to study their chemosensitivity, radiosensitivity, immunosensitivity, expression of oncogenes, tumour markers, surface markers, response to hormones and cytokines, growth behaviour, differentiation etc. Such cells may be immortalized and this has given rise to a large variety of cell lines allowing various areas of carcinogenesis to be studied, including mechanisms of (multi)drug resistance. A number of these cell lines exhibit characteristic features of peripheral airway cells (type II pneumocytes and Clara cells) [73]. The most widely utilized cell line is the A549 cell line, with cells that do not, however, appear to have much in common with the real type II cells.

Various procedures for the isolation and primary culture of type II cells have been described for various mammalian species, including humans, either from fetuses or surgical lung specimens [74-76].

Applications

The A549 cell line has been used for the *in vitro* study of the response to toxic compounds, such as cadmium, a known pneumotoxic metal [77-79], or SO_2 [80]. In a recent study [81] it was shown that A549 cells exposed to various carcinogenic or non-carcinogenic amines exhibited enhanced DNA single-strand breaks when the amines had been previously exposed to ambient levels of ozone. The mutagenic effects were not mediated by cellular biotransformation, since the A459 cells are not equipped with the necessary enzymes. McLemore *et al.* [82] have evaluated the expression and inducibility of the P450-1A1 gene in various pulmonary cancer cell-derived cell lines.

Studies with primary cultures of human alveolar type II cells have mainly focused on the physiology of this cell, e.g. the synthesis and secretion of surfactant [76,83]. However, as yet, few toxicological studies appear to have been carried out using primary cultures of human alveolar type II cells, neither in the area of inhaled pollutants nor in relation to systemic pneumotoxins.

One famous instance of pulmonary injury by a blood-borne chemical is paraquat-lung. Paraquat is a contact herbicide which is concentrated in the lung of mammals by being transported actively by an uptake system located mainly in alveolar epithelial cells [84]. This uptake system apparently has as endogenous substrates oligoamines, such as putrescine, spermidine and spermine, as well as the sulfhydryl cystamine. Following its uptake into the target cells, paraquat undergoes a 'futile' cycle of reduction by NADPH reductase and oxidation by molecular oxygen with the concomitant production of superoxide anion and further toxic species, such as hydroxyl radicals. The depletion of NADPH and the continuous production of toxic oxygen metabolites result in a severe imbalance in the oxidant-antioxidant balance of the cells and hence cell death. We have recently shown that the uptake system for paraquat/putrescine, which had been well characterized in animal lung tissue and isolated type II cells, is also present in human lung tissue slices [85] and in isolated human type II cells [86]. The kinetics of uptake appeared to be roughly similar between human and rat or hamster lung.

Other pulmonary cells

For the sake of completeness, it must be acknowledged that other cell types than the ones reviewed above have been isolated from the human lung: e.g. pulmonary endothelial cells [87], bronchial and pulmonary fibroblasts [34,88-91], lung dendritic cells [92], airway smooth muscle cells [35,93,94] and pleural mesothelial cells [95,96].

Conclusion

Research into the mechanisms by which chemicals interact with the respiratory system is important both to understand the health consequences of environmental exposure and to develop effective pharmacologic treatment for respiratory diseases. Studying the behaviour and response of human lung cells will undoubtedly contribute to progress in both areas.

The rationale - and great expectation - when carrying out *in vitro* experimentation with human material is to perform a valid 'parallelogram-type reasoning' whereby the knowledge of the 'animal *in vitro-in vivo* limb' and the 'animal *in vitro* - human *in vitro* comparison' may lead to a valid 'human *in vitro-in vivo* limb'. Leikauff and Driscoll [97] have recently summarized very aptly the advantages and drawbacks of using cells in culture for the study of responses to adverse environmental agents. One of the main advantages is that cells in culture offer the potential for investigating chemicals in a longer time frame than e.g. subcellular fractions or lung slices; one of the main drawbacks, however, is that the isolation and culture procedures may severely affect the response of the cells. Considerable research efforts are still needed to establish, among other problems, the validity of *in vitro* model systems. It may be anticipated that significant progress will be made through a collaborative research programme involving eight European teams and partly supported by the Commission of the European Communities within the BIOMED framework (BHM1-92-1229).

References

1. Gardner D.E., Crapo J.D. and McClellan R.O. Toxicology of the Lung, 2nd Ed. Raven Press, New York, 1993:1-672.
2. Cooper J.A.D., White D.A. and Matthay R.A. Drug-induced pulmonary disease. Part 1: Cytotoxic drugs. American Review of Respiratory Disease 1986;133:321-340.
3. Cooper J.A.D., White D.A. and Matthay R.A. Drug-induced pulmonary disease. Part 2: Noncytotoxic drugs. American Review of Respiratory Disease 1986;133:488-505.
4. Nemery B. and Hoet P.H.M. Use of isolated lung cells in pulmonary toxicology. Toxicology in Vitro 1993 (in press).
5. Smith L.L. and Nemery B. Cellular specific toxicity in the lung. In: Selectivity and molecular mechanisms of toxicity (De Matteis F. and Lock E.A., eds.) MacMillan Press, London, 1987: 3-26.
6. Smith L.L. and Nemery B. The lung as a target organ for toxicity. In: Target organ toxicity, 2nd Ed. (Cohen G.M., ed.) CRC Press, Boca Raton, Florida, 1986:45-80.
7. Breeze R. and Turk M. Cellular structure, function and organization in the lower respiratory tract. Environmental Health Perspectives 1984;55:3-24.
8. Devalia J.L., Sapsford R.J., Wells C.W., Richman P. and Davies R.J. Culture and comparison of human bronchial and nasal epithelial cells *in vitro*. Respiratory Medicine 1990;84:303-312.
9. Rossi G.A., Sacco O., Balbi B., Oddera S., Mattioni T., Corte G., Ravazzoni C. and Allegra L. Human ciliated bronchial epithelial cells: Expression of the HLA-DR antigens and of the HLA-DR alpha gene, modulation of the HLA-DR antigens by gamma-interferon and antigen-presenting function in the mixed leukocyte reaction. American Journal of Respiratory Cell and Molecular Biology 1990;3:431-439.
10. Kelsen S.G., Mardini I.A., Zhou S., Benovic J.L. and Higgins N.C. A technique to harvest viable tracheobronchial epithelial cells from living human donors. American Journal of Respiratory Cell and Molecular Biology 1992;7:66-72.
11. Jorissen M., Van Der Schueren B., Van Den Berghe H. and Cassiman J.J. Contribution of *in vitro* culture methods for respiratory epithelial cells to the study of the physiology of the respiratory tract. European Respiratory Journal 1991;4:210-217.
12. Gruenert D.C., Basbaum C.B. and Widdicombe J.H. Long-term culture of normal and cystic fibrosis epithelial cells grown under serum-free conditions. In Vitro Cellular and Developmental Biology 1990;26:411-418.
13. Yamaya M., Finkbeiner W.E. and Widdicombe J.H. Ion transport by cultures of human tracheobronchial submucosal glands. American Journal of Physiology 1991;261:L485-L490.

14. Devalia J.L. and Davies R.J. Human nasal and bronchial epithelial cells in culture: an overview of their characteristics and function. Allergy Proceedings 1991;12:71-79.
15. Devalia J.L., Sapsford R.J., Rusznak C., Toumbis M.J. and Davies R.J. The effects of salmeterol and salbutamol on ciliary beat frequency of cultured human bronchial epithelial cells, in vitro. Pulmonary Pharmacology 1992;5:257-263.
16. Devalia J.L., Sapsford R.J., Rusznack C. and Davies R.J. The effect of human eosinophils on cultured human nasal epithelial cell activity and the influence of nedocromil sodium in vitro. American Journal of Respiratory Cell and Molecular Biology 1992;7:270-277.
17. Wu R., Martin W.R., Robinson C.B., St.George J.A., Plopper C.G., Kurland G., Last J.A., Cross C.E., McDonald R.J. and Boucher R. Expression of mucin synthesis and secretion in human tracheobronchial epithelial cells grown in culture. American Journal of Respiratory Cell and Molecular Biology 1990;3:467-478.
18. Benali R., Tournier J.M., Chevillard M., Zahm J.M., Klossek J.M., Hinnrasky J., Gaillard D., Maquart F.X. and Puchelle E. Tubule formation by human surface respiratory epithelial cells cultured in a three-dimensional collagen lattice. American Journal of Physiology 1993;264:L183-L192.
19. Sommerhof C.P. and Finkbeiner W.E. Human tracheobronchial submucosal gland cells in culture. American Journal of Respiratory Cell and Molecular Biology 1990;2:41-50.
20. Tournier J.M., Merten M., Meckler Y., Hinnrasky J., Fuchey C. and Puchelle E. Culture and characterization of human tracheal gland cells. American Review of Respiratory Disease 1990;141:1280-1288.
21. Merten M.D., Tournier J.M., Meckler Y. and Figarella C. Secretory proteins and glycoconjugates synthesized by human tracheal gland cells in culture. American Journal of Respiratory Cell and Molecular Biology 1992;7:598-605.
22. Merten M.D. and Figarella C. Constitutive hypersecretion and insensitivity to neurotransmitters by cystic fibrosis tracheal gland cells. American Journal of Physiology 1993;264:L93-L99.
23. Noah T.L., Paradiso A.M., Madden M.C., McKinnon K.P. and Devlin R.B. The response of a human bronchial epithelial cell line to histamine: intracellular calcium changes and extracellular release of inflammatory mediators. American Journal of Respiratory Cell and Molecular Biology 1991;5:484-492.
24. Plopper C.G. Comparative morphologic features of bronchiolar epithelial cells. American Review of Respiratory Disease 1983;128:S37-S41.
25. Plopper C.G., Macklin J., Nishio S.J., Hyde D.M. and Buckpitt A.R. Relationship of cytochrome P-450 activity to Clara cell cytotoxicity. III. Morphometric comparison of changes in the epithelial populations of terminal bronchioles and lobar bronchi in mice, hamsters, and rats after parenteral administration of naphthalene. Laboratory Investigation 1992;67:553-565.
26. Bingle L., Bull T.B., Fox B., Guz A., Richards R.J. and Tetley T.D. Type II pneumocytes in mixed cell culture of human lung: a light and electron microscopic study. Environmental Health Perspectives 1990;85:71-80.

27. Salari H. and Chan-Yeung M. Release of 15-hydroxyeicosatetraenoic acid (15-HETE) and prostaglandin E2 (PGE2) by cultured human bronchial epithelial cells. American Journal of Respiratory Cell and Molecular Biology 1989;1:245-250.
28. Churchill L., Chilton F.H., Resau J.H., Bascom R., Hubbard W.C. and Proud D. Cyclooxygenase metabolism of endogenous arachidonic acid by cultured human tracheal epithelial cells. American Review of Respiratory Disease 1989;140:449-459.
29. Mattoli S., Masiero M., Calabro F., Mezzetti M., Plebani M. and Allegra L. Eicosanoid release from human bronchial epithelial cells upon exposure to toluene diisocyanate in vitro. Journal of Cellular Physiology 1990;142:379-385.
30. Mattoli S., Mezzetti M., Fasoli A., Patalano F. and Allegra L. Nedocromil sodium prevents the release of 15-hydroxyeicosatetraenoic acid from human bronchial epithelial cells exposed to toluene diisocyanate in vitro. International Archives of Allergy and Applied Immunology 1990;92:16-22.
31. Wu T., Mullol J., Rieves R.D., Logun C., Hausfield J., Kaliner M.A. and Shelhamer J.H. Endothelin-1 stimulates eicosanoid production in cultured human nasal mucosa. American Journal of Respiratory Cell and Molecular Biology 1992;6:168-174.
32. Becker S., Soukup J. and Yankaskas J.R. Respiratory syncytial virus infection of human primary nasal and bronchial epithelial cell cultures and bronchoalveolar macrophages. American Journal of Respiratory Cell and Molecular Biology 1992;6:369-374.
33. Shoji S., Rickard K.A., Ertl R.F., Robbins R.A., Linder J. and Rennard S.I. Bronchial epithelial cells produce lung fibroblast chemotactic factor: fibronectin. American Journal of Respiratory Cell and Molecular Biology 1989;1:13-20.
34. Shoji S., Rickard K.A., Takizawa H., Ertl R.F., Linder J. and Rennard S.I. Lung fibroblasts produce growth stimulatory activity for bronchial epithelial cells. American Review of Respiratory Disease 1990;141:433-439.
35. Mattoli S., Mezzetti M., Riva G., Allegra L. and Fasoli A. Specific binding of endothelin on human bronchial smooth muscle cells in culture and secretion of endothelin-like material from bronchial epithelial cells. American Journal of Respiratory Cell and Molecular Biology 1990;3:145-151.
36. Mattoli S., Colotta F., Fincato G., Mezzetti M., Mantovani A., Patalano F. and Fasoli A. Time course of IL1 and IL6 synthesis and release in human bronchial epithelial cell cultures exposed to toluene diisocyanate. Journal of Cellular Physiology 1991;149:260-268.
37. Ohtoshi T., Vancheri C., Cox G., Gauldie J., Dolovich J., Denburg J.A. and Jordana M. Monocyte-macrophage differentiation induced by human upper airway epithelial cells. American Journal of Respiratory Cell and Molecular Biology 1991;4:255-263.
38. Cox G., Ohtoshi T., Vancheri C., Denburg J.A., Dolovich J., Gauldie J. and Jordana M. Promotion of eosinophil survival by human bronchial epithelial cells and its modulation by steroids. American Journal of Respiratory Cell and Molecular Biology 1991;4:525-531.

39. Cox G., Gauldie J. and Jordana M. Bronchial epithelial cell-derived cytokines (G-CSF and GM-CSF) promote the survival of peripheral blood neutrophils *in vitro*. American Journal of Respiratory Cell and Molecular Biology 1992;7:507-513.
40. Marini M., Soloperto M., Mezzetti M., Fasoli A. and Mattoli S. Interleukin-1 binds to specific receptors on human bronchial epithelial cells and upregulates granulocyte/macrophage colony-stimulating factor synthesis and release. American Journal of Respiratory Cell and Molecular Biology 1991;4:519-524.
41. Marini M., Soloperto M., Zheng Y., Mezzetti M. and Mattoli S. Protective effect of nedocromil sodium on the IL1- induced release of GM-CSF from cultured human bronchial epithelial cells. Pulmonary Pharmacology 1992;5:61-65.
42. Xing Z., Ohtoshi T., Ralph P., Gauldie J. and Jordana M. Human upper airway structural cell-derived cytokines support human peripheral blood monocyte survival: a potential mechanism for monocyte/macrophage accumulation in the tissue. American Journal of Respiratory Cell and Molecular Biology 1992;6:212-218.
43. Tosi M.F., Stark J.M., Smith W., Hamedani A., Gruenert D.C. and Infeld M.D. Induction of ICAM-1 expression on human airway epithelial cells by inflammatory cytokines: Effects on neutrophil-epithelial cell adhesion. American Journal of Respiratory Cell and Molecular Biology 1992;7:214-221.
44. Mezzetti M., Soloperto M., Fasoli A. and Mattoli S. Human bronchial epithelial cells modulate CD3 and mitogen-induced DNA synthesis in T cells but function poorly as antigen- presenting cells compared to pulmonary macrophages. Journal of Allergy and Clinical Immunology 1991;87:930-938.
45. Ayars G.H., Altman L.C., McManus M.M., Agosti J.M., Baker C.B., Luchtel D.L., Loegering D.A. and Gleich G.J. Injurious effect of the eosinophil peroxide-hydrogen peroxide-halide system and major basic protein on human nasal epithelium *in vitro*. American Review of Respiratory Disease. 1989;140:125-131.
46. Kercsmar C.M. and Davis P.B. Resistance of human tracheal epithelial cells to killing by neutrophils, neutrophil elastase, and Pseudomonas elastase. American Journal of Respiratory Cell and Molecular Biology 1993;8:56-62.
47. Zahm J.M., Chevillard M. and Puchelle E. Wound repair of human surface respiratory epithelium. American Journal of Respiratory Cell and Molecular Biology 1991;5:242-248.
48. Davis P.B., Silski C.L. and Liedtke C.M. Amiloride antagonizes β-adrenergic stimulation of cAMP synthesis and Cl$^-$ secretion in human tracheal epithelial cells. American Journal of Respiratory Cell and Molecular Biology 1992;6:140-145.
49. Schleimer R.P. Potential regulation of inflammation in the lung by local metabolism of hydrocortisone. American Journal of Respiratory Cell and Molecular Biology 1991;4:166-173.

50. Samet J.M., Noah T.L., Devlin R.B., Yankaskas J.R., McKinnon K., Dailey L.A. and Friedman M. Effect of ozone on platelet-activating factor production in phorbol- differentiated HL60 cells, a human bronchial epithelial cell line (BEAS S6), and primary human bronchial epithelial cells. American Journal of Respiratory Cell and Molecular Biology 1992;7:514-522.
51. McKinnon K.P., Madden M.C., Noah T.L. and Devlin R.B. In vitro ozone exposure increases release of arachidonic acid products from a human bronchial epithelial cell line. Toxicology and Applied Pharmacology 1993;118:215-223.
52. Mattoli S., Miante S., Calabro F., Mezzetti M., Fasoli A. and Allegra L. Bronchial epithelial cells exposed to isocyanates potentiate activation and proliferation of T- cells. American Journal of Physiology 1990;259:L320-L327.
53. Grafström R.C. In vitro studies of aldehyde effects related to human respiratory carcinogenesis. Mutation Research 1990;238:17:5-184.
54. Sibille Y. and Reynolds H.Y. Macrophages and polymorphonuclear neutrophils in lung defense and injury. American Review of Respiratory Disease 1990;141:471-501.
55. Klech H. and Pohl W. Technical recommendations and guidelines for bronchoalveolar lavage (BAL). Report of the European Society of Pneumology Task Group on BAL. European Respiratory Journal 1989;2:561-585.
56. Thomassen M.J., Barna B.P., Wiedemann H.P., Farmer M. and Ahmad M. Human alveolar macrophage function: differences between smokers and nonsmokers. Journal of Leukocyte Biology 1988;44:313-318.
57. Linden M., Wieslander E., Eklund A., Larsson K. and Brattsand R. Effects of oral N-acetylcysteine on cell content and macrophage function in bronchoalveolar lavage from healthy smokers. European Respiratory Journal 1988;1:645-650.
58. Tardif J., Borgeat P. and Laviolette M. Inhibition of human alveolar macrophage production of leukotriene B4 by acute in vitro and in vivo exposure to tobacco smoke. American Journal of Respiratory Cell and Molecular Biology 1990;2:155-161.
59. Wallaert B., Gressier B., Aerts C., Mizon C., Voisin C. and Mizon J. Oxidative inactivation of alpha 1-proteinase inhibitor by alveolar macrophages from healthy smokers requires the presence of myeloperoxidase. American Journal of Respiratory Cell and Molecular Biology 1991;5:437-444.
60. Rom W.N., Bitterman P.B., Rennard S.I. and Crystal R.G. Characterization of the lower respiratory tract inflammation of nonsmoking individuals with interstitial lung disease associated with chronic inhalation of inorganic dusts. American Review of Respiratory Disease 1987;136:1429-1434.
61. Wallaert B., Lassalle P., Fortin F., Aerts C., Bart F., Fournier E. and Voisin C. Superoxide anion generation by alveolar inflammatory cells in simple pneumoconiosis and in progressive massive fibrosis of nonsmoking coal workers. American Review of Respiratory Disease 1990;141:129-133.
62. Lassalle P., Gosset P., Aerts C., Fournier E., Lafitte J.J., Degreef J.M., Wallaert B., Tonnel A.B. and Voisin C. Abnormal secretion of interleukin-1 and tumor necrosis factor alpha by alveolar macrophages in coal workers pneumoconiosis: comparison between simple pneumoconiosis and progressive massive fibrosis. Experimental Lung Research 1990;16:73-80.

63. Rom W.N. Relationship of inflammatory cell cytokines to disease severity in individuals with occupational inorganic dust exposure. American Journal of Industrial Medicine 1991;19:15-27.
64. Gosset P., Lassalle P., Vanhee D., Wallaert B., Aerts C., Voisin C. and Tonnel A.B. Production of tumor necrosis factor-alpha and interleukin-6 by human alveolar macrophages exposed *in vitro* to coal mine dust. American Journal of Respiratory Cell and Molecular Biology 1991;5:431-436.
65. Perkins R.C., Scheule R.K. and Holian A. *In vitro* bioactivity of asbestos for the human alveolar macrophage and its modification by IgG. American Journal of Respiratory Cell and Molecular Biology 1991;4:532-537.
66. Koren H.S., Devlin R.B., Graham D.E., Mann R., McGee M.P., Horstmann D.H., Kozumbo W.J., Becker S., House D.E., McDonnell W.F. and Bromberg P.A. Ozone-induced inflammation in the lower airways of human subjects. American Review of Respiratory Disease 1989;139:407-415.
67. Devlin R.B., McDonnell W.F., Mann R., Becker S., House D.E., Schreinemachers D. and Koren H.S. Exposure of humans to ambient levels of ozone for 6.6 hours causes cellular and biochemical changes in the lung. American Journal of Respiratory Cell and Molecular Biology 1991;4:72-81.
68. Wallaert B. and Voisin C. *In vitro* study of gas effects on alveolar macrophages. Cell Biology and Toxicology 1992;8:151-156.
69. Harris C.C., Hsu I.C., Stoner G.D., Trump B.F. and Selkirk J.K. Human pulmonary alveolar macrophages metabolise benzo(a)pyrene to proximate and ultimate mutagens. Nature 1978;272:633-634.
70. McLemore T.L., Martin R.R., Wray N.P., Cantrell E.T. and Busbee D.L. Dissociation between aryl hydrocarbon hydroxylase activity in cultured pulmonary macrophages and blood lymphocytes from lung cancer patients. Cancer Research 1978;38:3805-3811.
71. Petrilli F.L., Rossi G.A., Camoirano A., Romano M., Serra D., Bennicelli C., De Flora A. and De Flora S. Metabolic reduction of chromium by alveolar macrophages and its relation to cigarette smoke. Journal of Clinical Investigation 1986;77:1917-1924.
72. Bond J.A. Metabolism of xenobiotics by the respiratory tract. In: Toxicology of the lung, 2nd Ed. (Gardner D.E., Crapo J.D. and McClellan R.O., eds.) Raven Press, New York, 1993:187-215.
73. Gazdar A.F., Linnoila R.I., Kurita Y., Oie H.K., Mulshine J.L., Clark J.C. and Whitsett J.A. Peripheral airway cell differentiation in human lung cancer cell lines. Cancer Research 1990;50:5481-5487.
74. Dobbs L.G. Isolation and culture of alveolar type II cells. American Journal of Physiology 1990;258:L134-L147.
75. Massey T.E. Isolation and use of lung cells in toxicology. In: *In vitro* toxicology: model systems and methods (McQueen C.A., ed.) Telford Press, Caldwell, 1989; 35-66.
76. Robinson P.C., Voelker D.R. and Mason R.J. Isolation and culture of human alveolar type II epithelial cells. Characterization of their phospholipid secretion. American Review of Respiratory Disease. 1984;130:1156-1160.

77. Kang Y.J., Clapper J.A. and Enger M.D. Enhanced cadmium cytotoxicity in A549 cells with reduced glutathione levels is due to neither enhanced cadmium accumulation nor reduced metallothionein synthesis. Cell Biology and Toxicology 1989;5:249-259.
78. Kang Y.J., Liu M.S. and Enger M.D. Diamide reduces cadmium accumulation by human lung carcinoma A549 cells. Toxicology 1990;62:53-58.
79. Kang Y.J., Nuutero S.T., Clapper J.A., Jenkins P. and Enger M.D. Cellular cadmium responses in subpopulations T20 and T27 of human lung carcinoma A549 cells. Toxicology 1990;61:195-203.
80. Keller D.A. and Menzel D.B. Effects of sulfite on glutathione S-sulfonate and the glutathione status of lung cells. Chemico-Biological Interactions 1989;70:145-156.
81. Kozumbo W.J. and Agarwal S. Induction of DNA damage in cultured human lung cells by tobacco smoke arylamines exposed to ambient levels of ozone. American Journal of Respiratory Cell and Molecular Biology. 1990;3:611-618.
82. McLemore T.L., Adelberg S., Czerwinski M., Hubbard W.C., Yu S.J., Storeng R., Wood T.G., Hines R.N. and Boyd M.R. Altered regulation of the cytochrome P4501A1 gene: novel inducer-independent gene expression in pulmonary carcinoma cell lines. Journal of the National Cancer Institute 1989;81:1787-1794.
83. Ballard P.L., Liley H.G., Gonzales L.W., Odom M.W., Ammann A.J., Benson B., White R.T. and Williams M.C. Interferon- gamma and synthesis of surfactant components by cultured human fetal lung. American Journal of Respiratory Cell and Molecular Biology 1990;2:137-143.
84. Lewis C.P.L. and Nemery B. Physiopathology and biochemical mechanisms of paraquat toxicity. In: Human toxicology of paraquat (Bismuth C. and Hall A.H., eds) M. Dekker, New York, 1993 (in press).
85. Hoet P.H.M., Dinsdale D., Lewis C.P.L., Verbeken E.K., Lauweryns J.M. and Nemery B. Active uptake of putrescine by human lung tissue. Kinetic parameters and cellular localisation. Thorax 1993 (submitted for publication).
86. Hoet P.H.M., Lewis C.P.L. and Nemery B. The uptake of putrescine in isolated human pulmonary type II cells (abstract). European Respiratory Journal 1992;5:70s.
87. Carley W.W., Niedbala M.J. and Gerritsen M.E. Isolation, cultivation, and partial characterization of microvascular endothelium derived from human lung. American Journal of Respiratory Cell and Molecular Biology 1992;7:620-630.
88. Atzori L., Dypbukt J.M., Sundqvist K., Cotgreave I., Edman C.C., Moldéus P. and Grafström R.C. Growth-associated modifications of low-molecular-weight thiols and protein sulfhydryls in human bronchial fibroblasts. Journal of Cellular Physiology 1990;143:165-171.
89. Akamine A., Raghu G. and Narayanan A.S. Human lung fibroblast subpopulations with different C1q binding and functional properties. American Journal of Respiratory Cell and Molecular Biology 1992;6:382-389.
90. David G., Lories V., Heremans A., Van Der Schueren B., Cassiman J.J. and Van Den Berghe H. Membrane-associated chondroitin sulfate proteoglycans of human lung fibroblasts. Journal of Cellular Biology 1989;108:1165-1173.

91. Mayer D. and Branscheid D. Exposure of human lung fibroblasts to ozone: cell mortality and hyaluronan metabolism. Journal of Toxicology and Environmental Health 1992;35:235-246.
92. Nicod L.P., Lipscomb M.F., Weissler J.C., Lyons C.R., Albertson J. and Toews G.B. Mononuclear cells in human lung parenchyma. American Review of Respiratory Disease 1987;136:818-823.
93. Hirst S.J., Barnes P.J. and Twort C.H. Quantifying proliferation of cultured human and rabbit airway smooth muscle cells in response to serum and platelet-derived growth factor. American Journal of Respiratory Cell and Molecular Biology 1992;7:574-581.
94. Mattoli S., Soloperto M., Mezzetti M. and Fasoli A. Mechanisms of calcium mobilization and phosphoinositide hydrolysis in human bronchial smooth muscle cells by endothelin 1. American Journal of Respiratory Cell and Molecular Biology 1991;5:424-430.
95. Idell S., Zwieb C., Kumar A., Koenig K.B. and Johnson A.R. Pathways of fibrin turnover of human pleural mesothelial cells *in vitro*. American Journal of Respiratory Cell and Molecular Biology 1992;7:414-426.
96. Jaurand M.C., Buard A., Zeng L., Laurent P., Fleury J. and Kheuang L. The mesothelial cell *in vitro:* contribution to the study of mesothelioma. European Respiratory Review 1993;3:126-131.
97. Leikauf G. and Driscoll K. Cellular approaches in respiratory tract toxicology. In: Toxicology of the lung, 2nd Ed. (Gardner D.E., Crapo J.D. and McClellan R.O., eds.) Raven Press, New York, 1993:335-370.

15

Research and testing in pharmaco-toxicology with human intestinal cells

F. Zucco* and A. Stammati**

* Istituto di Tecnologie Biomediche, C.N.R., Via G.B. Morgagni 30/E, 00161 Roma (Italy).
** Istituto Superiore di Sanità, Lab. Tossicologia Comparata ed Ecotossicologia, Viale Regina Elena 299, 00161 Roma (Italy).

Introduction

Over the last two decades a rapid evolution of *in vitro* pharmaco-toxicology has been recorded. At the same time cellular models of the gastrointestinal tract have been set up and carefully analyzed, so that very specialized functions can be studied *in vitro* thanks to technological progress and our increased knowledge in the field of biology.
Nonetheless, intestinal cells are not yet widely used in pharmaco-toxicological research, except in antitumoral drug studies and testing. Most of the intestinal cellular models of human origin are indeed tumoral established cell lines which have been characterized, only recently, for specific intestinal structures and/or functions [1]. Studies with freshly isolated cells are quite rare, probably due to the difficulties encountered in preparations and maintainance of pure functional epithelial cells from intestine in culture. This review deals with human intestinal cell lines mainly derived from colorectal tumors. For some of these, detailed data are available concerning their degree of differentiation and their ability to perform specific functions in relation to their polarization, such as the transport and secretion of various molecules.

Intestinal cell lines and their characteristics.

The human intestinal cell lines mostly utilized in the field of pharmaco-toxicology are listed in Table I.

Caco-2 :	derived from a human colon adenocarcinoma, moderately differentiated; hypertetraploid; specific subclones exist.
HT 29 :	derived from a human colon adenocarcinoma, moderately differentiated: hypertriploid; specific subclones exist.
T84 :	derived from a lung metastasis of a human colon carcinoma; poorly differentiated but polarizing.
HCT 8 :	derived from an ileocoecal human carcinoma; partially differentiating; pseudodiploid.
HRT 18 :	derived from a human rectal adenocarcinoma; partially differentiating; pseudodiploid.
INT 407 :	derived from a human embryo; aneuploid; tumorigenic; HeLa markers.
LoVo :	derived from supraclavicular metastasis of a colon carcinoma; hyperdiploid; high malignancy features.
WiDr :	derived from a human colon adenocarcinoma: high malignancy features; hypertriploid.

Table I :
Intestinal cells in pharmaco-toxicological research

a) The Caco-2 cell line was established by Fogh [2] from a human colon carcinoma. In culture it is able to differentiate for both, the morphological aspect and the functional pattern [3-6]. The Caco-2 cell line is to date the only cell line able to differentiate spontaneously in culture [7,8]. After the 7th day of culture, the cells in the confluent monolayer stop dividing and 'domes' appear, indicating a polarization of the cells arranged in a barrier which performs a transepithelial ionic transport [3] (Fig. 1). This has been confirmed by transmission and scanning electron microscopy. The cells have been shown to be asymmetric, with tight junctions and microvilli on the upper side. Several enzymatic activities, typical of the small intestine brush border, have been measured during the in vitro differentiation: alkaline phosphatase, sucrase-isomaltase, aminopeptidase N and lactase. Their levels increase after 9 days, reaching quite high levels after 19-21 days, towards the end of the culture. These

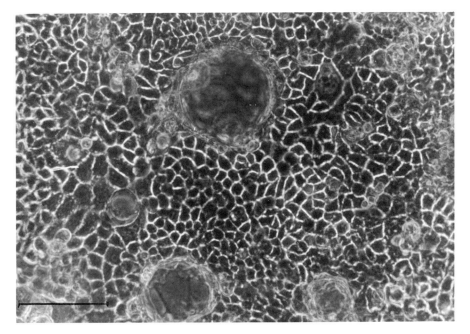

Figure 1 :
"Domes" in Caco-2 cell monolayer at the 19th day of culture.
⊢⎯⎯⎯⊣ = 100 μm

values are close to those observed in the normal small intestine. Glycosoaminoglycan synthesis and structure also undergo changes during the differentiation process. Heparan sulfate and chondroitin sulfate increase in chain length and sulfation [5,6]. The protein kinase C has a modulating effect on the latter, which is gradually lost when the cells become differentiated. This enzyme and its role as regulator of various cellular events has been also investigated by Rydell et al.[9]. The Caco-2 cell line has the (Vitamin A) retinol-binding protein II and the related enzymatic activities [10]. Vitamin A is usually required in normal intestinal absorption: the data concerning its binding and esterification in Caco-2 are only slightly lower than in vivo. The undifferentiated/differentiated Caco-2 cells may offer a model to study not only the properties and differentiation of the intestinal epithelial cells, but may also mimic closely the in vivo situation: immature crypt cells actively divide and contribute in this way to the renewal of the intestinal epithelium. Once the differentiation process starts the cells migrate along the villi, reaching the highest degree of differentiation at their tip.

Clones of Caco-2 have been recently isolated, displaying a high taurocholic acid transport [11]; other clones with more or less sucrase-isomaltase expression have been isolated by Beaulieu and Quaroni [12].

Despite their origin, being the adult human colon, the differentiated cells express some characteristics, such as electrical parameters, ion conductance and permeability, which are very similar to those of colonic crypt cells [13,14] and also typical features of normal small intestinal villus (membrane hydrolases) which are present only for a short period in the human foetal colon [15].

b) The HT29 cell line derives from a human colon adenocarcinoma [16]. Of particular interest is its ability to differentiate and polarize under different experimental conditions, i.e. replacement of glucose by galactose in Dulbecco's Modified Eagle Medium (DMEM) [17], removal of all sugars [18], replacement of DMEM by Roswel Park Memorial Institute medium (RPMI) [19,20], and treatment with appropiate salt solutions [21]. The main difference between Caco-2 and HT29 is that the latter cell line does not spontaneously differentiate in culture. Moreover, even when induced to differentiate in inosine-supplemented glucose-free medium, the cells do not display any lactase activity [7], while the other brush border enzymes are present but at much lower levels than in the normal small intestine [17,18]. Finally, they are only partially polarized, never form 'domes' and require a longer time to undergo *in vitro* differentiation (30 days). Only at a later stage clones were isolated, showing full polarization and 'dome' formation with chloride secretion [22]. Moreover, Huet *et al.* [23] were able to isolate from the HT29-18 clone two subclones characterized by 'absorptive cells' (HT29-18-Cl), with a well organized brush border, and 'cells containing mucous granules' (HT29-18-N2). Both of the subclones are able to keep most of their differentiated properties even in a glucose-containing medium.

HT29 cells have a high rate of glucose consumption and a low glycogen storage while for Caco-2 cells the situation is reversed. A possible relation between the glucose metabolism and the modulation of differentiation versus dedifferentiation is currently explored and HT29 cells represent a good model for this type of approach [22].

c) The T84 cell line is derived from a human colon carcinoma transplantable in Balb/c nude mice and originally derived from a lung metastasis of a patient with colonic carcinoma. When confluent, these cells are able to polarize and express microvilli on the apical membrane, tight junctions and desmosomes between adjacent cells, being thus morphologically very similar to intestinal cells *in vivo*. The presence of hormone and neurotransmitter receptors has also been demonstrated, together with the capacity of transepithelial electrolyte transport [24,25].

d) HCT-8 and HRT-18 cells are derived from an ileocoecal and rectal human adenocarcinoma, respectively, and are able to form microvilli and tight junctions [26]. They have been mainly used for studies and preparations of carcino-embryonic antigens (CEA), for diagnostic purposes and immunological studies.

e) The intestine 407 cell line is derived from the jejunum and ileum of a human embryo and has an epithelial-like morphology [27]. It has been shown to be sensitive to a broad spectrum of viruses, although not as sensitive as HeLa cells.

f) LoVo cells have been established from a human adenocarcinoma. They are cuboidal and columnar in morphology with desmosomes between cells, large terminal bars (tight junctions) and numerous microvilli at the free border of cells lining the lumen of the acinar organization they undergo in culture. Like other intestinal cells, they are able to produce CEA [28].

Biotransforming capabilities.

An extensive characterization of intestinal cell lines regarding their biotransformation capabilities is of fundamental importance if one wants to know the extent to which these experimental models can metabolize toxic compounds.

Until some years ago most efforts were devoted to the characterization of liver cells, which are derived from the liver playing the leading role in the biotransformation of xenobiotics. Only recently has the attention of researchers shifted to cells derived from organs other than the liver, mainly to the skin and the intestine. Regarding the latter, quite a good description of the *in vivo* situation is available in the literature [29,30], but very little has to date been done *in vitro*. Furthermore, the majority of the existing studies have been performed on Caco-2 cells, either for phase I or Phase II metabolism.

A number of cytochrome P450-dependent reactions have been recorded in microsomal preparations of Caco-2 cells, cultured between 7 and 35 days, by using specific substrates of different cytochrome P450 iso-enzymes (P450IA1, P450IA2, P450IIA and P450IIIA): 7-ethoxyresorufin (EROD), phenacetin, coumarin and nifedipine, respectively. EROD activity could be detected from the 7th day of culture on and its basal activity increased till the 20th day, after which it decreased until the

35th day of culture. The EROD activity had the same behaviour as both differentiation markers, alkaline phosphatase and sucrase-isomaltase, whose maximum activity was detected on the 20th day of culture. Moreover, the EROD activity was inhibited by α-naphthoflavone (specific inhibitor of cytochrome P450IA1) and induced by 3-methylcholanthrene, β-naphtoflavone and dioxin (inducers of cytochrome P450IA1), thus demonstrating that it is related to the cytochrome P450IA1 isoenzyme. The other activities tested, phenacetin-O-deethylation, nifedipine oxydation and coumarin 7-hydroxylation were very low or situated under the detection limit [31].

The presence of cytochrome P450 activity has also been demonstrated in Caco-2 cells by Peters and Roelofs [32]. It was estimated to be 1.52 units/mg protein, which is more or less the same as the value found in SW1116, another human colon carcinoma cell line (2.08 units/mg protein). Two isoenzymes of cytochrome P450 (P450IA1 or A2 and P450IIE1) were also found in the human colon cell line 65 174T [33]. The cytochrome P450IA1 or A2 activity increased after induction with benzanthracene.

While investigating the possible correlation between glutathione S-transferase (GST) activity and drug resistance Peters and Roelofs [34] have examined Caco-2 cells for the presence of enzymes involved in phase II metabolism, e.g. GST. Only placental GST is present in freshly seeded cells and in cells until 8 days after confluency, remaining practically stable until the 32nd day of culture. However, at the 8th day after confluency, the GST-alpha class (intestinal) starts to be expressed. At the same time microvilli are developed and increases continue till the 32nd day after confluency. The authors could not detect GST's of the alpha class either in normal human colon specimens or in colon carcinomas, whereas large amounts of alpha class have been found in normal mucosa, from the human small intestine. This demonstrates, in accordance with morphologic features, that Caco-2 cells, even if derived from human colon, express characteristics of small-intestine epithelial cells. Placental GST's were found in small amounts, while the GST alpha class was not detected in the SW1116 adenocarcinoma cell line [32]. Both intestinal cell lines were investigated for the presence of glutathione (GSH) content and detoxifying enzymes, such as selenium-dependent and -independent GSH peroxidase and UDP-glucuronyl transferase [32]. UDP-glucuronyl transferase was also detected in Caco-2 cells by Bjorge et al. [35] using p-nitrophenol as substrate with a radioactive flow detection (RFD) liquid chromatography methods. In the same cells no activity could be detected at 7, 14 and 21 days of culture, using three different methods: colorimetric, radiochemical (p-nitrophenol as substrate) and spectrofluorimetric (1-naphtol as substrate) assays were performed by Baranczyk-Kuzma *et al.* [36]. On the other hand, the same authors were able to detect phenol sulphotransferase in Caco-2 cells using p-nitrophenol and dopamine as substrates. The enzyme activity was much higher for dopamine than for paranitrophenol and, for both substrates, its specific activity increased with cell age.

Transport and uptake of nutrients.

All the cell lines previously mentioned are able to form an epithelial-like barrier when cultured on filters to confluency. This is due to the presence of tight junctions between the cells.
This culture system favours the cell polarization and the subsequent layer organization and allows more precise transport studies of both, the apical (corresponding to the intestinal lumen) and the basolateral (connected with blood vessels) exposure sites of the cells (Fig. 2).
However, in setting up this system, several aspects must be taken into account [37], such as the seeding density of the cells, the different

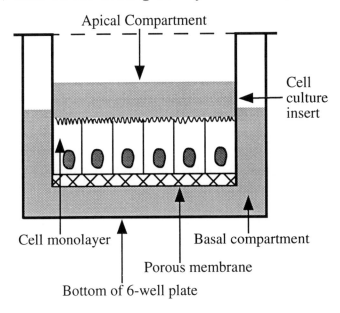

Figure 2 :
Reproduction of the transwell filter culture system

requirements for media components and extracellular matrix according to the cell type used and the properties of the microporous membrane. The permeable support may indeed influence the transport across the layer. Nicklin and coworkers [38] have shown that, when Caco-2 cells are cultured on nitrocellulose filters, the transport of taurocholic acid is higher than when the cells are grown on aluminium oxide filters. These filters are translucent and permit the microscopic inspection of the cells, which also display a higher transepithelial electrical resistance (TER) and form characteristic 'domes'. It is suggested that the different inserts may favour the growth of different cellular subpopulations. It is also known that the size and distribution of pores on the membrane may influence the formation of the cellular barrier and therefore the transport mechanisms [39].

Attention should be given to the aqueous boundary layer present on the apical side of the cells, which may affect the permeability of lipophylic compounds. The layer is formed in the microenvironment, determined by the extruding components of the glycocalyx and other macromolecules they entrap. The thickness and the influence of this layer on drug absorption have been recently characterized in Caco-2 cells by Hidalgo and coworkers [40] and Karlsson and Artursson [41]. The Caco-2 cells are the experimental model mostly used in transport studies. Grown on a collagen-coated polycarbonate membrane they represent a 'valuable transport model system for the small intestinal epithelium' [42]. The system has also been used to study nutrient transport and accumulation in Caco-2 cells. The Vitamin B12 [43] and Vitamin D-regulated calcium transcellular transports [44] have been elucidated in Caco-2 cells cultured on filters. Moreover, the expression of 25-hydroxyvitamin D3-24-hydroxylase, the first enzyme in Vitamin D catabolism, was induced on exposure [45] to actinomycin D, α-amanitin and cycloheximide, suggesting that mRNA and protein synthesis are required.

A large neutral aminoacid (phenylalanine) is transported by a carrier-mediated system from the apical to the basolateral side and requires Na^+-ions. The mechanism seems to be shared by large neutral and cationic aminoacids, and exhibits stereospecificity towards L-stereoisomers [46,47]. Moreover, the basolateral efflux is the rate-limiting step in the transcellular transport of phenylalanine. It has also been shown that bile acid transport is carrier-mediated and follows the apical to basolateral route [48,49].

Other examples consist of the iron absorption [50] and the folic acid uptake by Caco-2 cells cultured as monolayers on plastic [51].

Toxicological studies

Only recently, intestinal cells have been considered as models in toxicological investigations. A number of compounds have been tested using this model (Table II). Besides the measurement of basic cell functions end-points were often related to the specific potentialities of the cells in culture.
- Since the intestine is the main site of absorption of zinc and copper, both differentiated and undifferentiated Caco-2 cells have been used to investigate their effects. The interferences with protein synthesis at toxic and non toxic concentrations have been studied and inhibition of protein synthesis was especially pronounced in undifferentiated cells [52]. The induction of metallothionein (MT) has been followed [53], as this protein is involved in the regulation of the homeostasis of heavy metals. It was found that MT synthesis increased slightly from 6 to 18 h after copper addition, while, during zinc exposure, it was already detectable after 6h and it increased till 18h. Protein synthesis was inhibited in a similar manner for both heavy metals.
- Other studies involving a variety of substances have been performed using Caco-2 cells. A typical example also consists of the effect of furazolidone. It is a chemical belonging to the nitrofuran family. It was found to seriously affect the proliferating Caco-2 cells, while differentiated cells appeared to be more resistant [54].
- The effect of orellanine (3,3',4,4'-tetrahydroxy-2,2'-dipyridyl-1,1'dioxide), a fungal toxin of *Cortinarius Orellanus* and *C. orellanoides*, has also been investigated in Caco-2 cells by measuring the changes in alkaline phosphatase (AP) activity, an enzyme present in the brush border of differentiated cells [55]. Specific inhibition of alkaline phosphatase was also observed in the renal epithelial cell line, LLC-PK1. *In vitro* kinetic investigations have shown that intestinal AP is competitively inhibited by orellanine, which on the contrary acts as a noncompetitive inhibitor for renal AP.
- As far as toxicological studies on T84 cells are concerned, the effect of Toxin A, derived from *Clostridium difficile*, has been followed in order to detect which cell types were the toxicological targets [56]. This intestinal epithelial T84 cell line was chosen as *in vitro* model for its well characterized permeability capacities. *In vivo*, it was already clearly shown that Toxin A could provoke severe injury associated with haemorrhages and fluid secretion when it was injected into rabbit ileal loops. When T84 cells were exposed *in vitro*, dramatic changes in

CELLS	CHEMICALS	PARAMETERS OBSERVED	REFERENCES
Caco-2	$ZnSO_4$ $CuSO_4$	MT synthesis	Scarino et al. 1991
"	$ZnSO_4$ $CuSO_4$	MT induction; protein synthesis	Scarino et al. 1992
"	Furazolidone	Cell survival and proliferation; alkaline phosphatase; O_2 consumption	Vincentini et al. 1993
"	Orellanine	Alkaline phosphatase	Ruedl et al. 1989
I-407	Asbestos samples	Cell survival (colony-forming ability)	Reiss et al. 1980
"	Chrysotile Amosite	Cell suvival (colony-forming ability)	Reiss et al. 1980
"	Beverages (dried preparations)	Cell survival	Itagaki et al. 1992
T_{84}	Toxin A (Clostridium difficile)	Flux alteration; transephitelial resistance; LDH and ^{51}Cr release; morphology	Hecht et al. 1988
"	Quercetin, Koempferol Myricetin	Effect on secretion; cell. protein phosphorilation; cAMP	Nguyen et al. 1991
HT 29	1-methyl-2-nitrosoimidazole (INO)	Cell survival colony-forming ability); GSH determination	Mulcahy et al. 1989
HCT-8	Non-steroidal anti-inflammatory drugs	Mitochondrial function (MTT); Viability (neutral red)	Allen et al. 1991
Colonocytes (primary cultures)	Deoxycholic, oleic, palmitic and linoleic acids	Cell growth	Bruset et al. 1990

Table II :

Chemicals tested and parameters used in toxicological investigations in intestinal human cell lines.

transepithelial resistance were recorded. These were related to a change in tight junction permeability, but not to cell death, membrane damage or morphological alterations.

- In another study T84 cells were treated with three flavonols widely present in plants: koempferol, quercetin and myricetin which are mono, di-, and trihydroxylated, respectively, on the phenyl ring, [57]. Quercetin was the most active in inducing the secretion by the T84 cells, followed by koempferol, while myricetin did not exert any activity. Quercetin-induced secretion was not mediated by reactive oxygen species generated through auto-oxidation and/or redox cycling. Moreover, a slight increase in cAMP and phosphorylation of endogenous protein substrates for cAMP-dependent protein kinase was observed in cells treated with quercetin. For this reason it seems to behave as other secretagogues known to stimulate T84 cells via cAMP.

- The toxic potential of eight non-steroidal anti-inflammatory drugs (NSAID), covering the major chemical groups, was investigated using the HTC-8 intestinal epithelial cell line [58]. As NSAID are supposed to cause ATP reduction in isolated gastric mucosa, a marker of the mitochondrial function was examined. A modification of the MTT assay was used. The effect on cell viability was also recorded by measuring the uptake of the vital dye neutral red (NR) into lysosomes of viable cells. Between both assays, MTT was shown to be the most sensitive, while NR discriminated better between the various NSAID. Some similarities could be found in ranking of the compounds when rat *in vivo* data were compared to the available human *in vitro* data in HTC-8 cells. The results further showed that a rather good prediction of the *in vivo* ulcerogenic and haemorrhagic potential in the rat may be expected, better than the prediction of injuries occurring in man during chronic exposure.

- Other interesting studies have been published. The biological effect of 1-methyl-2-nitrosoimidazole (INO), the reduction product of 1-methyl-2-nitroimidazole, has been investigated in the HT29 cell line [59]. INO was highly toxic for these cells both under aerobic and anaerobic conditions. The amount of damage was related to the cell number: the higher the cell concentration, the lower the damage. GSH content was also measured and an initial dose-dependent depletion was observed, followed by a plateau phase when GSH content of INO-treated cells reached approximately 8% of the control levels. HT29 cells pretreated with buthionine sulfoximine (BSO), an inhibitor of GSH synthesis, were more sensitive to INO exposure. On the basis of these results the authors suggested that the nitroso-reduction product of 2-nitroimidazoles might be responsible for the cytotoxicity observed and the GSH depletion associated with hypoxic exposure to these compounds

In another study by Reiss et al.[60], the inhibition of the colony-forming ability of human embryonic intestine-derived epithelial (I-407) cells was utilized to assay the toxic potential of six coded samples, consisting of particulates, including three samples of particulates from drinking water of different regions. In a previous study, the same authors [61] tested amosite, crocidolite and chrysotile in the same cells and in cells derived from rat liver (ARL-6) and mouse colon (MCE-1) They found that the intestinal I-407 cells were the most sensitive ones. This simple test was thus useful for the screening of particulates from drinking water and was also sensitive enough to discriminate between samples of similar densities. Moreover, the toxicity observed correlated well with the asbestos content of the samples tested.

- The effect on the survival of I-407 cells of dried preparations of nine beverages has been studied by Itagaki et al.[62]. Instant coffee and green tea were found to be the most toxic. Since the mutagenicity of instant coffee seemed to be related to oxygen-dependent generation of hydrogen peroxide in coffee solution, the cytotoxicity mechanism was studied in more detail by examining the effect of several enzymes. Peroxidase completely inhibited the toxic effect by instant coffee on intestinal cells, while this was only partially true in the presence of catalase. On the contrary, superoxide dismutase, which increased the amount of hydrogen peroxide in coffee solutions, enhanced its toxicity. These results suggest that instant coffee probably exerts both its toxic and mutagenic effects by a common action mechanism.

- Finally, the modulatory action of $CaCl_2$ on the toxicity exerted by endogenous compounds such as deoxycholic, oleic, palmitic and linolenic acids on primary monolayer cultures of normal colonocytes derived from adult subjects has been studied by Buset et al.[63]. In this study the hypothesis is made that free calcium blocks the toxic effects of free fatty acids and bile acids on cell growth. Using the quantitative assay of H^3 thymidine incorporation on colonocytes, ionized calcium has been shown to have a protective effect against the lytic action of bile and fatty acids..

Pharmacological studies

Antitumoral drugs

Colorectal tumors are very common in human adults and are particularly resistant to various therapies, even to combined treatments, shown to have an improved effectiveness. This observation probably has encouraged the investigation of the cytotoxic effects of antitumoral drugs on intestinal human colon adenocarcinoma cell lines and of related resistance mechanisms. In recent years many papers have been published. As it is impossible to describe in detail all the cellular models and the related antitumoral drug studies, only a few examples will be reported here in order to show some of the more recent approaches.
- Adriamycin is a widely used antitumoral drug which is practically ineffective against intestinal cancer. Different mechanisms may be involved, such as protection from the quinone moiety of the drug during redox cycling by GSH, a free radical scavenger. Lai et al. [64] have shown that the tripeptide and glutathione dependent enzymes are responsible for the detoxification of adriamycin in at least one human colon cancer cell line. The same conclusion was reached by Peters and Roelofs [32], who correlated the Caco-2 resistance to metoxantrone and adriamycin with the high levels of glutathione S-transferases present in those cells.
Lai and coworkers [64,65] have shown the involvement of the P-glycoprotein (P-gp) expression in the resistance to adriamycin in some human colon carcinoma cell lines by using competitive inhibitors of P-gp.
P-gp is the product of the multidrug resistance gene mdr 1. It is involved as a pumping component controlling the energy-dependent drug efflux. Tetracycline resistance due to energy-dependent extrusion mechanisms has also been shown by Grandi and Giuliani [66] in LoVo cells. The resistance was partially reversible following verapamil exposure, a Ca^{2+}-channel blocker. A correlation between the presence of P-gp and the intrinsic resistance of various wild-type colon cancer cells has been suggested by Spoelstra et al. [67]. It was based on the effects of verapamil and other resistance modifiers on daunorubicin toxicity.
- Since antitumoral drugs are obviously used to prevent cellular replication, the mechanism of their interaction with DNA and the enzymes involved has been widely investigated. DNA damage by 1-methyl-2-nitrosoimidazole, a reductive metabolite of 1-methyl-2-nitro-imidazole was studied in HT29 cells by Gipp et al. [68]. A concentration

dependent induction was found supporting the hypothesis of the existence of a nitroso intermediate, responsible for the cytotoxic effect. However, in some cases a poor correlation between drug retention, DNA damage and cytotoxicity was oberved, suggesting that various mechanisms might be involved.

- This was also the case for LoVo cells treated with doxorubicin and daunorubicin derivatives. Different toxic effects were recorded which were not related to the DNA-single strand break production [69]. On HTC cells activities of DNA cross-link repair might account for the resistance observed to chlorozotocin [70].

- Etoposide and teniposide are anticancer drugs which are able to stabilize the transient covalent intermediate formed by topoisomerase II and the DNA. Long and coworkers [71] have tried to identify the possible mechanism of resistance in HTC cells. A subclone showing no difference in mdr-1 gene, mdr-1 mRNA or P-gp protein but with low levels of topoisomerase II mRNA was 6-9 fold more resistant to the drug than the parental cell line. However, another clone displayed an even higher resistance. By comparing the results with those obtained in human lung carcinoma cells, the authors conclude that low resistance is mainly related to one specific mechanism, namely the action on topoisomerase, while high resistance probably implies the action of more than one mechanism.

- Another mechanism widely studied in human colon tumoral cells is the well-known 'Thymineless-death'. When anticancer agents, such as 5-fluorouracil or 5-fluorodeoxyuridine (FdUra), are given to cells the common metabolite FdUra-monophosphate (FdUMP) strongly inhibits thymidylate synthase in the presence of the folate cofactor thus inhibiting DNA synthesis. DNA fragmentation has been associated with the toxicity observed. In HT29 cells, the formation of a high molecular weight DNA fragment has been demonstrated [72]. Since the fragmentation sites were not randomly distributed (when compared to those produced in other cells), it seemed that the event leading from thymidine starvation to the final lethal effect, was related to the cell type. Concomitant exposure to folinic acid was able to enhance the toxicity on WiDr cells [73], confirming the role of the cofactor in ternary complex formation with thymidylate synthase and FdUMP. Resistance to FUra may be shown by cells able to perform thymidine salvage. Indeed, by using a thymidine kinase deficient human colon carcinoma cell line, which is not able to use the thymidine salvage pathway, Radparvar *et al.* [74] have shown that

FUra is highly toxic to the cells exposed.
Resistance to 5-FUra may be also achieved in clones of human colon cancer cell lines selected for overexpression of thymidylate synthase [75].

Drug transport.

- The elucidation of specific transport mechanisms may help in designing new drugs which may cross the intestinal barrier more efficiently without loosing their therapeutic properties. The Caco-2 cell line has been widely explored as a possible model of intestinal epithelium when cultured at confluency on permeable filters [39,42,76].
Artursson [77] has studied the passive diffusion of six beta-blocking agents with a 2000-fold lipophilicity range in the same model. The permeability coefficients of these homologous series have been determined and compared with *in vivo* data reported in the literature. The more lipophilic drugs were transported more rapidly than the less lipophilic ones, with only one exception, probably related to the bulky chemical structure of the compound. Lipophilic drugs pass the intestinal barrier by the transcellular route, being able to cross the cell membrane. The junctional complex is a dynamic structure which may modulate permeability following microenvironmental variations. By using the same beta-adrenergic antagonists [77] the contribution of the paracellular route to the transport of the less lypophilic drugs following variations in extracellular calcium concentration was studied in Caco-2 cells [78]. In a further study on 20 drugs and peptides, a correlation between oral drug absorption in man and permeability coefficients has been demonstrated [79]. Thus, the Caco-2 cell line appears to be a good model for screening drugs to evaluate their *in vivo* absorption.
- Traber and coworkers [80,81] measured the uptake of d-alpha-tocopheryl-polyethylene glycol 1000 succinate in Caco-2 cells cultured on filters. The compound is a water miscible form of Vitamin E, used as a therapeutic agent in children with cholestatic liver disease. They have shown that the presence of bile and amphipathic lipids facilitated micelle formation and uptake by the cells.
- Another interesting example is given by L-α-methyldopa, an antihypertensive drug with a poor systemic bioavailability. As it is known that the drug is not processed at the level of the intestinal lumen and is transported by the carrier of the large neutral aminoacids. Hu and Brochardt [82] investigated the possibility of a poor membrane permeability by using the Caco-2 cell line. The transport system was shown to be

energy-dependent and was found to be slower than the one observed for aminoacids (caused probably by a lower affinity of α-methyldopa). Moreover, the transport was markedly increased by prolonging the postfeeding time, indicating a competition for the carrier between the drug and the large neutral aminoacids.

- In the same cell line different transport systems for different antimicrobial agents have been demonstrated recently by Ranaldi and coworkers [83]. A canine renal epithelial cell line (MDCK) was also used to assess the specificity of the drug transport. The drugs involved had different physicochemical and pharmacokinetic characteristics. By this approach, the *in vitro* model was shown to be predictive of the oral bioavailability, being in agreement with *in vivo* absorption characteristics. Of the drugs examined, two were shown not to be transported across the cell layer, three were passively transported, two probably used the paracellular route, and trimetoprin and D-cycloserine were specifically and actively transported only by the Caco-2 cells.

- An active transport mechanism by a dipeptide carrier has been shown to be involved in the uptake of cephalosporin and cephalexin in Caco-2 cells [84]. The transport mechanism is energy- and proton-dependent and is competitively inhibited by dipeptides. The carrier exhibited stereospecificity and closely resembled the intestinal transporter. This cell line may therefore also be considered as a good model to study active transport mechanisms.

The rectal administration of drugs is also an effective therapeutic route, but no *in vitro* studies are currently available on this topic; only one human rectal carcinoma cell line, namely HRT-18, has been established and is able to partially differentiate. It may be a useful tool for further explorations in this field.

References

1. Rutzky L.P. The biology of human colon tumor cells in culture. Advances in Cell Culture 1985;4:47-83.
2. Fogh J., Wright W.C. and Loveless J.D. Absence of HeLa cell contamination in 169 cell lines derived from human tumors. Journal of the National Cancer Institute 1977;21:393-408.
3. Pinto M., Robine-Leon S., Appay M.-D., Kedinger M., Triadou N., Dussaulx E., Lacroix B., Simon-Assman P., Haffen K., Fogh J. and Zweibaum A. Enterocyte-like differentiation and polarization of the human colon carcinoma cell line Caco-2 in culture. Biology of the Cell 1983;47:323-330.

4. Matsumoto H., Erickson R.H., Gum J.R., Yoshioka M., Gum E. and Kim Y.S. Biosynthesis of alkaline phosphatase during differentiation of the human colon cancer cell line Caco-2. Gastroenterology 1990;98:1199-1207.
5. Levy P., Cherqui G., Robert A., Wicek D. and Picard J. Changes in glycosoaminoglycan sulfation and protein kinase C subcellular distribution during differentiation of the human colon tumor cell line Caco-2. Experientia 1989;45:588-591.
6. Levy P., Robert A. and Picard J. Biosynthesis of glycosoaminoglycans in the human colonic tumor cell line Caco-2: structural changes occurring with the morphological differentiation of the cells. Biology of the Cell 1988;62:255-264.
7. Chantret I., Barbat A., Dussaulx E., Brattain M.G. and Zweibaum A. Epithelial polarity, villin expression, and enterocytic differentiation of cultured human colon carcinoma cells: a survey of twenty cell lines. Cancer Research 1988;48:1936-1942.
8. Rousset M. The human colon carcinoma cell lines HT29 and Caco-2: two *in vitro* models for the study of intestinal differentiation. Biochimie 1986;68:1035-1040.
9. Rydell E., Magnusson K.-E., Sjo A. and Axelsson K. Protein kinase C and casein kinase II activities in two human colon carcinoma cell lines, HT29 and Caco-2: possible correlation with differentiation. Bioscience Reports 1990;10:293-299.
10. Quick T.C. and Ong D.E. Vitamin A metabolism in the human intestinal Caco-2 cell line. Biochemistry 1990;29:11116-11123
11. Woodcock S., Williamson I., Hassan I. and Mackay M. Isolation and characterisation of clones from the Caco-2 cell line displaying increased taurocholic acid transport. Journal of Cell Science 1991;98:323-332.
12. Beaulieu J.-F. and Quaroni A. Clonal analysis of sucrase-isomaltase expression in the human colon adenocarcinoma Caco-2 cells. Biochemical Journal 1991;280:599-608.
13. Grasset E., Pinto M., Dussaulx E., Zweibaum A. and Desjeux J-F. Epithelial properties of human colonic carcinoma cell line Caco-2: electrical perameters. American Journal of Physiology 1984;247:C260-C267.
14. Grasset E., Bernabeu J. and Pinto M. Epithelial properties of human colonic carcinoma cell line Caco-2: effect of secretagogues. American Journal of Physiology 1985;248:C410-C418.
15. Neutra M. and Louvard D. Differentiation of intestinal cells *in vitro*. In: Functional epithelial cells in culture (Mathin K.S. and Valurtich J.D., eds.) Alan R.Liss Inc., New York, 1989:363-398.
16. Fogh J. and Trempe C. New human tumor cell lines. In: Human tumor cells *in vitro* (Fogh J., ed.) Plenum Publishing Corporation, New York, 1975:115-141.
17. Pinto M., Appay M.D., Simon-Assman P., Chevalier G., Dracopoli N., Fogh J. and Zweibaum A. Enterocytic differentiation of cultured human colon cancer cells by replacement of glucose by galactose in the medium. Biology of the Cell 1982;44:193-196.

18. Zweibaum A., Pinto M., Chevalier G., Dussaulx E., Triadou N., Lacroix B., Haffer K., Brun J.L. and Rousset M. Enterocytic differentiation of a subpopulation of the human colon tumor cell line HT29 selected for growth in sugar free medium and its inhibition by glucose. Journal of Cellular Physiology 1985;122:21-29.
19. Polak-Charcon S., Hekmati M. and Ben-Shaul Y. The effect of modifying the culture medium on cell polarity in a human colon carcinoma cell line. Cell Differentiation and Development 1989;26:119-131.
20. Hekmati M., Polak-Charcon S. and Ben-Shaul Y. A morphological study of a human adenocarcinoma cell line (HT29) differentiating in culture. Similarities to intestinal embryonic development. Cell Differentiation and Development 1990;31:207-218.
21. Faff O., Mitreiter R., Muckter H., Ben-Shaul Y. and Bacher A. Rapid formation of tight junctions in HT29 human adenocarcinoma cells by hypertonic salt solutions. Experimental Cell Research 1988;177:60-72.
22. Rousset M., Paris H., Chevalier G., Terrain B., Murat J-C. and Zweibaum A. Growth-related enzymatic control of glycogen metabolism in cultured human tumor cells. Cancer Research 1984;44:154-160.
23. Huet C., Sahuquillo-Merino C., Coudrier E. and Louvard D. Absorptive and mucus-secreting subclones isolated from a mutlipotent intestinal cell line (HT29) provide new models for cell polarity and terminal differentiation. The Journal of Cell Biology 1987;105:345-357.
24. Dharmasathaphorn K., Mandel K.G., McRoberts J.A., Tisdale L.D. and Masui H. A human colonic tumor cell line that maintains vectorial electrolyte transport. American Journal of Physiology 1984;246:G204-G208.
25. Madara J.L. and Dharmsathaphorn K. Occluding junction structure-function relationship in a cultured epithelial monolayer. The Journal of Cell Biology 1985;101:2124-2133
26. Tompinks A.F., Watrach A.M., Schmale J.D., Schultz R.M. and Harris J.A. Cultural and antigenic properties of newly established cell strains derived from adenocarcinomas of the human colon and rectum. Journal of the National Cancer Institute 1974;52:1101-1110.
27. Henle G. and Deinhardt F. The establishment of strains of human cells in tissue culture. Journal of Immunology 1957;79:54-67.
28. Drewinko B., Romsdhal M.M., Yang L.Y., Ahearn M.J. and Trujillo J.M. Establishment of a human carcinoembryonic antigen-producing colon adenocarcinoma cell line. Cancer Research 1976;36:467-475.
29. Kaminski 1.S. and Fasco M.J. Small intestinal cytochrome P450. CRC Critical Reviews in Toxicology 1992;21:407-422.
30. Stralka D.J. and Strobel H.W. Cytochrome P450 activity and distribution in the human colon mucosa. Cancer 1989;64:2111-2116.
31. Boulenc X., Bourrie M., Fabre I., Roque C., Joyeux H., Berger Y. and Fabre G. Regulation of cytochrome P450IA1 gene expression in a human intestinal cell line , Caco-2. Journal of Pharmacology and Experimental Therapeutics 1992;263:1471-1478.

32. Peters W.H.M. and Roelofs H.M.J. Biochemical characterization of resistance to mitoxantrone and adriamycin in Caco-2 human colon adenocarcinoma cells: a possible role of glutathione-S-transferase. Cancer Research 1992;52:1886-1890.
33. Withe T.B., Hammond D.K., Vasquez H. and Strobel H.W. Expression of two cytochromes P450 involved in carcinogen activation in a human colon cell line. Molecular and Cellular Biochemistry 1991;102:61-69.
34. Peters W.H.N. and Roelofs H.M.J. Time-dependent activity and expression of glutathione S-transferases in the human colon adenocarcinoma cell line Caco-2. Biochemical Journal 1989;264:613-616.
35. Bjorge S., Hamelehle K.L., Homan R., Rose S.E., Turluck D.A. and Wright D.S. Evidence for glucuronide conjugation of p-nitrophenol in the Caco-2 cell model. Pharmaceutical Research 1991;8:1441-1443
36. Baranczyk-Kuzma A., Garren J.A., Hidalgo I.J. and Borchardt R.T. Substrate specificity and some properties of phenol sulfotransferase from human intestinal Caco-2 cells. Life Sciences 1991;49:1197-1206.
37. Wilson G. Cell culture techniques for the study of drug transport. European Journal of Drug Metabolism and Pharmacokinetics 1990;15:159-163.
38. Nicklin P., Irwin B., Hassan I., Williamson I. and Mackay M. Permeable support type influences the transport of compounds across Caco-2 cells. International Journal of Pharmaceutics 1992;83:197-209.
39. Audus K.L., Bartel R.L., Hidalgo I.J. and Borchardt R.T. The use of cultured epithelial and endothelial cells for drug transport and metabolism studies. Pharmaceutical Research 1990;7:435-451.
40. Hidalgo I.J., Hillgren K.M., Grass G.M. and Borchardt R.T. Characterization of the unstirred water layer in Caco-2 cell monolayers using a novel diffusion apparatus. Pharmaceutical Research 1991;8:222-227.
41. Karlsson J. and Artursson P. A method for the determination of cellular permeability coefficients and aqueous boundary layer thickness in monolayers of intestinal epithelial (Caco-2) cells grown in permeable filter chambers. International Journal of Pharmaceutics 1991;71:55-64.
42. Hidalgo I.J., Raub T.J. and Borchardt R.T. Characterization of the human colon carcinoma cell line (Caco-2) as a model system for intestinal epithelial permeability. Gastroenterology 1989;96:736-749.
43. Dix C.J., Hassan I.F., Obray H.Y., Shah R. and Wilson G. The transport of vitamin B12 through polarized monolayers of Caco-2 cells. Gastroenterology 1990;98:1272-1279.
44. Giuliano A.R. and Wood R.J. Vitamin D-regulated calcium transport in Caco-2 cells: unique *in vitro* model. American Journal of Physiology 1991;260:G207-G212.
45. Tomon M., Tenenhouse H.S. and Jones G. Expression of 25-hydroxyvitamin D3-24-hydroxylase activity in Caco-2 cells. An *in vitro* model of intestinal vitamin D catabolism. Endocrinology 1990;126:2868-2875.
46. Hidalgo I.J. and Borchardt R.T. Transport of a large neutral aminoacid (phenylalanine) in a human intestinal epithelial cell line: Caco-2. Biochimica et Biophysica Acta 1990;1028:25-30.

47. Hu M. and Borchardt R.T. Transport of a large neutral aminoacid in a human intestinal epithelial cell line (Caco-2): uptake and efflux of phenylalanine. Biochimica et Biophysica Acta 1992;1135:233-244.
48. Hidalgo I.J. and Borchardt R.T. Transport of bile acids in a human intestinal epithelial cell line, Caco-2. Biochimica et Biophysica Acta 1990;1035:97-103.
49. Hidalgo I.J. and Borchardt R.T. Carrier-mediated transport of bile acids and aminoacids in Caco-2 cells. In: Pharmaceutical applications of cell and tissue culture to drug transport (Wilson G., Illum L. and Davies S.S., eds.) Plenum Press, New York, 1991:77-91
50. Helleux C. and Schneider Y.-J. Iron absorption by intestinal epithelial cells: 1. Caco-2 cells cultivated in serum-free medium, on polyethylene-terephthalate microporous membranes, as an *in vitro* model. In Vitro Cellular and Developmental Biology 1991;27A:293-302.
51. Vincent M.L., Russell R.M. and Sasak V. Folic acid uptake characteristics of a human colon carcinoma cell line, Caco-2. A newly-described cellular model for small intestinal epithelium. Human Nutrition: Clinical Nutrition 1985;39C:355-360.
52. Scarino M.L., Poverini R., Di Lullo G. and Bises G. Inhibition of protein synthesis after exposure of Caco-2 cells to heavy metals. ATLA 1992;20:325-333.
53. Scarino M.L., Poverini R., Di Lullo G. and Bises G. Metallothionein gene expression in the intestinal cell: modulation of mRNA on protein synthesis by copper and zinc. Biochemical Society Transactions 1991;19:238S.
54. Vincentini O., De Angelis I., Stammati A. and Zucco F. Functional alterations induced by the food contaminant furazolidone on the human tumoral intestinal cell line Caco-2. Toxicology in Vitro 1993;7 (in press).
55. Ruedl C., Gstraunthaler G. and Moser M. Differential inhibitory action of the fungal toxin orellanine on alkaline phosphatase isoenzymes. Biochimica et Biophysica Acta 1989;991:280-283.
56. Hecht G., Pothoulakis C., LaMont J.T. and Madara J.L. *Clostridium difficile* toxin A perturbs cytoskeletal structure and tight junction permeability of cultured human intestinal epithelial monolayers. The Journal of Clinical Investigations 1988;82:1516-1524.
57. Nguyen T.D., Canada A.T., Heintz G.G., Gettys T.W. and Cohn J.A. Stimulation of secretion by the T_{84} colonic epithelial cell line with dietary flavonols. Biochemical Pharmacology 1991;41:1879-1886.
58. Allen C.N., Harpur E.S., Gray T.J.B. and Hirst B.H. Toxic effects of non-steroidal anti-inflammatory drugs in a human intestinal epithelial cell line (HCT-8), as assessed by the MTT and neutral red assay. Toxicology in Vitro 1991;5:183-191.
59. Mulcahy R.T., Gipp J.J., Ublacker G.A., Panicucci R. and McClelland R.A. Cytotoxicity and glutathione depletion by 1-methyl-2-nitrosoimidazole in human colon cancer cells. Biochemical Pharmacology 1989;38:1667-1671.
60. Reiss B., Solomon S., Weisburger J.H. and Williams G.M. Comparative toxicities of different forms of asbestos in a cell culture assay. Environmental Research 1980;22:109-129.

61. Reiss B., Millette J.R. and Williams G.M. The activity of environmental samples in a cell culture test for asbestos toxicity. Environmental Research 1980;22:315-321.
62. Itagaki S.K., Kobayashi T., Kitagawa Y. Iwata S., Suwa Y., Nukaya H. and Tsuji K. Cytotoxicity of coffee in human intestinal cells in vitro and its inhibition by peroxidase. Toxicology in Vitro 1992;6:417-421.
63. Buset M., Galand P., Lipkin M., Winawer S. and Friedman E. Injury induced by fatty acids or bile acid in isolated human colonocytes prevented by calcium. Cancer Letters 1990;50:221-226.
64. Lai G.-M., Moscow J.A., Alvarez M.G., Fojo A.T. and Bates S.E. Contribution of glutathione and glutathione-dependent enzymes in the reversal of adriamycin resistance in colon carcinoma cell lines. International Journal of Cancer 1991;49:688-695.
65. Lai G.-M., Chen Y.-N., Mickley L.A., Fojo A.T. and Bates S.E. P-glycoprotein expression and schedule dependence of adriamycin cytotoxicity in human colon carcinoma cell lines. International Journal of Cancer 1991;49:696-703.
66. Grandi M. and Giuliani F.C. Reduced cytotoxicity of tetracyclines to a multidrug resistant human cell line. Biochemical Pharmacology 1988;37:3038-3041.
67. Spoelstra E.C., Dekker H., Schuurhuis G.J., Broxterman H.J. and Lankelma J. P-glycoprotein drug efflux pump involved in the mechanisms of intrinsic drug resistance in various colon cancer cell lines. Evidence for a saturation of active daunorubicin transport. Biochemical Pharmacology 1991;41:349-359.
68. Gipp J.J., McClelland R.A. and Mulcahy R.T. DNA damage Induced in HT-29 colon cancer cells by exposure to 1-methyl-2-nitrosoimidazole, a reductive metabolite of 1-methyl-2-nitroimidazole. Biochemical Pharmacology 1991;42:S127-S133.
69. Belvedere G., Suarato A., Geroni C., Giuliani F.C. and D'Incalci M. Comparison of intracellular drug retention, DNA damage and cytotoxicity of derivatives of doxorubicin and daunorubicin in a human colonadenocarcinoma cell line (LoVo). Biochemical Pharmacology 1989;38:3717-3721.
70. Srivenugopal K.S. Formation and disappearance of DNA interstrand crosslinks in human colon tumor cell lines with different levels of resistance to chlorozotocin. Biochemical Pharmacology 1992;43:1159-1163.
71. Long B.H., Wang L., Lorico A., Wang R.C.C., Brattain M.G. and Casazza A.M. Mechanism of resistance to etoposide and teniposide in acquired resistant human colon and lung carcinoma cell lines. Cancer Research 1991;51:5275-5284.
72. Dusenbury C.E., Davis M.A., Lawrence T.S. and Maybaum J. Induction of megabase DNA fragments by 5-fluorodeoxyuridine in human colorectal tumor (HT29) cells. Molecular Pharmacology 1991;39:285-289.
73. Moran R.G. and Scanlon K.L. Schedule-dependent enhancement of the cytotoxicity of fluoropyrimidines to human carcinoma cells in the presence of folinic acid. Cancer Research 1991;51:4618-4623.

74. Radparvar S., Houghton P.J., Germain G., Pennington J., Rahman A. and Houghton J.A. Cellular pharmacology of 5-fluorouracil in a human colon adenocarcinoma cell line selected for thymidine kinase deficincy. Biochemical Pharmacology 1990;39:1759-1765.
75. Chu E., Drake J.C., Koeller D.M., Zinn S., Jamis-Dow C.A., Chao Yeh G. and Allegra C.J. Induction of thymidylate synthase associated with multidrug resistance in human breast and colon cancer cell lines. Molecular Pharmacology 1991;39:136-143.
76. Artursson P. Cell cultures as models for drug absorption across the intestinal mucosa. Critical Reviews in Therapeutic Drug Carrier Systems 1991;8:305-330.
77. Artursson P. Epithelial transport of drugs in cell culture. I: A model for studying the passive diffusion of drugs over intestinal absorptive (Caco-2) cells. Journal of Pharmaceutical Sciences 1990;79:476-482.
78. Artursson P. and Magnusson C. Epithelial transport of drugs in cell culture. II: Effect of extracellular calcium concentration on the paracellular transport of drugs of different lipophilicities across monolayers of intestinal epithelial (Caco-2) cells. Journal of Pharmaceutical Sciences 1990;79:595-600.
79. Artursson P. and Karlsson J. Correlation between oral drug absorption in humans and apparent drug permeability coefficients in human intestinal epithelial (Caco-2) cells. Biochemical and Biophysical Research Communications 1991;175:880-885.
80. Traber M.G., Thellman C.A., Rindler M.J. and Kayden H.J. Uptake of intact TPGS (d-alpha-tocopheryl polyethylene glycol 1000 succinate) a water-miscible form of Vitamin E by human cells *in vitro*. The American Journal of Clinical Nutrition 1988;48:605-611.
81. Traber M.G., Goldberg I., Davidson E., Lagmay N. and Kayden H.J. Vitamin E uptake by human intestinal cells during lipolysis *in vitro*. Gastroenterology 1990;98:96-103.
82. Hu M. and Borchardt R.T. Mechanism of L-a-methyldopa transport through a monolayer of polarized human intestinal epithelial cells (Caco-2). Pharmaceutical Research 1990;7:1313-1319.
83. Ranaldi G., Islam K. and Sambuy Y. Epithelial cells in culture as a model for intestinal transport of antimicrobial agents. Antimicrobial Agents and Chemotherapy 1992;36:1374-1381.
84. Dantzig A.H. and Bergin L. Uptake of cephalosporin, cephalexin, by a dipeptide transport carrier in the human intestinal cell line, Caco-2. Biochimica et Biophysica Acta 1990;1027:211-217.

16

Legislation and regulation on the use of cells from human origin in pharmaco-toxicology

A. Vercruysse

Vrije Universiteit Brussel, Department of Toxicology, Laarbeeklaan 103, 1090 Brussels (Belgium).

The use of *in vitro* systems in pharmacology, in toxicology and in fundamental research has expanded enormously in the last 15 years. This has occurred partly due to the increasing public pressure to reduce the use of animals for toxicity testing.
Other reasons for using *in vitro* methods to screen for the cytotoxicity and mutagenicity of compounds are that such methods are more rapid and probably cheaper than *in vivo* tests. In the fields of pharmacology and toxicology, cell, organ and tissue culture systems are essential tools for the study and the understanding of biological and toxicological processes. It is much easier to study the mechanisms of toxicity and the pathways of biotransformation in *in vitro* cell systems than in the whole organism.
Pharmaco-toxicology is essentially a predictive science: the *in vitro* tests and models are used to assess the nature and the degree of the toxic effect and the risk to man.
In vitro systems use all kinds of cells and tissues from different species and the methodology developed can be extended to man. In cellular systems of human origin, assessment of toxicity and risk to man can be more directly undertaken. This is in contrast to the *in vivo* animal model where extrapolation of results to man is difficult and sometimes impossible.
However, many laboratories experience serious difficulties in obtaining tissues and cells of human origin for research and pharmaco-toxicological testing. These difficulties, which are of a social, cultural, religious,

emotional, medical and economic origin are also encountered in obtaining organs for transplantation. Because of the substantial increase in organ transplantation and tissue grafting, the World Health Organization (WHO) and the Committee of Ministers of the Council of Europe have adopted Guidlines on human organ transplantation.

In 1978 the Committee of Ministers of the Council of Europe adopted a Resolution [1] on the harmonisation of the legislation of member States related to removal, grafting and transplantation of human organs. The WHO adopted in 1987, on the occasion of the Fortieth World Health Assembly, a resolution WH A 40.13 [2]: 'Development of guiding principles for human organ transplants'. This Resolution and the Guidelines provide a framework for regulating the different aspects for the acquisition and the transplantation of human organs for therapeutic purposes. The term 'human organs' in the context of the Guidelines and the Resolution is always defined as : all organs and tissues with the exception of reproductive tissues and blood and blood constituents.

The general and principal recommendations in the Resolution and the Guidelines made are :
   1. a requirement of a consent. There are two systems: the "opting in/ contracting in" (explicit consent) system and the "opting out/ contracting out " (presumed consent) system.
   2. an exact described procedure for the determination of the criteria of death of the potential donor.
   3. a free consent for living donors, minors are excluded from donation.
   4. a prohibition of traffic, any commercial (profit-making) interest and advertisement.

Throughout the world a large number of States have adopted regulations and legislation on the acquisition and the use of human organs in accordance with this Guidelines and the Resolution.

In Europe most of the member States have passed legislation. The United Kingdom and Northern Ireland adopted The Human organ Transplant Act (1989) [3], Belgium The Law On The Removal And Transplantation Of Organs (1986) [4], Denmark The Law On The Examination Of Cadavers, Autopsies And Transplantation (1990) [5], France The Law On The Removal Of Organs (1976) [6], Greece The Law On The Removal And Transplantation Of Human Tissues And Organs (1983) [7], Italy The Law Regulating The Removal Of Parts Of Cadavers For The Purpose Of Therapeutic Transplantation And Prescribing Rules Governing The Removal Of The Pituitary Gland From Cadavers With A View To Produce Extracts For Therapeutic Purpose

(1975) [8], Luxembourg The Law Regulating The Removal Of Substances Of Human Origin (1982), Spain The Law On The Removal And Transplantation Of Organs (1979) [9]. Other European countries have similar legislation (Austria, Finland, Hungary, Liechtenstein, Malta, Switzerland, Turkey). Germany, Ireland and the Netherlands do not yet have formal legislation on organ transplantation. In these countries unofficial codes exist and legislation is in preparation at the level of ethical commissions or in parliament. In Germany legislation will be oficially adopted on the first of January 1994 [11].

In the United States organs and tissues for transplantation and research are covered by the Uniform Anatomical Gift Act (UAGA) (1984) [10].

As a consequence of the above legislation, many countries are now preparing regulations and laws concerning the installation of tissue banks. The modality of accreditation, the supervision and the quality control are the main topics of interest.

In nearly all the national legislation provision has only been made for the removal of human organs (on death or during surgery) for transplantation or therapeutic use.

Some exceptions exist: the French legislation allows removal of organs for therapeutic or scientific purposes; the Turkish legislation makes provision for the use of organs and tissues for therapeutic, diagnostic and scientific purposes; and, in the U.S.A. [10] organs and tissues for research can be utilised under the UAGA. Every Organ Procurement Organisation provide on their consent forms the possibility to use organs and tissues on the condition that these cannot be utilised for transplantation.

Although there is no competition with the use of human organs for research and education, the number of organs available for transplantation is for many reasons still limited. In several European countries there is a shortage of post mortem organ donations.

Despite the difficulty in obtaining sufficient organs for transplantation the use of organ donation for research purposes is still not regulated in many countries.

Creating the possibility of obtaining organs and tissues from humans on a legal base is the *sine qua non* condition for further development and practical application of this very valuable instrument in pharmacotoxicology and other areas of research. Therefore we formulate the following proposals for such a legislation:

　1. the existing legislation on organ removal for transplantation can practically always be extended to their use in research.

2. the organs or tissues can be used for research if they are not utilised for transplantation.
3. the same restrictions concerning consent and age can be adopted.
4. the organs cannot be sold or bought.
5. the organs have to be used by certified and qualified researchers or research institutions.
6. research tissue banks work on a non-profit base and are certified.

It is essential that European and National legislators create a legal framework whereby human cells and tissues can be obtained for research purposes. It is also of the utmost importance that the public be kept informed of current progress and developments in this important area of research.

References

1. Resolution (78) 29 adopted by the Committee of Ministers of the Council of Europe (11 May 1978) and exploratory Memorandum. Council of Europe.
2. International Digest of Health Legislation 1991;42(3):390-394.
3. International Digest of Health Legislation 1989;40(4):840-842.
4. Belgisch Staatsblad-Moniteur Belge, 10 February 1987;32:2129-2132.
5. International Digest of Health Legislation 1991;42(1):30-32.
6. Journal Officiel de la République Française, 22 December 1976, 7365.
7. International Digest of Health Legislation 1984;35(3):601-602.
8. International Digest of Health Legislation 1977;28(3):626-627.
9. International Digest of Health Legislation 1979;30(2):298-300.
10. Cowen, D.H. et al.(ed.) Human organ transplantation: societal, regulatory end reimbursement issues. Health Administration Press, Ann Arbor, Michigan, 1987:416-432.
11. Becker H. Das neue Transplantations-gesetz. Berliner Ärzte 1993;7:30-31.

17
Pharmaceutical research initiatives of the EC[1]

G.N. Fracchia

Commission of the European Communities DG XII-E - Life Sciences and Technologies, Rue de la loi 200, 1049 Brussels (Belgium).

The Community has recently started a series of pharmaceutical research activities.
At the initiative of the European Parliament, a special line was created in the 1992 budget in order to start research into the efficacy and safety of new medicines in the Directorate General XII (Science, Research and Development) of the Commission of the European Communities.
The rising costs of pharmaceutical Research and Development, the pressing request for innovative drugs for patients suffering from a variety of still incurable and costly diseases, the concern for the safety of new medicines, the uncontrollable rise in public health expenditures Europewide and the concern about the excessive number of animals used in preclinical research are some of the background issues on which seven different ad hoc expert meetings were held in 1992 (Table I).
Experts participating in these meetings were representatives of the scientific world, the pharmaceutical industry, the regulatory authorities and officials from both DG XII and the Directorate General III (Internal Market and Industrial Affairs).
Some of the participants prepared a series of working documents on the current state of the area concerned, existing methodological approaches and comments regarding future directions.
The analysis was particularly focused on possible bottlenecks or obstacles

---

1. The content of this publication reflects the opinion of the author, and not necessarily the official views of the institutions of the Community.

to scientific progress in the different areas. These working documents were prepared in advance and served the purpose of fuelling discussions during the meeting.

The main objective of each meeting was to draft recommendations for future research and to suggest priorities for future community research programmes.

These recommendations were taken into consideration by the EC Commission services in the preparation of the proposal for the Fourth Framework Programme (1994-1998).

All Community research activities are undertaken under a five year Research Programme called the Framework Programme, an instrument for medium-term planning in Research and Development based on the Single European Act and expanded in the Maastricht Treaty. The Framework Programme sets general objectives and priorities as well as providing an overall financial allocation and its breakdown between the different major specific programmes.

The current Third Framework Programme runs from 1990 to 1994 and is endowed with a provision of 5,7 billion ECU for this period. At the end of 1992, the Council reached a common position with regards to granting an additional 900 million ECU to the Third Framework Programme. The total provision represents less than 5% of the total amount spent by the Member States on civilian Research and Development [1].

The expert meetings mentioned in Table I have been successful in

Venue	Title	Date 1992
Brussels	Euro A.D.R. - Pharmacovigilance and Research	26-27 May
Brussels	Research and Development of *in vitro* Pharmacotoxicology	9-10 July
Edinburgh	Transgenic Animals as models for Human Diseases	29-30 Oct.
Brussels	Safety and Efficacy of Cytokines for Human Therapy	3-4 Nov.
Bergamo	Research Perspectives for a European Clinical Trials Network	11-12 Nov.
Lille	Safety and Efficacy of Second Generation Vaccines	19-20 Nov.
Paris	Safety and Efficacy of Monoclonal Antibodies for Human Therapy	7-8 Dec.

Table I :
EC expert meetings on Pharmaceutical Research.

defining clear recommendations for research at Community level. These recommendations have been included in final reports which took into account the discussion results. All seven final reports have been accepted for publication in different peer-reviewed Journals [2-8].

In a few cases, the experts expressed the wish to have the report submitted to more than one Journal for publication in order to reach a wider spectrum of readers. Simultaneous appearance of a paper within different Journals was possible thanks to the cooperation of the publishers.

On the basis of the recommendations expressed by the experts, it was possible to start twenty-five pilot research actions (1992-1993), mainly in the fields of pharmacovigilance and pharmacotoxicology. The list of the pharmacotoxicology actions is reported in Table II, including the names of the leaders responsible for the projects. These pilot actions are of limited scope and duration (one year) in order to continue the work of the expert groups on very specific points that were identified as needing urgent action in order to allow progress in that field. The results of these actions will be published in peer-reviewed scientific journals and will also be evaluated by the EC Commission services. Ideally, these actions should prepare and precede a more strategic and systematic approach under the framework of a formal EC research programme.

The consideration of the needs and opportunities existing in the pharmaceutical research sector of the Community seems to have occurred on a very opportune moment.

On one hand, the EC Commission is on the verge of establishing a European Medicines Evaluation Agency whose tasks will entail marketing authorisation for the whole territory of the Community. The Agency will need to refer constantly to the latest advances in science and technology and to integrate them in its regulations; hence the importance of the existence of a visible and reliable research programme to serve these needs. Similarly, the International Conference on Harmonization (ICH) initiative has provided a forum for the regulatory authorities of the EC, USA and Japan to install a dialogue aimed at achieving greater harmonization of regulatory requirements for the registration of medicines.

On the other hand, there is a growing concern at Community level about consumer and patient protection and animal welfare. Safety of the patients must be guaranteed while at the same time reducing animal experimentation. This represents a challenge to the research community which it is hoped will lead to the development of a research-based and

Receptor and transductional expression in cultured and co-cultured renal cells for studies in chronic nephropathies.	Dr. P. Bach Polytechnic of East London
Inventory of the use, within Europe, of human cells in toxicological research on drugs. A first step in the creation of human cell banks for long-term projects.	Prof. Vera Rogiers Vrije Universiteit Brussel
Development of an *in vitro* embryotoxicity assay using the differentiation of embryonic mouse stem cells into hematopoetic cells.	Prof. Horst Spielmann Institut fur Veterinarmedizin im Bundesgesundheitsamt - Berlin
Comparison of different oncogenes for the immortalization of rabbit articular chondrocytes. Development of a model for the *in vitro* evaluation of pharmaceuticals.	Prof. Monique Adolphe Lab. de Pharmacologie Cellulaire Ecole Pratique des Hauts Etudes - Paris
Establishment of hepatic cell lines derived from transgenic animals for hepatotoxicity assessments.	Prof. Dieter Paul Heinrich-Pette-Institut - Universitat Hamburg
Utilization of *in vitro* techniques in the evaluation of phototoxicity of new compounds.	Prof. Louis Dubertret Unité INSERM 312 Hôpital St. Louis - Paris
Development of an *in vitro* neuronal culture system for the evaluation of learning and memory impairment by new drugs.	Prof. Jacopo Meldolesi H. S. Raffaele - Milano
In vitro studies on cell recognition systems as endpoints for developmental pharmaco-toxicology.	Dr. Ciaran Regan University College of Dublin
Specific effects of immunosuppressive drugs on human cell populations.	Dr. Dominique Latinne University of Louvain
Primary culture of proximal tubular cells from normal rat and porcine kidney as an *in vitro* model to study the mechanisms of nephrotoxicity.	Dr. J.F. Nagelkerke Sylvius Laboratories - Leiden
Use of renal cells *in vitro* to study mechanisms of nephrotoxicity induced by aminosides and cephalosporins.	Prof. Claude Amiel INSERM Unit 251 - Université Paris 7
Apoptosis and programmed cell death in *in vitro* immunotoxicity testing of new compounds.	Prof. Marcel Roberfroid Université Catholique de Louvain
Modelling human sensitivity to toxins in transgenic animals.	Prof. Richard Lathe University of Edinburgh

Table II :
Pharmacotoxicology pilot actions

scientifically sound discipline of modern pharmacotoxicology in the next decade. As a contribution towards this goal, the Commission created in November 1991 a Center for the Validation of Alternative Test Methods (ECVAM) to cater for the needs identified by the Council, the European Parliament and the Commission. Previously in November 1986 the Council of the European Communities adopted Directive 86/609/EEC on the approximation of the laws, regulations and administrative provisions of the Member States regarding the protection of animals used for experimental and other scientific purposes. Article 23 of this Directive calls on the Commission and Member States to encourage the development and validation of alternative techniques which could provide the same level of information as those used at present but which involve fewer animals or entail less painful procedures. Equally, the European Parliament called on the Commission to provide a mechanism for the validation of alternative testing methods including, where necessary, the provision of financial support to the participating laboratories. This led the Commission in 1988 to propose a framework for the evaluation and validation of alternative test procedures, hence the setting-up of ECVAM. The primary task of ECVAM will be to coordinate the validation of alternative test methods at Community level. Meetings such as Human Cells in *In Vitro* Pharmaco-Toxicology have been organised within the framework of one of the pilot actions referred to above and are important in bringing forward this field and preparing for future collaboration with ECVAM.

The development of cheaper, faster and more significant methods for the testing of the toxicity of new compounds should contribute to the accelerated development of efficient drugs, especially those required for the treatment of chronic and degenerative diseases such as cancer, AIDS, cardiovascular diseases and neurological and mental disorders. Such diseases account for the biggest share of public health expenditures. The cost of disease is an unbearable burden in terms of both human suffering and economic resources, yet pharmaceutical innovation can contribute considerably to their alleviation. It is our role as Community actors to facilitate a more rapid access to safe and effective drugs whilst at the same time contributing to the containment of European spending on health.

References

1. Sôete L., The Scientific and Technological Challenge Facing Europe between Now and the End of the 20th Century. Background Paper for the International Workshop organised by the Committee on Energy, Research and Technology of the European Parliament STOA and MERIT. Brussels, 14-15 April, 1992.
2. Rawlins M.D., Fracchia G.N. and Rodriguez-Farré E. Euro-A.D.R. - Pharmacovigilance and Research Pharmacoepidemiology and Drug Safety 1992;1,5:261-268.
3. Rodriguez-Farré E., Roberfroid M. and Fracchia G.N. Research and Development of *in vitro* pharmacotoxicology. A European Perspective. ATLA 1993;21:285-293.
4. Lathe R. and Mullins J.J. Transgenic Animals as models for human disease. Report of an EC study group. Transgenic Research (in press).
5. Stryckmans P. and Fracchia G.N. Safety and Efficacy of second generation vaccines. A European Study Group Report. Cytokines and European Journal of Haematology (in press).
6. Garattini S. and Fracchia G.N. Research perspectives for a European Clinical Trials Network. Clinical Trials and Meta-analysis (in press).
7. Capron A. and Fracchia G.N. Safety and Efficacy of second generation vaccines. A European Study Group Report. Vaccine (in press).
8. Bach J.F. and Fracchia G.N. Safety and efficacy of monoclonal antibodies for human therapy. A European Study Group Report. Immunology Today (in press).

18
Obtaining human tissues for research and testing : practical problems and public attitudes in Britain

J. Gurney and M. Balls*

FRAME (Fund for the replacement of Animals in Medical Experiments), 34 Stoney Street, Nottingham NG1 1NB, UK.
* Present address : ECVAM, JRC Environment Institute, 21020 Ispra, Va (Italy).

Introduction

There are sound scientific reasons why, if *in vitro* systems are to be developed for predicting likely pharmaceutical and toxic effects in human beings, *human*, rather than *animal* cells and tissues should be used wherever possible:

> The applicability of animal data to the assessment of human risk will always be limited by species differences, just as *in vitro* data will always have limited direct applicability to *in vivo* situations. This leads to the logical and unavoidable conclusion that, when human beings are the objects of concern, *in vitro* systems employing animal cells will suffer from the problems of both species differences and *in vitro*/ *in vivo* extrapolation [1] (Fig. 1).

Moreover, the effects of a compound in man may sometimes be more accurately predicted from *in vitro* studies on human tissue than from *in vivo* studies on intact animals. An example is hepatotoxicity due to paracetamol: the rat is relatively insensitive to this effect, which could have been predicted from *in vitro* experiments on human liver.

The increased use of human tissue for *in vitro* studies at an early stage of compound development could have two further advantages. First, it could expedite the identification of human metabolic pathways, so that further research could concentrate on those animal species which handle the compound in similar ways to man. Second, it could facilitate the recognition of those compounds that will be toxic in man, so that they need not be studied further in intact animals.

Thus, an increase in the use of human tissue is desirable on grounds of scientific accuracy, human safety, humanitarianism and cost effectiveness. Therefore, greater effort should be focused on solving the ethical, legal, logistical, technical and safety problems associated with obtaining human material for use in *in vitro* systems. However, the magnitude of these difficulties should not be underestimated.

In this paper we summarise the results of a survey of the position in Great Britain in the late 1980s and of a survey of public opinion, both conducted for FRAME with the support of a grant from the Home Office.

Sources of human tissue

Healthy Volunteers

Samples of blood, skin and hair can sometimes be taken from other workers in the same laboratory, with their informed consent. Also blood which has been taken for transfusion, but has not been needed before its expiry date, may be useful for some purposes. There are no major legal questions here, but the safety of volunteers, and of those who take or use the samples, must be protected.

Tissue from Surgical Patients

Tissue being removed for the patient's benefit. This includes organs which may be removed in their entirety because of a lesion, such as a tumour, in part of the organ. Examples are lung, kidney and uterus. Also the excision of diseased tissue sometimes necessitates, for surgical reasons, the concurrent excision of adjacent healthy tissue which may be suitable for research. This tissue is most likely to be available from the following organs:

1. *Skin* - large amounts of skin are removed in the course of an apronectomy. More frequently, smaller amounts are excised to facilitate neat skin closure after removal of an underlying mass, e.g. a tumour or a breast.
2. *Gastrointestinal tract* - some normal tissue may be removed from above or below a lesion, for surgical reasons.

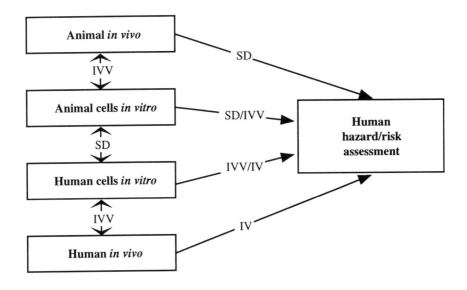

Figure 1 :
Types of extrapolation and their limiting factors.
SD = Species differences; IVV = *in vivo/in vitro*; IV = individual variation

3. *Liver* - liver tissue may be removed after major trauma and for diagnostic biopsy. However, neither of these are likely to prove satisfactory as major sources of tissue for research, for several reasons: first, both procedures are performed only rarely; second, following major trauma, the excised tissue is likely to be badly damaged; and third, for diagnostic biopsy, the amount of tissue removed is too small for most research purposes, though it could conceivably be of use in population surveys of differences in enzyme levels.

4. *Placenta* - placental tissue may be available from some centres and can be used for research in the UK. However, it is of limited value, because it is a highly specialised tissue and because it degrades very rapidly after delivery.

The following points also apply to the use of tissue from surgical patients:

Legally, tissue continues to be the property of the patient after surgical removal. Thus, if it is to be used for research, the patient's consent should be sought pre-operatively. In the opinion of the Medical Protection Society, it is adequate for oral permission to be obtained and recorded in the patient's notes.

Ethically, since the use of tissue in research is not generally perceived as being substantially different from normal histological examination, there is a case for not risking unnecessary distress to a patient by discussing the disposal of organs that are to be removed at operation. However, should patients raise the subject spontaneously, then their wishes should be respected.

Technically, tissue that is removed to facilitate the excision of adjacent diseased tissue may not be strictly normal. For instance, lung tissue adjacent to a carcinoma may show pre-cancerous changes, though this may be advantageous if pre-cancerous changes are the object of the research. Additional effects on tissue may occur from compression due to a large tumour, from the trauma of surgery, and from the effects of anaesthetics and other drugs.

Tissue that has been removed surgically for the patient's benefit has considerable potential for use in research, since it could become more readily available than tissue from most of the other sources described.

Tissue that is not being removed for the patient's benefit. This source of tissue has only been considered for liver, since the removal of other tissues, such as pancreas, would entail an unacceptable risk of severe complications.

A survey of the literature was undertaken to try to determine the risk that the taking of liver samples would pose to the patient. All the large surveys examined described either percutaneous or transvenous liver biopsy. Complications arose from unexpected movement (tear leading to haemorrhage); from lack of visualisation of the biopsy site (puncture of other viscera); or from liver disease itself (haemorrhage). Although these complications were rare, they occurred too often for the use of these procedures to be acceptable as a method of obtaining samples for research. However, they could all be avoided during intra-operative biopsy.

This leads to the conclusion that intra-operative liver biopsy would be safe, a conclusion that was confirmed by all the practising surgeons whose opinion was asked. However, in practice, most surgeons are reluctant to accept the responsibility for taking a liver sample for research from patients undergoing intra-abdominal surgery to an organ other than the liver.

The only Hospital Ethical Committee that was asked for its consent to this procedure, refused to give it. However, the Royal College of Physicians Committee on Ethical Issues in Medicine consider that "it is ethically acceptable to remove a sample of liver or other tissue from patients undergoing abdominal surgery, provided the patient has previously given consent".

Regarding consent, it should, perhaps, be pointed out that obtaining informed consent would not absolve the surgeon of responsibility for undertaking the procedure. This is because: first, most patients have too little understanding of medicine and surgery to be truly fully informed; second, some patients will do whatever their clinicians say; and third, since the surgeon is in a powerful position in relation to the patient, there can never be certainty that the patient did not feel compelled to agree to the proposal against his of her better judgement.

It may sometimes be possible to obtain consent by methods similar to those used for obtaining the consent of healthy volunteers for research without implied psychological pressure. This could entail the use of posters or leaflets to inform patients about the possibility of organ donation, while leaving the initiative for volunteering to the patient.

Tissues from donors of other organs for transplantation

It is important to point out that it has never been our intention to try to obtain for research tissue that would otherwise be used for transplantation. Even with this proviso, patients who are donating organs for transplantation could provide much valuable tissue for research. Organ donors are, by definition, healthy until the occurrence of the acute episode which caused brain death; and their organs are, so far as can be determined, clinically normal. Moreover, since organ donors have been declared dead, there need be no concern about the possibility of their suffering complications from the removal of all or part of their vital organs.

Virtually all those individuals who are concerned with the harvesting of organs for transplantation have appeared to recognise the potential value of donor tissue in research. Moreover, there are sufficient kidney donors in the UK each year to provide ample amounts of liver tissue. Furthermore it is generally agreed, amongst those who deal with relatives of organ donors, that organ donation can, by making the death seem less than totally pointless, confer some help to the bereaved when coming to terms with their loss.

However, in practice, it has been impossible to obtain more than a very limited, and quite inadequate, amount of liver from kidney donors. Some of the difficulties encountered are described below.

Legal considerations. In the UK, the *Human Tissue Act 1961*, applies to the removal of organs for transplantation or for research. This Act states that, unless a person has recorded his wishes in writing, permission for the removal of organs must be obtained from the owner of the body. A body in a National Health Service hospital is owned by the local Health Authority until it is claimed by the coroner, executor or next of kin. If no next of kin can be found, then the Health Authority can give permission for the removal of organs. However, if the circumstances of the death necessitate a coroner's inquest, as is frequently the case with organ donors, then, legally, the coroner can grant permission for the removal of organs without the consent of the next of kin. However, it is generally agreed by transplant teams that there is an ethical requirement to ask for consent from the next of kin and to respect their wishes.

A code of practice on the use of cadaveric organs for transplantation states that it is sufficient to obtain the relatives consent verbally and to record the fact in the patient's notes. If the next of kin are asked to sign a form, then this should be worded in terms of lack of objection, rather than consent.

Obtaining consent from relatives. Potential organ donors are nearly always young people whose death is sudden and unexpected, and their close relatives are stressed to the point of being mentally unbalanced. It can be very difficult to ask consent to remove organs for transplantation; and even harder to ask for consent to use tissue in research, which is a more complex concept and less easily portrayed as potentially life-saving. Some of the transplant teams that do harvest tissue for research simply ask the relatives consent for removal of organs, without specifying the use to which they will be put; others ask them to sign a consent form on which research is mentioned. One transplant surgeon, who often asks specifically for consent to use organs in research, said that it is extremely rare to obtain consent to the use of organs for transplantation, but not for research.

Ethically, it can be argued that the priority of the medical team in charge of a potential donor is to help the relatives to come to terms with the donor's death. Some people feel, very deeply, that the body of the dead should be respected, and therefore left intact. However, others believe that organ donation can be positively beneficial to the relatives by enabling them to feel that some good, however inadequate, has resulted from the death. A high proportion of organ donations originate from the relatives themselves asking for organs to be used.

Views of relatives on organ donation. In order to investigate further the feelings of relatives about organ donation, six close relatives of previous organ donors were interviewed in depth. These were all parents of sons who had died as the result of an accident: two were the parents of a seven-year old boy; one the mother of a teenage boy; and the sons of the remaining three had died as young adults.

All of those interviewed stressed that, while in no way compensating for their loss, organ donation gave them considerable help in coming to terms with their grief, by enabling them to feel that some good had resulted from their son's death. They all felt that this beneficial effect should receive more emphasis in discussions about the moral implications of organ donation.

The interviewees were also agreed about the value of having discussed the principle of donating organs for transplantation before their sons received their fatal injuries. They felt that this would be even more important with the more complex concept of donating organs for research.

The final recommendation to emerge from these interviews was the importance of being seen to treat donor tissue with respect.

Organ donor cards. A possible means of increasing the availability of donor organs for research is by the addition of 'research' to the organ donor card or to one of the computers on which people can record their wish to donate organs for transplantation in the event of their death.

Donor cards are not carried by all those who wish to donate their organs for transplantation. Two independent surveys found that, whereas 75-80% of the population wished to donate organs, only slightly over 20% normally carried donor cards and a further 7% claimed that they had signed a card but had lost it, left it at home, etc. A further limitation arises because of the distribution of cards, to hospitals, libraries, etc., which are seldom visited by certain sections of the population, so that many people claim never to have seen a donor card. Moreover, when an unconscious or badly injured patient is admitted to hospital, their handbag or wallet may be handed to a friend or relative without the presence of a donor card being noted.

Despite these qualifications, it was generally agreed that organ donor cards do provide a useful service by publicising the need for organ donors and, more importantly, by encouraging people to discuss the matter, so that, if possibility of organ donation arises, relatives are already aware of the patient's wishes. These advantages would also apply to the addition of 'research' to the card.

However, the DHSS have refused to add 'research' to the organ donor card. The reason given was that the mention of research would deter people from donating organs for transplantation. This fear conflicts with the experience of the transplant surgeons, mentioned above, who actually ask relatives for permission to remove organs for research and who find refusal extremely rare. Moreover it was found, in the survey to be described later, that some people have a strong positive wish to donate tissue for research and resent the fact that they found this hard to do.

Although it would theoretically be possible for an organisation such as FRAME to distribute their own donor cards, giving consent to remove organs for research, enormous resources would be needed to distribute such cards throughout the general population in sufficient numbers to have any useful effect.

Practical difficulties with harvesting. Virtually all the transplant teams approached with a request for liver samples, expressed willingness to provide them wherever possible, but never actually did so. This is analogous to the situation encountered by transplant teams who approach consultants in charge of intensive care units, asking to be provided with organs for transplantation. They are often given verbal support, but are not actually offered organs.

Among those few transplant teams who were reluctant to help, the reasons given were: first, that the tissue was used by their own research teams; second, that an additional request to use tissue for research could cause the relatives to refuse consent for the harvesting of organs for transplantation; and, third, previous experience had taught them that the difficulties in contacting research scientists at the time when tissue became available were virtually insurmountable. This last comment was, unfortunately, confirmed by our experience.

When a suitable donor becomes available, the transplant team is extremely busy arranging the transplantation of suitable organs. Any extra work entailed in donating additional tissue for research must, therefore, be minimal. It seemed that this extra work could be confined to one brief telephone call to the research team, but in practice this proved not to be the case.

Since the telephone call offering tissue would arise unexpectedly, and at any time of day or night, the research scientist concerned carried a British Telecom bleep. But failures in communication were frequent.

Few failures were in any way the fault of the scientists concerned - even though calls arrived very infrequently and it becomes difficult, after a bleep has not been used for several weeks, to maintain a high standard of readiness to respond. Even brief trips outside the area covered by the bleep could result in a call being missed, and a further difficulty is that tissue may become available when the investigator requiring it is about to fulfil other commitments. Other failures occurred as a result of critical delays of up to ten minutes spent waiting for the hospital switchboard to answer the phone; and because British Telecom disconnected the bleep without warning, because the bill, which has been sent to the wrong address, had not been paid.

It was hoped that the UK Transplant Service (UKTS), who are on call 24 hours every day and who have considerable expertise in the rapid transport of tissue from cadaveric organ donors, would be willing to arrange for tissue to be taken to a collection point. However, the UKTS Management Committee "felt that this was not a proper role for the UKTS". They also felt that "local arrangements were the best way of handling this issue". However local arrangements necessarily limit research on human tissue to centres which are suitable located. Other centres, no matter how excellent, are unable to participate.

Transport. The number of cells that could be recovered from any specimen decreased with an increase in the time taken from excision to its use in the laboratory and this time became critical after a few hours. For this reason the initial arrangement, in which scientists travelled to the donating hospital, collected the tissue, and returned to the laboratory to set up their equipment, was abandoned.

A more satisfactory arrangement was for the transplant teams to be provided with suitable containers, clearly labelled with the name of the scientist and the laboratory. These containers were transported to the laboratory by motorcycle couriers, while the scientists set up their equipment.

Characteristics of donors. Patients who are considered suitable to donate organs for transplantation are typically young and healthy until they have suffered a sudden catastrophe, such as an accident or spontaneous intra-cranial haemorrhage, which has led to admission to an Intensive Care Unit and subsequently to brain-stem death. They therefore do not represent a complete cross-section of the community. However, they do probably represent the closest approximation to clinical normality that can, in practice, be obtained for samples of organs such as the liver and pancreas.

Hepatitis and AIDS. Testing for hepatitis (HBsAg) and AIDS antibodies is normally carried out on all potential organ donors before transplantation. However, it cannot be guaranteed that tissue received by the laboratory will be negative for these tests, since the results of the tests may not be available at the time of harvesting. Further, some transplant centres will use HBsAg-positive organs for transplantation into HBsAg-positive recipients.

However, the consensus of opinion among pathologists is: first, that the risk of contracting hepatitis from such tissue is far greater than the risk of acquiring AIDS; and, second, that, provided the appropriate safety recommendations are followed, the handling of tissue from organ donors should be acceptably safe.

Tissues Obtained at Post-mortem

Post-mortem tissue can be more readily obtained than tissue from transplant organ donors. The harvesting of tissues can proceed at a relatively leisurely pace and during working hours. Moreover, post-mortem tissue can be obtained from donors whose death, possibly from old age or disease, has been expected, so that relatives have had the time to come to terms with the death and to consider the implications of organ donation.

However, the value of post-mortem tissue in research is limited by the fact that post-mortem examinations are generally conducted a day or more after death, when enzymatic degradation is too far advanced for the tissues to be used for investigations into normal metabolism or into responses to foreign substances.

However, organs obtained at post-mortem can be useful for certain lines of research. For example, at the Cambridge Brain Bank, brains harvested at post-mortem have been used for studies of the concentrations of substances such as noradrenaline and GABA in the brains of patients with dementia, schizophrenia, Parkinson's disease and Huntington's chorea.

Attitudes of the general public

In 1986, FRAME commissioned the Harris Research Centre to carry out a survey to determine the attitudes of the general public to the donation of human tissue for research.[2]

A questionnaire was sent to 1000 names drawn from the electoral register and 200 of these were completed and returned. This response rate was slightly lower than usual for a postal survey, possibly because of the complexity and nature of the subject, and because the questionnaire was sent out shortly before Christmas. However, the respondents were similar to the general population in age and sex, though they showed a slightly higher proportion of females and of younger adults. Of the respondents, 29% said that they normally carry a kidney donor card. A similar figure was found in a 1986 Gallup survey, in which 21% were carrying a card and 7% claimed they had left them at home.

Asked if they would be prepared to carry a card to permit the removal, after death, of their tissues for use in research, 108 (54%) of respondents said they would be willing to do this, and 51 (26%) said they would not. Answers to the two questions following suggested that the decision was less affected by the particular organ taken than by the use to which it was put. About half of the respondents were willing to leave any of the organs listed for research into the prevention and cure of disease, but only one third were prepared to leave the same organs for research into the safety testing of pesticides, cosmetics and household chemicals. Under 'further comments', four respondents expressed the opinion that it should be easier to arrange to leave one's body for research.

A similar differentiation between medical research and safety testing was reflected in responses to questions relating to the use of animals in experiments. For medical research, 73 (37%) were *against* or *strongly against* the use of laboratory animals; whereas 128 (65%) were *against* or *strongly against* their use for the safety testing of pesticides, cosmetics and household chemicals. An analysis of the additional comments made by respondents showed that approval or disapproval of animal experiments was also affected by the amount of pain and suffering caused to the animals and by the absence of alternative techniques.

Asked about the use of various animal species in the laboratory, slightly more than half of the respondents thought that cats and dogs should not be used, while one third thought the use of mice and rats was unjustified. Replies about the other species listed - which included rabbits, monkeys, snakes and fish - ranged between these two extremes.

When asked for further comments on the use of laboratory animals, six respondents felt it was wrong to differentiate between species in this way, and a further two said that only laboratory-bred animals should be used in experiments.

The next group of questions asked respondents whether they agreed: first, with the principle of tissue donation while the donor was still alive, provided that the appropriate tissue could be painlessly removed and, second, whether they themselves would consider being a donor in these circumstances. In principle, 69% of respondents either *agreed* or *strongly agreed* with live tissue donation for medical research. However, only 46% *agreed* or *strongly agreed* when the question related to the safety testing of new products. Over half of respondents reported willingness to donate their own tissue for use in research.

Conclusions

It would seem indisputable that, for scientific, ethical and financial reasons, the use of human tissue in research should be developed and expanded. However, if sufficient quantities of the right tissues, in a sufficiently normal state and with sufficient regularity and reliability, are to made available to scientists, not only in hospitals, but also in academic, industrial and contract testing laboratories, then there are two major problems to overcome.

First is the fear, among individuals who could contribute to the provision of human tissue for research, of upsetting potential organ donors or their relatives. However, there is ample evidence that some individuals actively wish to donate tissue for this purpose: relatives of brain-dead organ donors report consolation from organ donation; the Harris survey has shown a strong desire in some individuals to donate tissue; medical schools have more bodies than they can use; and organisations dealing with organ or tissue donation, such as the medical schools and the Blood Transfusion Service, report much distress and difficulty with individuals or relatives of individuals who are unable to donate for some reason.

Some individuals undoubtedly have a strong intuitive repugnance to the concept of organ donation. While it is right that their desire not to have their organs used should be respected, it is equally important that those who believe that human tissues should be used in research can donate their organs if they wish to do so.

Thus, while the fear of upsetting potential tissue donors or their relatives may have some justification, it is important that this fear should be contained within the provision of adequate safeguards for donors or potential donors, and not be allowed to overwhelm the wishes of individuals who *do* wish to donate or the benefits that their donations could provide.

The second major problem in expanding the use of human tissue in research is the practical difficulty of maintaining an efficient tissue transport system on 24-hour alert. From our experience, and that of others, it would seem that this cannot in practice, be undertaken effectively by the scientists involved in the research. Moreover, transplant teams who repeatedly fail to make contact promptly with scientists when tissue becomes available, are liable to refuse to make further attempts to offer tissue, either to those scientists or to others. Thus, if the use of human tissue is to be expanded as it should, it is essential to enlist the help of an organisation that is already on 24-hour alert and, preferably, one that already has expertise in the rapid transportation of human tissue.

If there is to be an increase in the availability and use of human tissue culture, for the benefit of both human beings and animals, then three essential steps need to be taken:

First, public education is needed, so that, coupled with a reassurance that any removal of tissues would be properly conducted and properly controlled, any apprehension would be replaced by willingness to collaborate. There is no intrinsic reason why, given similar safeguards, donation of tissue should not be as widely available to the public as donation of blood.

Second, a transport system should be established, so that, as human organs and tissues become available, they can be properly handled in order to maintain the quality needed for their use in *in vitro* procedures. This would need to be coupled with the setting up of registers of approved users, with contact telephone numbers and details of tissues required, etc.

Third, the problem of storing human cells and tissues needs to be overcome, so that viable and relatively-normal cells and tissues can be stored, distributed and used in more ideal circumstances than at present.

Until these three steps are taken, the present unsatisfactory solution will continue. Those who have secured their own sources of supply will jealously guard them, and those without such a supply will feel that their scientific progress is being frustrated. Meanwhile, those of us who repeatedly call for the greater use of human tissue culture systems as a logical replacement for animal studies, will merely be wasting our breath.

Acknowledgements

This article is based on conclusions resulting from a survey, conducted for, and with the financial support of, the Home Office, London, and on the results of a public opinion survey, conducted for FRAME by Harris Research Centre, Richmond, Surrey, UK.

References

1. Balls M., Garle M. and Clothier R. H. Future developments in *in vitro* methodology. In: Animals and alternatives in toxicology - present status and future prospects (Balls M., Bridges J. and Southee J., eds.) Macmillan, London, 1991:313-339.
2. Anon. Human tissue as an alternative in biomedical research. ATLA (Alternatives to Laboratory Animals) 1987;14:375-385.